Multiple Sclerosis Handbook

Multiple Sclerosis Handbook

Editor: Floyd Freemont

AMERICAN
MEDICAL PUBLISHERS
www.americanmedicalpublishers.com

AMERICAN
MEDICAL PUBLISHERS
www.americanmedicalpublishers.com

Cataloging-in-publication Data

Multiple sclerosis handbook / edited by Floyd Freemont.
p. cm.
Includes bibliographical references and index.
ISBN 979-8-88740-281-9
1. Multiple sclerosis. 2. Multiple sclerosis--Pathogenesis. 3. Multiple sclerosis--Diagnosis.
4. Multiple sclerosis--Treatment. 5. Neurology. I. Freemont, Floyd.
RC377 .M85 2023
616.834--dc23

American Medical Publishers,
41 Flatbush Avenue,
1st Floor, New York,
NY 11217, USA

ISBN 979-8-88740-281-9 (Hardback)

Contents

Preface

In my initial years as a student, I used to run to the library at every possible instance to grab a book and learn something new. Books were my primary source of knowledge and I would not have come such a long way without all that I learnt from them. Thus, when I was approached to edit this book; I became understandably nostalgic. It was an absolute honor to be considered worthy of guiding the current generation as well as those to come. I put all my knowledge and hard work into making this book most beneficial for its readers.

Multiple sclerosis (MS) is a serious disease that worsens over time. The immune system harms the fatty coverings called myelin sheaths that are present around nerve cells in the central nervous system (CNS). This disease affects people differently and can cause problems with their bodies, eyesight, speech, and minds. Various risk factors associated with MS include lack of vitamins in the body, taking too much stress, smoking habits, being sick frequently as a youngster, and genetics of the person. In MS, infiltration of immune cells results in inflammation within the CNS, leading to the loss of the protective insulator known as "demyelination". People with MS frequently experience severe pain and fatigue. They have weak muscles and have difficulty in moving and balancing. Their speech and vision can deteriorate over time. A doctor can assist a person with MS in managing their symptoms once they have been diagnosed. This book brings forth some of the most innovative concepts and elucidates the unexplored aspects of multiple sclerosis. Those in search of information to further their knowledge will be greatly assisted by it.

I wish to thank my publisher for supporting me at every step. I would also like to thank all the authors who have contributed their researches in this book. I hope this book will be a valuable contribution to the progress of the field.

Editor

1

Neuroprotection: A New Therapeutic Approach of Relapsing Remitting Multiple Sclerosis

Juan Espinosa-Parrilla, Marco Pugliese,
Nicole Mahy and Manuel J Rodríguez

Abstract

Neurodegenerative changes occurring early from primary acute immune-mediated inflammation support the hypothesis that multiple sclerosis (MS) is a complex disease. Axonal loss progresses with the disease course and represents the principal driver of disability. In this context, the pursuit of neuroprotective therapies in multiple sclerosis provides new valid alternatives that could significantly impact on disease progression and neurodegenerative changes, including the promotion of restoration of myelin sheaths through the remyelination process. This chapter reviews promising drugs with proposed neuroprotective or neuroregenerative effects that are currently approved or in clinical trials for the treatment of multiple sclerosis. Although the chapter highlights the diazoxide action on neuroinflammation and the results of a clinical trial with this drug, the review also includes other molecules with oral or parenteral administration.

Keywords: relapsing-remitting multiple sclerosis, disease-modifying drugs, neuroprotection, neuroregeneration, neuroinflammation, central nervous system

1. Introduction

Immunosuppressive and immunomodulatory drugs have been designed for years to treat multiple sclerosis (MS), as it was considered the most appropriate approach to balance the effects of the patients' immune reaction. However, the new data recently offered by basic and clinical research increase our understanding of this complex disease, allowing changes in its therapeutic approach. As a consequence, the first disease-modifying drug with a suggested neuroprotective mechanism of action has been recently approved, broadening and improving the therapeutic landscape against MS.

In this chapter, we review new drugs with proposed neuroprotective or neuroregenerative effects that are currently approved or in clinical trials for MS treatment. Although we highlight the diazoxide action on neuroinflammation and the results of a clinical trial with this drug, the review also includes other molecules with oral or parenteral administration.

The articles analysed for this review were selected using PubMed database filtered by English language. Clinical trials were selected at the ClinicalTrials.gov database. Studies in the database labelled as "unknown status" were excluded. The initial search was done in December 2015.

2. Treating neurodegeneration in multiple sclerosis

MS is an autoimmune disease in which elements of the neuronal myelin sheath are recognized as antigens by the immune system. Focal inflammatory and immune actions against neuronal cover cause a neurodegenerative process that leads to neurological impairment. The difficulty to characterize the neurodegenerative process supports the hypothesis that MS is a complex disease, with high variations among individuals. In any case, as a consequence of the immune aggression, an axonal loss progresses with the disease and represents the principal driver of disability in the chronic course of MS [1]. In this context, multiple mechanisms could contribute to demyelination and axonal injury including energy imbalance, ion accumulation, neuroinflammation and astroglial response to oxidative and metabolic stress.

2.1. Chronic neurodegenerative processes in multiple sclerosis

About 85% of MS patients present the so-called relapsing-remitting (RR) form, characterized by unpredictable relapses related to inflammatory activity, followed by periods of months to years of relative quietness. During the remitting period, patients present no new signs of disease activity and, occasionally, partial remissions of symptoms associated with reparative processes are observed [2]. Progressive forms are less frequent forms of initial MS, but about 55–65% of relapsing-remitting multiple sclerosis (RRMS) patients develop a secondary progressive course [1].

At the pathophysiological level, the neurological impairment develops due to focal inflammatory and immune attacks against the neuronal cover, which cause a chronic neurodegenerative process. The reason why and where these focal demyelinating inflammatory lesions appear within the central nervous system (CNS) remains unknown. Current hypothesis establish that CD4-positive T lymphocytes are mainly responsible for the initial autoimmune attack, but with a secondary role in chronic neuronal damage [3]. Resident microglia and astrocytes, and infiltrated macrophages, B lymphocytes, natural killer (NK)-positive and CD8-positive T cells would be the major players in the neurodegenerative process [4, 5].

At the subcellular level, a plethora of inflammatory effectors mediating myelin and neuronal damage have been described. These effectors include molecules such as nitric oxide (NO), reactive oxygen species (ROS), tumour necrosis factor α (TNF-α), interferon γ (IFNγ), granzymes, perforin and matrix metalloproteinases, and also molecular processes such as activation of the complement, antibody secretion and phagocytosis [4, 6, 7]. Furthermore, as a concomitant event, glutamate release from damaged axons will trigger excitotoxicity, which leads to ion imbalance and mitochondrial metabolic stress, feeding neuronal damage and neuroinflammation [8, 9]. Thus, inflammatory damage leads to oligodendrocyte death, axon demyelination, axonal damage, neuronal death and the formation of glial scars. Progressive axonal injury and neuronal loss increase with the course of MS and represent the principal driver of disability.

Key elements that mediate inflammation in MS are microglial cells. Microglia are often considered to be macrophages of the CNS, but a series of recent findings in the mouse have established that they are a unique cell population distinct from macrophages [10]. In normal conditions, microglia present a surveillance state and important roles in normal development, connectivity and plasticity of the CNS. However, they are transformed and activated by a range of signals, such as neuronal death, mechanical injury and toxins [11]. Once activated, they form the first line of defense against infection or injury to the CNS [12]. As a consequence, microglia mediate and trigger a neuroinflammatory response to injury. In MS, this microglial reaction is an early event that often precedes and triggers demyelination and neurodegeneration [13].

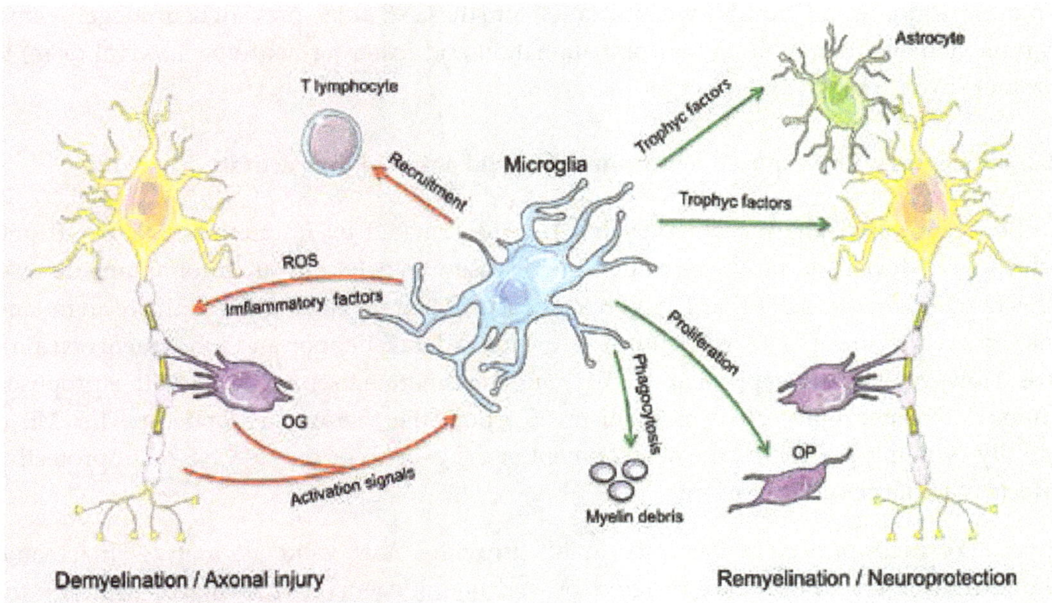

Figure 1. Dual role of microglia in MS. Reactive microglia mediate different pro-inflammatory (red arrows) and neuroprotective processes (green arrows) according to the diversity of signals from the lesioned axons and oligodendrocytes. OG, oligodendrocytes; OP, oligodendrocyte precursors; ROS, reactive oxygen species. (Cell drawings are from SERVIER Medical Art.)

Perivascular microglia are the antigen-presenting cells that recruit myelin-specific T cells and promote the inflammatory process inside the CNS. This process then activates parenchymal microglia by secreting pro-inflammatory and neurotoxic factors such as TNF-α, prostaglandins, interleukin-6 (IL-6), NO or ROS, which elicit myelin damage and neurodegeneration [11, 14]. Whether microglia adopt a phenotype that mostly exacerbates tissue injury or one that promotes brain repair is likely to depend on the diversity of signals from the lesion environment and the response capacity of the cell (**Figure 1**).

As a response to the inflammatory aggression, reparative and regenerative processes are activated and originate MS remissions. This neuroprotective response is led by the activation of microglia and TH2-IL-10 lymphocyte pathways, and results in inhibition of the inflammatory process, up-regulation of antioxidant mechanisms, and secretion of neurotrophic factors. These processes promote remyelination by surviving oligodendrocytes and precursors [15–17]. According to this, the progression of MS symptoms depends on a delicate balance between neuroinflammation and the regenerative process. However, neuronal regeneration is not an easy and common process within the CNS, especially for large myelinated neurons. Although myelin sheath can be partially restored, oligodendrocytes regenerated and axons repaired, and if the inflammatory insult persists, the degenerative damage becomes chronic and cannot be counteracted.

According to these processes, the therapeutic approaches for MS should follow three different but not exclusive strategies: (a) to suppress the autoimmune reaction by inhibiting the initial immune response and lymphocyte infiltration into the CNS, (b) to prevent neurodegenerative chronic damage by inhibiting neuroinflammation and fostering neuronal survival or (c) to promote myelin repair and neuroregeneration.

2.2. Molecules with proposed neuroprotective and antioxidative activity

Until recently, MS pharmacotherapy has been dominated by immunomodulatory drugs, which were developed on the basis that the disease was primarily an autoimmune disease. This hypothesis postulates that T lymphocytes specific for myelin antigens initiate an inflammatory reaction in the CNS, which ultimately leads to demyelination and subsequent neuronal loss. However, since the approval of oral dimethyl fumarate to treat RRMS, with a proposed antioxidative neuroprotective mechanism of action, the therapeutic landscape for MS is rapidly evolving. Currently, the development of drugs with primarily CNS neuroprotective effects is a pharmaceutical priority.

Pursuit of neuroprotective therapies in MS provides new valid alternatives that could significantly impact on disease progression and neurodegenerative changes, including the promotion of myelin sheath restoration through the remyelination process [18]. Thus, fingolimod, laquinimod, Anti-LINGO antibody, (-)-epigallotechin-3-gallate (EGCG) and diazoxide emerge as neuroprotective drugs for the treatment of MS (**Table 1**). Nevertheless, the neuroprotective effect of these compounds has not been fully established and requires further investigation.

Compound	Proposed mechanism of action	Effects	Clinical phase	Key adverse effects
Dimethyl fumarate	Nrf2 up-regulation Induction of IL-4-Th2 response	Anti-inflammatory activity Decreased lymphocyte entry into CNSProtective effects on oligodendrocytes, myelin, axons and neurons	Phase III: DEFINE and CONFIRM Approved	Moderate infections Elevated liver enzymes Leucopenia
Fingolimod	Decreased expression of S1p1 on lymphocytes and other cells	Decrease of T lymphocytes infiltrated in the CNS Anti-inflammatory and neuroprotective microglia phenotypes	Phase III: TRANSFORMS and FREEDOMS Approved	Bradycardia and AV block Severe viral infections Macular oedema
Laquinimod	Unknown Inhibition of NF-kB activation? Inhibition of IL-17expression?	Decreased lymphocyte entry into CNS Axon protection Decrease of pro-inflammatory cytokines Increased BDNF levels	Phase III studies CONCERTO Results expected by 2017	Elevated liver enzymes Infections
Anti-LINGO antibody BIIB033	Blockade of Nogo signaling	promotes axonal integrity/remyelination functional recovery	Phase I NCT01052506 NCT01244139 Phase II: SYNERGY Results expected by 2016	Hypersensitivity reactions Elevated liver enzymes
(−)-Epigallotechin-3-galeate	Inhibition of NF-kB activation Free radical scavenger.	Improves muscle metabolism during moderate exercise in MS patients	Phase II SuniMS completed. No results available NCT01417312 completes	Elevated liver enzymes (1 case)
Diazoxide	Activation of K_{ATP} channels Maintenance of mitochondrial homeostasis and function	Anti-inflammatory activity Neuronal, axonal and myelin protection Modulation of antigen presentation	Phase II: NEUROADVAN completed	Autoimmune hypothyroidism (1 case)

Table 1. Neuroprotective drugs for the treatment of RRMS.

2.2.1. Dimethyl fumarate

Fumaric acid esters (FAEs) are a group of simple low-molecular structured compounds that has been used for long time in the treatment of moderate to severe psoriasis [19]. Due to their immunomodulatory potential, FAEs were also evaluated as a potential treatment for RRMS. At preclinical stages, FAEs showed promising results in myelin oligodendrocyte glycoprotein (MOG)-induced experimental autoimmune encephalomyelitis (MOG-EAE) mice, ameliorating the disease course [20]. In vivo, the mechanism of action of dimethyl fumarate is not completely understood. For some authors, fumarate treatment induces IL-4-producing Th2 dendritic cells [21]. In the human and mice, type II dendritic cells subsequently produce the anti-inflammatory cytokines IL-10 and IL-4 instead of pro-inflammatory IL-12 and IL-23 [21]. This anti-inflammatory activity also causes apoptosis of activated T cells preserving the CNS from influx of activated lymphocytes.

Regarding the neuroprotective role of fumarate, other authors found in vitro and in vivo effects, potentially via up-regulation of the nuclear factor (erythroid-derived 2)-like 2 (Nrf2). Dimethyl fumarate also exerts protective effects on oligodendrocytes, myelin, axons and neurons, and reduces oxidative stress as measured by protein nitrosylation [22]. Nonetheless, as recently shown, the protective effect of dimethyl fumarate could depend on pre-existing tissue expression of Nrf2. Actually, Nrf2 is intrinsically higher in astrocytes and macrophages from active MS lesions and increased Nrf2 levels have been recently reported in oligodendrocytes from active MS lesions [23].

Two randomized, placebo- and active-controlled, double-blind, parallel-group Phase III studies (DEFINE and CONFIRM) of dimethyl fumarate (Code name BG-12) have been conducted (funded by Biogen Idec). The primary end point of these studies was the proportion of patients who had a 2-year relapse. Secondary end points included the annualized relapse rate (ARR), the time to confirmed progression of disability as measured by Expanded Disability Status Scale (EDSS), and findings on brain magnetic resonance imaging scan (MRI) such as the number of gadolinium-enhancing lesions. Both studies described highly significant superiority of BG-12 to placebo on almost all end points in patients with RRMS [24]. In the DEFINE and CONFIRM extension study (ENDORSE), a minimum of 5 years of treatment with the drug was associated with continued benefit and no new/worsening tolerability signals. Thus, in March 2013, the Food and Drug Administration (FDA) approved dimethyl fumarate as a new first-line oral treatment for patients with RRMS. In September 2013, it was also approved in Canada and Australia and, in 2014, the European Commission has approved the use of the drug for the treatment of RRMS in Europe.

2.2.2. Fingolimod

Fingolimod became the first drug approved for relapsing forms of MS in the USA in 2010. However, some safety issues were identified during the drug development process, after completion of trials and in the first months of clinical use in the United States. These issues led to the approval of fingolimod as a second-line drug by the European Medicines Agency (EMA) after the FDA had licensed it as a first-line agent. In addition, contradictory results regarding efficacy on progression of disability in MS patients were found in the two pivotal Phase III trials that allowed fingolimod marketing in most countries [18].

Although fingolimod was primarily believed to be a pure immunosuppressive compound, recent findings revealed direct effects on the CNS [25]. When incorporated to the organism, fingolimod is rapidly phosphorylated by sphingosine kinases [26] and the product of this phosphorylation, phosphofingolimod, is a potent modulator of S1P receptors. Administration of fingolimod and similar S1P1 modulators produce marked beneficial effects on different animal models of MS, especially when administered preventively. The proposed mechanism of action for fingolimod is the inhibition of encephalitogenic T-cell responses and/or their migration into the CNS [27, 28]. According to this, EAE animals treated with fingolimod showed a dramatic decrease of T lymphocytes infiltrated in the CNS and even a reversible peripheral lymphocytopaenia. These animals also showed better myelin preservation and decrease of pro-inflammatory cytokine production [29].

In the CNS, both neurons and glia profusely express S1P receptors. Some of the beneficial effects of fingolimod in EAE and MS could be attributed to SP1 receptor modulation in these cells and result in neuroprotection. Activation of neuronal S1P1 and S1P3 receptors promotes neurogenesis and increases neurite outgrowth, although high and continuous activation of neuronal S1P receptors could lead to overactivation of the glutamatergic system with deleterious effects [30]. In microglia, fingolimod promotes anti-inflammatory and neuroprotective phenotypes, but the exact mechanism of action involved remains unclear [31]. Furthermore, one of the most discussed direct effects of fingolimod on the CNS is on myelin repair and oligodendrocyte regeneration [32, 33].

One Phase II study, followed by an active extension, and two clinical Phase III placebo-controlled and active comparator-controlled clinical trials (named TRANSFORMS and FREEDOMS, sponsored by Novartis) have been performed with fingolimod in patients with RRMS. These studies have demonstrated the efficacy of fingolimod in treating RRMS [34, 35]. More recently, FREEDOMS II, a third Phase III trial of fingolimod, was conducted predominantly in USA and Canada. The trial replicated the findings of FREEDOMS regarding the ARR and MRI outcomes, but the significant effect on reducing EDSS score progression was not confirmed. On the other hand, disability showed a statistically significant change in favour of fingolimod treatment in the FREEDOMS II study [36]. Finally, the recently completed INFORMS trial showed no significant benefit of fingolimod on neurological disability in primary progressive MS patients treated for at least 3 years [37].

2.2.3. *Laquinimod*

Laquinimod (N-ethyl-N-phenyl-5-chloro-1,2-dihydroxy-1-methyl-2-oxo-quinoline-3-carboxamide) is structurally related to linomide, which was tested for efficacy in MS more than one decade ago, and discontinued after serious adverse events occurred in a Phase III trial [38, 39]. After an extensive screening of a large number of chemically modified quinoline-3-carboxamides, laquinimod was selected to have less toxicity and better efficacy than linomide in various experimental autoimmune inflammatory-mediated animal models, including experimental autoimmune neuritis in Lewis rats [40].

The precise mechanism by which laquinimod induces these beneficial effects is yet to be fully elucidated. Preclinical studies in EAE mice have shown that laquinimod might protect myelin and axons by decreasing pro-inflammatory cytokines such as IL-17 by T cells [41]. In addition, suppression of the nuclear factor-kappaB (NF-κB) pathway that concordantly led to the activation of apoptosis of immunocompetent cells was also induced by laquinimod, proving the anti-inflammatory potency of the drug [42]. Regarding the effects in the CNS, laquinimod treatment prevented the loss of brain-derived neurotrophic factor (BDNF) induced by the disease process. In EAE mice, laquinimod induced an elevation of BDNF expression in various brain regions to reach similar BDNF concentration as that of naïve controls [43]. In the human, a Phase II study undergoing laquinimod treatment showed a significant and specific elevation of serum BDNF levels compared to the placebo group after 3 months of treatment [44]. Whether laquinimod directly affects BDNF expression within the neurons, or induces bystander mechanisms that arrest the inflammatory progression and facilitates neuroprotection, needs to be further clarified.

Two Phase III clinical trials of laquinimod in RRMS (the ALLEGRO and BRAVO trial sponsored by TEVA) have been completed. In the first one, treatment with laquinimod as compared with placebo was associated with a modest reduction in ARR, decreased the risk of disability progression and reduced the number of gadolinium-enhancing lesions detected by MRI. However, the failure to meet primary end point in the BRAVO study led the manufacturer to delay requesting FDA approval. On May 2013, laquinimod was approved in Russia as a treatment for RRMS.

Nevertheless, in 2013 Teva Pharmaceutical and Active Biotech started the third Phase III trial of laquinimod in patients with RRMS. The study is designed to evaluate the safety and efficacy of laquinimod with a primary end point of time to confirmed disability progression, as measured by the EDSS (CONCERTO trial, ClinicalTrials.gov Identifier: NCT01707992). CONCERTO results are expected to be available towards mid-2017.

2.2.4. *Anti-LINGO antibody*

Nogo receptor-interacting protein (LINGO-1) is a transmembrane signal-transducing molecule, selectively expressed by oligodendrocytes and neurons and that associates with the Nogo-66 receptor (NgR1) complex [45]. NgR1 binds myelin-associated inhibitors of axonal regeneration such as Nogo-A, myelin-associated glycoprotein and oligodendrocyte myelin glycoprotein [46]. In response to CNS injury and demyelination, oligodendrocyte precursor cells and stem cells from the white matter become activated, migrate to the demyelinated area, proliferate and differentiate into oligodendrocytes that will remyelinate damaged axons. In chronic MS lesions, despite the presence of oligodendrocyte precursors in demyelinated plaques and the close proximity between pre-myelinating oligodendrocytes and demyelinated axons, axonal remyelination failed. This suggests that the differentiation process may be locally blocked by inhibitory factors [47].

In animal models, LINGO-1 expression is up-regulated in rat spinal cord injury, experimental EAE, 6-hydroxydopamine neurotoxic lesions and glaucoma models [48, 49]. Several works have reported the blockade of Nogo signalling as a therapeutic approach for neurological disorders such as spinal cord injury, traumatic brain injury, stroke, schizophrenia, amyotrophic lateral sclerosis and MS [50]. Animal models provide evidence that LINGO-1 is a potent inhibitor of axonal remyelination and regeneration in vivo. For example, transgenic mice overexpressing full-length LINGO-1 under the neuronal promoter of synapsin showed a significant reduction in the number of myelinated axons in the spinal cord and brain at P8 [51]. Other authors showed that neurite outgrowth inhibitor Nogo-A is involved in autoimmune-mediated demyelination in vivo [52].

BIIB033 is a monoclonal antibody that inhibits LINGO-1 and promotes axonal integrity/ remyelination in MOG-EAE mice [49]. In preclinical experiments, LINGO-1 antagonist antibodies did not alter EAE onset but did significantly mitigate disease severity across all stages of disease progression. This functional recovery in EAE correlates with improved axonal integrity as determined by magnetic resonance diffusion tensor imaging, and with newly formed myelin sheaths as determined by electron microscopy [53].

Biogen Idec Inc. started two different human studies with BIIB033 in 2010 (ClinicalTrials.gov Identifier: NCT01244139 and NCT01052506, respectively). Both studies finished in 2012 and BIIB033 showed favourable safety profile, desirable pharmacokinetic in healthy adults and MS patients and predicted brain penetration [53]. Based on these promising results, in 2013, Biogen started a Phase II dose-response study to assess the efficacy, safety, tolerability and pharmacokinetics of BIIB033 in 400 RRMS patients when used concurrently with Interferon β-1a (Avonex®) (SYNERGY, ClinicalTrials.gov Identifier: NCT01864148). SYNERGY results are expected to be available along 2016.

2.2.5. (−)-Epigallotechin-3-gallate

Green tea consumption has been associated to differences in the incidence of some diseases such as different kinds of cancer or cardiovascular pathologies [54]. Its composition includes, among other bioactive molecules, vitamins, pro-vitamins and antioxidants. Some of the more abundant components are tea polyphenols, also known as catechins, especially the (-)-epigallotechin-3-gallate (EGCG) [55]. EGCG has been profusely studied as an anticancer compound, as long as it can cause apoptosis and arrest cell cycle of tumoural cells [56]. As long as EGCG presents antioxidative properties, it can act as a chelator of neurotoxic metals and inhibit pro-inflammatory processes [57].

Efficacy studies in the EAE models for MS have shown that, alone or in combination with approved treatments for MS, oral EGCG ameliorated disease course and decreases EAE severity, preventing and reversing disability. This positive effect has been mainly attributed to the inhibition of NF-κB-mediated inflammation, cell proliferation, TNF-α secretion and Th1/ Th2 response. EGCG enhanced axonal preservation and inhibited neuronal apoptosis in treated animals [58]. The neuroprotective profile of EGCG has been attributed to its activity as a free radical scavenger [58]. Although this effect may be related with the inhibition of NF-κB pathway and glial reactivity, this indirect neuroprotection is also of main interest for the treatment of MS and other neurodegenerative diseases.

Several epidemiologic studies and clinical trials have been performed to test the preventive and therapeutic effects of EGCG in neurodegenerative diseases such as Alzheimer's, Parkinson's or Huntington's diseases [59]. In general, these studies show no EGCG-related prevention of neuronal and glial cell death in patients [59]. In 2013, a multicentric Phase II national study to investigate the anti-inflammatory and neuroprotective effects of EGCG in 120 RRMS patients was started (SuniMS Study, ClinicalTrials.gov identifier: NCT00525668, sponsored by Charite University, Berlin, Germany). At the moment, no results are available for this study.

Finally, to analyse the metabolic effects of EGCG and to assess the importance of lipid oxidation in fuel muscle's energy metabolism and its relationship with muscle weakness and fatigue in RRMS patients, the same institution completed a clinical research trial in 2013 (ClinicalTrials.gov identifier: NCT01417312). Results showed that EGCG given to MS patients over 12 weeks improves muscle metabolism during moderate exercise to a greater extent in men than in women, possibly because of sex-specific effects on autonomic and endocrine control. These results indicate that EGCG could be a promising treatment for MS, with a good- and well-known safety profile and an interesting combinability with other treatments. However, as the EGCG pass through the blood-brain barrier in humans is still controversial, its bioavailability remains to be characterized [60].

3. Effects of diazoxide in multiple sclerosis

3.1. K_{ATP} channels and neuroinflammation

Adenosine triphosphate (ATP)-dependent potassium (K_{ATP}) channels play important roles in many cellular functions by coupling cell metabolism to electrical activity. First detected in cardiac myocytes, they are also expressed in a wide number of cell types such as pancreatic β-cells, skeletal and smooth myocytes, neurons and microglia. In these cells, K_{ATP} channels regulate potassium fluxes across the cell membrane when glucose is available in sufficient conditions, which couple the electrical activity of the cell to energy metabolism [61, 62]. An increase in the cellular ATP concentration leads to channel closure and membrane depolarization. On the contrary, metabolic inhibition opens K_{ATP} channels and suppresses electrical activity.

Functional K_{ATP} channels in the cell membrane are assembled as a heterooctameric complex [63] from two structurally distinct subunits: the regulatory sulphonylurea receptor (SUR) and the pore-forming inwardly rectifying potassium channel (Kir) subunit 6.1 or 6.2. While ATP inhibits the K_{ATP} channel by directly binding to the cytoplasmic Kir6 domains, activators, such as potassium channel openers (KCOs), and inhibitors, such as sulphonylurea drugs [64], bind SUR to modulate the channel. Similar K_{ATP} channels have also been described in the mitochondria, located on the inner membrane of these organelles where they play a crucial role in the maintenance of mitochondrial homeostasis and function [65].

In recent years, K_{ATP} channels have attracted increasing interest as targets for drug development. Their pivotal role in a plethora of physiological processes has been underscored by recent discoveries linking potassium channel mutations to various diseases. The second generation of KCOs with an improved in vitro or in vivo selectivity has broadened the chemical diversity of K_{ATP} channel ligands. On the other hand, considering the unique role that K_{ATP} channels play in the maintenance of cellular homeostasis, KCOs add their potential in promoting protection against metabolic stress to the already existing pharmacotherapy. Studies in animal models showed KCO effects in several pathological situations such as hypertension, cardiac ischaemia or asthma, which indicates a broad therapeutic potential for KCOs. For example, in the smooth muscle of blood vessels and pancreatic β-cells, diazoxide (7-chloro-3-methyl-4H-1,2,4-benzothiadiazine 1,1-dioxide) binds with similar affinities to SUR1 and SUR2B subunits of K_{ATP} channels, increases membrane permeability to potassium ions and induces hyperpolarization [64]. In these cells, diazoxide-induced hyperpolarization inhibits the opening of voltage-gated calcium channels, and results in vasorelaxation and inhibition of insulin secretion [66]. As a consequence, diazoxide has been used since the 1970s for treating malignant hypertension and hypoglycaemia in the United States, Canada, and most European countries [67].

Our laboratory has described the expression of K_{ATP} channels in microglia [68–70], through which they control the release of a diversity of inflammatory mediators, such as NO, IL-6 or TNF-α [71, 72]. We also evidenced that reactive microglia increase the expression of the K_{ATP}-channel components Kir6.1, Kir6.2, SUR1 and SUR2B [69, 73]. With this increased microglial expression, KCOs may modulate neuroinflammation. In this line, we and other authors have documented that pharmacological activation of K_{ATP} channels with diazoxide can exert CNS neuroprotective and anti-inflammatory effects against excitotoxicity, ischaemia, trauma and neurotoxicants [71, 72, 74, 75]. For example, any rat brain microinjection of glutamate analogues triggers a persistent process that leads to progressive atrophy with a widespread neuronal loss and a concomitant neuroinflammation [76]. This neurodegenerative process is reduced by diazoxide oral treatment, which ameliorated microglia-mediated inflammation and reduced neuronal loss [73].

Controlling the extent of microglial activation may offer prospective clinical therapeutic benefits for inflammation-related neurodegenerative disorders [73]. In this context, increased expression of K_{ATP} channels by activated microglia and the specific anti-inflammatory actions of diazoxide reveal the use of this drug as a therapeutic agent to treat MS inflammatory processes.

3.2. K_{ATP} channel openers and experimental autoimmune encephalomyelitis

We analysed the putative neuroprotective effects of diazoxide on an EAE murine model of MS by its oral administration in the classical EAE MOG35-55 mouse model for preclinical studies of MS [72]. The doses tested (0.8 and 0.05 mg/kg) were below those that induce blood glucose increase (>1 mg/kg) and both of them ameliorated clinical signs of EAE, being 0.8 mg/kg more effective [72]. Then, this dose was tested in two different experimental designs: (a) a preventive paradigm, in which diazoxide was administrated daily starting on the same day animals were immunized and (b) a palliative paradigm, in which mice were treated with diazoxide daily starting when they reached a clinical score of ≥1. In both cases, the treatment showed similar effectiveness and mice treated with diazoxide obtained a lower clinical score during the chronic phase of EAE. However, in the preventive paradigm, diazoxide could not delay EAE onset or reduce the number of animals developing EAE. This indicates that diazoxide effects could be mediated mainly by neuroprotection rather than by immunosuppression. The histopathological analysis of injured spinal cords confirmed that diazoxide elicited a significant reduction in myelin and axonal loss accompanied by a decrease in glial activation and neuronal damage, but it did not affect the number of infiltrating lymphocytes positive for CD3 and CD20.

We then analysed the neuroprotective properties of diazoxide in vitro and ex vivo [77]. In this study, diazoxide effectively protected NSC-34 motoneurons against oxidative, excitotoxic and inflammatory insults. It also enhanced the expression and nuclear translocation of Nrf2 in these cells as well as in the spinal cord of EAE animals orally administered with diazoxide. This demonstrated that one of the mechanisms of actions implied in the neuroprotective role of diazoxide is mediated by the activation of Nrf2 expression and nuclear translocation. Finally, diazoxide decreased neuronal death in organotypic hippocampal slice cultures after excitotoxicity and preserved myelin sheath in organotypic cerebellar cultures exposed to pro-inflammatory demyelinating damage. Thus, diazoxide is a neuroprotective agent against oxidative stress-induced damage and cellular dysfunction.

We finally studied the putative actions of diazoxide on autoimmune key processes during EAE such as antigen presentation and lymphocyte activation and proliferation [78]. For this, we analysed K_{ATP} channel expression in CD4-positive T cells and the proliferative of lymphocyte response in the EAE model. When we used whole splenocytes to test whether diazoxide could modulate lymphocyte proliferation, results showed a significant inhibition of the lymphocyte proliferative rate both in vitro and in vivo. Also, the expression of dendritic cell activation markers such as CD83, CD80, CD86 or major histocompatibility complex class II was reduced in cultures treated with diazoxide. However, we observed no inhibition of cell proliferation when isolated CD4-positive T lymphocytes were used instead of whole splenocytes. Diazoxide also failed to inhibit the expression of lymphocyte activation markers. These results suggest that although diazoxide does not directly suppress lymphocyte activation and proliferation, it could modulate lymphocyte activity by regulating antigen presentation. These discrete effects indicate again that diazoxide treatment attenuates EAE pathology with no immunosuppressive effects.

Taken together, at the doses studied, our results demonstrate novel actions of diazoxide as an anti-inflammatory drug that present beneficial effects on EAE through neuroprotection. At the functional level, diazoxide is a neuroprotective agent against oxidative stress-induced damage and cellular dysfunction (**Figure 2**). It attenuates EAE pathology not by causing lymphocyte suppression but by modulating immune communication, decreasing glial harmful activation and promoting myelin and neuronal protection. Thus, treatment with this widely used and well-tolerated drug may be a useful therapeutic intervention in ameliorating MS disease.

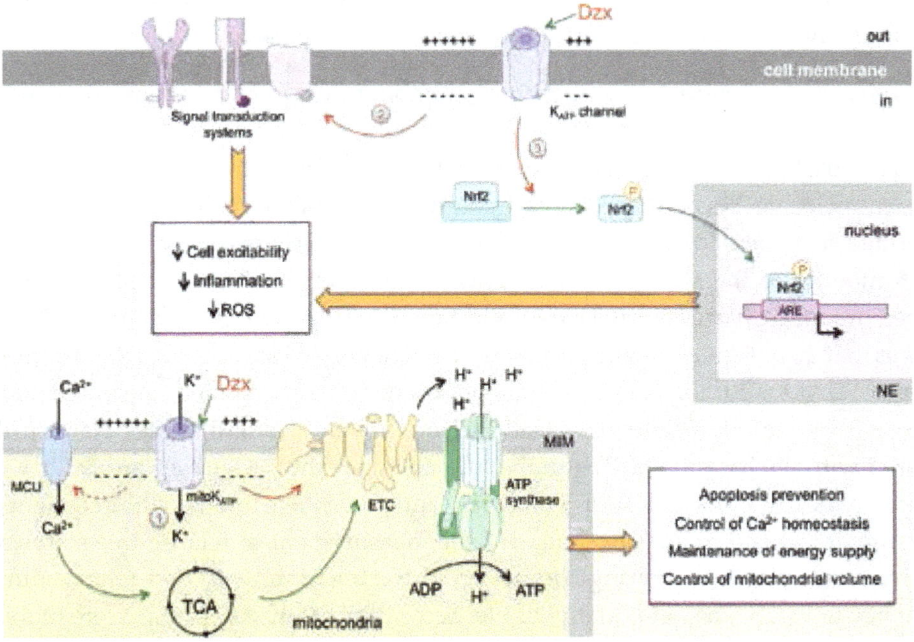

Figure 2. Diazoxide modifies microglial reactivity in brain. Drawing of the effects of diazoxide in the microglial reaction during MS. (1) Diazoxide (Dzx) binds to mitochondrial K_{ATP} channels, induces depolarization of the mitochondrial internal membrane (MIM) and potentiates the H^+ gradient generated by the electron transport chain (ETC). This enhances both ATP synthesis and calcium concentration by activation of ATP synthase and the mitochondrial calcium uniporter (MCU), respectively. Calcium in the mitochondria also increases the tricarboxylic acid cycle (TCA) flux by activation of deshydrogenases and enhances ATP production [73]. Dzx also activates K_{ATP} channels from the plasma membrane, which modifies the cell response to activation signals, (2) activates Nrf2 and (3) through a mechanism that remains to be described. ARE, antioxidant response element; NE, nuclear envelope.

3.3. Effects of diazoxide in MS patients

Based on the positive preclinical studies and considering that diazoxide has been on the market for decades with an excellent safety profile, two Spanish biotechnological companies, Neurotec Pharma and Advancell, performed a clinical development programme to assess diazoxide efficacy and safety in MS patients. NEUROADVAN trial (ClinicalTrials.gov identifier: NCT01428726) was initiated in 2011 and ended in 2014. NEUROADVAN was a Phase IIa, multinational, double-blind, placebo-controlled clinical trial to evaluate the efficacy and safety of diazoxide. The drug was orally administered at two different doses and compared in 103 patients with RRMS versus placebo (1:1:1). The total duration of the treatment was 6 months. Additionally, patients were allowed to continue during an optional extension period, in the same arm of the study, in a blinded way, until study finalization.

Men and women aged 18–55 years with RRMS (McDonald criteria 2010 [79]) and an EDSS score of 0–5.0 were eligible for the study. The inclusion criteria required at least one relapse in the previous 2 years or the presence of at least one Gad1 lesion in the previous year. During 24 weeks, patients received one daily oral tablet with 0.3 or 4 mg diazoxide. MRI scans were performed at baseline and every 4 weeks until the end of the study. Patients enrolled in the follow-up study were subjected to an additional scan at week 48.

The primary efficacy end point was that the number of new Gad1 lesions appeared on T1-weighted sequences from weeks 4 to 24. This end point has been validated in many previous 6-month MS trials and was based on the diazoxide effects on microglia activation and blood-brain barrier closing. Secondary MRI end points included cumulative number of lesions on T2-weighted sequences for all MRIs, cumulative number of lesions on T2-weighted sequences in the 6 months of the study (compared with the baseline MRI); cumulative number of combined unique active lesions (CUALs), addition of new or enlarged lesions on T2-weighted sequences that do not enhance with gadolinium and new Gad1 lesions for all MRIs; cumulative number of CUALs, addition of new or enlarged lesions on T2-weighted sequences that do not enhance with gadolinium and new Gad1 lesions in the 6 months after starting therapy (compared with the baseline MRI); number of patients without Gad1 lesions in T1-weighted sequences in the 6 months after starting therapy; and percentage brain volume change (PBVC). Secondary clinical end points also included the measurement of relapse-free status, relapse rate, number of relapses requiring corticosteroid treatment, time to first relapse during the trial, change in EDSS scale and quality of life. Secondary safety end points were monitorized during the 6 months of therapy up until 15 days after the last dose of diazoxide and included incidence, nature and severity of adverse events (AEs). Control of glucose levels, glycated haemoglobin and blood pressure were also monitorized.

The results of the clinical trial showed no differences in the diazoxide groups in the primary end point or in the other MRI variables associated with the presence of new lesions [80]. However, an interesting decrease in the PBVC in the patients who received diazoxide compared with placebo was found. The number of new T2/Proton Density lesions converting to black holes was not different between arms. Finally, in accordance with the small sample size of the trial, no differences were detected in clinical variables of relapse-free status, relapse rate, number of relapses requiring corticosteroid treatment, change in EDSS or quality of life.

There were six serious adverse events during the study but only a case with autoimmune hypothyroidism was considered to be related to the therapy that was not discontinued. Regarding the described clinical effects of diazoxide on glycaemia, the detected glucose blood levels were always within the limits of normality. This confirms that the diazoxide doses used in this trial were lower than those that induce hyperglycaemic and hypotensive effects.

As commented above, at the doses tested, diazoxide does not seem to have a significant effect that impedes the appearance of new Gad1 lesions. However, although patients were randomly distributed within the groups, at the beginning of the study those patients receiving diazoxide presented a higher number of Gad1 lesions than patients included in the placebo group. This initial higher disease activity in the group treated with diazoxide was maintained throughout the trial. These findings confirm the need to perform an extensive and accurate selection of patients, in terms of the activity of the disease, which must be carried out prior to the clinical trial.

Regarding the effects of diazoxide on brain atrophy, PBVC progressed more slowly in treated patients in a dose-dependent manner. This is consistent with a recent study that validates the measurement of brain atrophy as an outcome for Phase II trials in RRMS [81]. However, taking into account that treated patients had a more active disease, and that diazoxide presents vasodilator actions and peripheral resistance, the reduced atrophy found in patients treated with diazoxide may also be secondary to fluid shifts and not a true protection against brain injury. Nevertheless, the effects in slowing the progression of brain atrophy would require further validation.

To sum up, NEUROADVAN study indicates that diazoxide is a safe drug, well tolerated in patients with MS, but it was not possible to find evidence of efficacy in preventing the formation of new inflammatory lesions.

4. Conclusion

Neurodegenerative changes in MS such as demyelination and axonal loss take place early in the disease and independently from acute immuno-mediated inflammation. The reason why these focal demyelinating inflammatory lesions appear within the CNS still needs to be clarified, but diverse clinical presentations indicate the existence of different patterns of inflammation and neurodegeneration. Nevertheless, the molecular mechanisms underlying axonal damage in acute inflammation and chronic demyelination are potentially amenable to therapy. In this context, the pursuit of neuroprotective therapies in MS should provide new valid alternatives to significantly impact on disease progression. In this pursuit, the standard view of neuroprotection, which has long been mostly focused on neurons, is no longer valid. Instead, this view has been replaced by an integrative approach that recognizes the importance of dynamic interactions between immune cells, microglia, astrocytes and neurons.

A proper evaluation of neurodegenerative aspects in MS remains difficult. Also, for all mentioned drugs the neuroprotective effect has not been fully established. These issues could be better understood by applying well-established and new clinical and imaging parameters that require further preclinical and clinical investigations. Moreover, molecular characterization of the different MS clinical presentations must allow a pharmacogenomics classification of patients and development of personalized therapies. In this line, promising future approaches will combine high-throughput techniques such as proteomics and genomics to investigate further MS neurodegenerative processes, in particular neuroinflammation.

5. Disclosures

JFEP and MP have applied for a PCT application 'Diazoxide for use in the treatment of a central nervous system (CNS) autoimmune demyelinating disease' (application number PCT/EP2011/050049).

Acknowledgements

This research was supported by grant IPT-2012-0614-010000 from the Ministerio de Economía y Competitividad, and by grant 2014SGR1115 from the Generalitat de Catalunya, Spain.

Author details

Juan Espinosa-Parrilla, Marco Pugliese, Nicole Mahy and Manuel J Rodríguez*

*Address all correspondence to: marodriguez@ub.edu

Department of Biomedical Sciences, Institute of Neuroscience, IDIBAPS, University of Barcelona, and Center for Biomedical Research Network in Neurodegenerative Diseases (CIBERNED), Barcelona, Spain

References

[1] Katz Sand IB, Lublin FD. Diagnosis and differential diagnosis of multiple sclerosis. Continuum (Minneap Minn). 2013 Aug; 19(4 Multiple Sclerosis):922–43.

[2] Trapp BD, Nave K-A. Multiple sclerosis: an immune or neurodegenerative disorder? Annu Rev Neurosci. 2008 Jan; 31:247–69.

[3] Hohlfeld R, Dornmair K, Meinl E, Wekerle H. The search for the target antigens of multiple sclerosis, part 1: autoreactive CD4+ T lymphocytes as pathogenic effectors and therapeutic targets. Lancet Neurol. 2016 Feb; 15(2):198–209

[4] Krumbholz M, Derfuss T, Hohlfeld R, Meinl E. B cells and antibodies in multiple sclerosis pathogenesis and therapy. Nat Rev Neurol. 2012 Nov 5; 8(11):613–23.

[5] Losy J. Is MS an inflammatory or primary degenerative disease? J Neural Transm. 2013 Oct; 120(10):1459–62.

[6] Goverman J, Perchellet A, Huseby ES. The role of CD8(+) T cells in multiple sclerosis and its animal models. Curr Drug Targets Inflamm Allergy. 2005 Apr; 4(2):239–45.

[7] Lopez-Diego RS, Weiner HL. Novel therapeutic strategies for multiple sclerosis – a multifaceted adversary. Nat Rev Drug Discov. 2008 Nov; 7(11):909–25.

[8] Senanayake VK, Jin W, Mochizuki A, Chitou B, Goodenowe DB. Metabolic dysfunctions in multiple sclerosis: implications as to causation, early detection, and treatment, a case control study. BMC Neurol. 2015 Jan; 15:154.

[9] Luchtman D, Gollan R, Ellwardt E, Birkenstock J, Robohm K, Siffrin V, et al. In vivo and in vitro effects of multiple sclerosis immunomodulatory therapeutics on glutamatergic excitotoxicity. J Neurochem. 2016 Mar; 136(5):971–980

[10] Salter MW, Beggs S. Sublime microglia: expanding roles for the guardians of the CNS. Cell. 2014 Jul 3; 158(1):15–24.

[11] Block ML, Zecca L, Hong J-S. Microglia-mediated neurotoxicity: uncovering the molecular mechanisms. Nat Rev Neurosci. 2007 Jan; 8(1):57–69.

[12] Hellwig S, Heinrich A, Biber K. The brain's best friend: microglial neurotoxicity revisited. Front Cell Neurosci. 2013 Jan; 7:71.

[13] Lassmann H. Multiple sclerosis: is there neurodegeneration independent from inflammation? J Neurol Sci. 2007 Aug 15; 259(1–2):3–6.

[14] Ransohoff RM, Perry VH. Microglial physiology: unique stimuli, specialized responses. Annu Rev Immunol. 2009 Jan; 27:119–45.

[15] Kwilasz AJ, Grace PM, Serbedzija P, Maier SF, Watkins LR. The therapeutic potential of interleukin-10 in neuroimmune diseases. Neuropharmacology. 2015 Sep; 96(Pt A): 55–69.

[16] Tanaka T, Yoshida S. Mechanisms of remyelination: recent insight from experimental models. Biomol Concepts. 2014 Aug; 5(4):289–98.

[17] Vogel DY, Vereyken EJ, Glim JE, Heijnen PD, Moeton M, van der Valk P, et al. Macrophages in inflammatory multiple sclerosis lesions have an intermediate activation status. J Neuroinflamm. 2013 Jan; 10(1):35.

[18] Pugliese M, Espinosa-Parrilla JF, Bustos J, Campàs C, de Frias M, Sorrosal G. Novel therapeutic approaches to multiple sclerosis: neuroprotective drugs for relapsing-remitting multiple sclerosis. Adv Neuroimmune Biol. IOS Press; 2013; 4(3):187–204.

[19] Schweckendiek W. Treatment of psoriasis vulgaris. Med Monatsschr. 1959 Feb; 13(2): 103–4.

[20] Gold R, Linker RA, Stangel M. Fumaric acid and its esters: an emerging treatment for multiple sclerosis with antioxidative mechanism of action. Clin Immunol. 2012 Jan; 142(1):44–8.

[21] Ghoreschi K, Brück J, Kellerer C, Deng C, Peng H, Rothfuss O, et al. Fumarates improve psoriasis and multiple sclerosis by inducing type II dendritic cells. J Exp Med. 2011 Oct 24; 208(11):2291–303.

[22] Scannevin RH, Chollate S, Jung M, Shackett M, Patel H, Bista P, et al. Fumarates promote cytoprotection of central nervous system cells against oxidative stress via the nuclear factor (erythroid-derived 2)-like 2 pathway. J Pharmacol Exp Ther. 2012 Apr; 341(1):274–84.

[23] Licht-Mayer S, Wimmer I, Traffehn S, Metz I, Brück W, Bauer J, et al. Cell type-specific Nrf2 expression in multiple sclerosis lesions. Acta Neuropathol. 2015 Aug; 130(2):263–77.

[24] Gold R, Kappos L, Arnold DL, Bar-Or A, Giovannoni G, Selmaj K, et al. Placebo-controlled phase 3 study of oral BG-12 for relapsing multiple sclerosis. N Engl J Med. 2012 Sep 20; 367(12):1098–107.

[25] Groves A, Kihara Y, Chun J. Fingolimod: direct CNS effects of sphingosine 1-phosphate (S1P) receptor modulation and implications in multiple sclerosis therapy. J Neurol Sci. 2013 May 15; 328(1–2):9–18.

[26] Brinkmann V, Davis MD, Heise CE, Albert R, Cottens S, Hof R, et al. The immune modulator FTY720 targets sphingosine 1-phosphate receptors. J Biol Chem. 2002 Jun 14; 277(24):21453–7.

[27] Fujino M, Funeshima N, Kitazawa Y, Kimura H, Amemiya H, Suzuki S, et al. Amelioration of experimental autoimmune encephalomyelitis in Lewis rats by FTY720 treatment. J Pharmacol Exp Ther. 2003 Apr; 305(1):70–7.

[28] Kataoka H, Sugahara K, Shimano K, Teshima K, Koyama M, Fukunari A, et al. FTY720, sphingosine 1-phosphate receptor modulator, ameliorates experimental autoimmune encephalomyelitis by inhibition of T cell infiltration. Cell Mol Immunol. 2005 Dec; 2(6): 439–48.

[29] Rossi S, Lo Giudice T, De Chiara V, Musella A, Studer V, Motta C, et al. Oral fingolimod rescues the functional deficits of synapses in experimental autoimmune encephalomyelitis. Br J Pharmacol. 2012 Feb; 165(4):861–9.

[30] Cipriani R, Chara JC, Rodríguez-Antigüedad A, Matute C. FTY720 attenuates excitotoxicity and neuroinflammation. J Neuroinflammation. 2015 May 8; 12(1):86.

[31] Sato K, Ishikawa K, Ui M, Okajima F. Sphingosine 1-phosphate induces expression of early growth response-1 and fibroblast growth factor-2 through mechanism involving extracellular signal-regulated kinase in astroglial cells. Brain Res Mol Brain Res. 1999 Dec 10; 74(1–2):182–9.

[32] Choi JW, Gardell SE, Herr DR, Rivera R, Lee C-W, Noguchi K, et al. FTY720 (fingolimod) efficacy in an animal model of multiple sclerosis requires astrocyte sphingosine 1-phosphate receptor 1 (S1P1) modulation. Proc Natl Acad Sci U S A. 2011 Jan 11; 108(2): 751–6.

[33] Noda H, Takeuchi H, Mizuno T, Suzumura A. Fingolimod phosphate promotes the neuroprotective effects of microglia. J Neuroimmunol. 2013 Mar 15; 256(1–2):13–8.

[34] Cohen JA, Barkhof F, Comi G, Hartung H-P, Khatri BO, Montalban X, et al. Oral fingolimod or intramuscular interferon for relapsing multiple sclerosis. N Engl J Med. 2010 Feb 4; 362(5):402–15.

[35] Kappos L, Radue E-W, O'Connor P, Polman C, Hohlfeld R, Calabresi P, et al. A placebo-controlled trial of oral fingolimod in relapsing multiple sclerosis. N Engl J Med. 2010 Feb 4; 362(5):387–401.

[36] Calabresi PA, Radue E-W, Goodin D, Jeffery D, Rammohan KW, Reder AT, et al. Safety and efficacy of fingolimod in patients with relapsing-remitting multiple sclerosis (FREEDOMS II): a double-blind, randomised, placebo-controlled, phase 3 trial. Lancet Neurol. 2014 Jun; 13(6):545–56.

[37] Novartis. Novartis provides update on fingolimod Phase III trial in primary progressive MS (PPMS) [Accessed 2015-09-20]. Available from: https://www.novartis.com/news/media-releases/novartis-provides-update-fingolimod-phase-iii-trial-primary-progressive-ms-ppms.

[38] Wolinsky JS, Narayana PA, Noseworthy JH, Lublin FD, Whitaker JN, Linde A, et al. Linomide in relapsing and secondary progressive MS: part II: MRI results. MRI Analysis Center of the University of Texas-Houston, Health Science Center, and the North American Linomide Investigators. Neurology. 2000 May 9; 54(9):1734–41.

[39] Noseworthy JH, Wolinsky JS, Lublin FD, Whitaker JN, Linde A, Gjorstrup P, et al. Linomide in relapsing and secondary progressive MS: part I: trial design and clinical results. North American Linomide Investigators. Neurology. 2000 May 9; 54(9):1726–33.

[40] Yang J-S, Xu L-Y, Xiao B-G, Hedlund G, Link H. Laquinimod (ABR-215062) suppresses the development of experimental autoimmune encephalomyelitis, modulates the Th1/Th2 balance and induces the Th3 cytokine TGF-beta in Lewis rats. J Neuroimmunol. 2004 Nov; 156(1–2):3–9.

[41] Wegner C, Stadelmann C, Pförtner R, Raymond E, Feigelson S, Alon R, et al. Laquinimod interferes with migratory capacity of T cells and reduces IL-17 levels, inflammatory demyelination and acute axonal damage in mice with experimental autoimmune encephalomyelitis. J Neuroimmunol. 2010 Oct 8; 227(1–2):133–43.

[42] Gurevich M, Gritzman T, Orbach R, Tuller T, Feldman A, Achiron A. Laquinimod suppress antigen presentation in relapsing-remitting multiple sclerosis: in-vitro high-throughput gene expression study. J Neuroimmunol. 2010 Apr 15; 221(1–2):87–94.

[43] Aharoni R, Saada R, Eilam R, Hayardeny L, Sela M, Arnon R. Oral treatment with laquinimod augments regulatory T-cells and brain-derived neurotrophic factor expression and reduces injury in the CNS of mice with experimental autoimmune encephalomyelitis. J Neuroimmunol. 2012 Oct 15; 251(1–2):14–24.

[44] Thöne J, Ellrichmann G, Seubert S, Peruga I, Lee D-H, Conrad R, et al. Modulation of autoimmune demyelination by laquinimod via induction of brain-derived neurotrophic factor. Am J Pathol. 2012 Jan; 180(1):267–74.

[45] Mi S, Miller RH, Lee X, Scott ML, Shulag-Morskaya S, Shao Z, et al. LINGO-1 negatively regulates myelination by oligodendrocytes. Nat Neurosci. 2005 Jun; 8(6):745–51.

[46] Liu BP, Fournier A, GrandPré T, Strittmatter SM. Myelin-associated glycoprotein as a functional ligand for the Nogo-66 receptor. Science. 2002 Aug 16; 297(5584):1190–3.

[47] Kuhlmann T, Miron V, Cui Q, Cuo Q, Wegner C, Antel J, et al. Differentiation block of oligodendroglial progenitor cells as a cause for remyelination failure in chronic multiple sclerosis. Brain. 2008 Jul; 131(Pt 7):1749–58.

[48] Inoue H, Lin L, Lee X, Shao Z, Mendes S, Snodgrass-Belt P, et al. Inhibition of the leucine-rich repeat protein LINGO-1 enhances survival, structure, and function of dopaminergic neurons in Parkinson's disease models. Proc Natl Acad Sci U S A. 2007 Sep 4; 104(36):14430–5.

[49] Mi S, Hu B, Hahm K, Luo Y, Kam Hui ES, Yuan Q, et al. LINGO-1 antagonist promotes spinal cord remyelination and axonal integrity in MOG-induced experimental autoimmune encephalomyelitis. Nat Med. 2007 Oct; 13(10):1228–33.

[50] Petratos S, Ozturk E, Azari MF, Kenny R, Lee JY, Magee KA, et al. Limiting multiple sclerosis related axonopathy by blocking Nogo receptor and CRMP-2 phosphorylation. Brain. 2012 Jun; 135(Pt 6):1794–818.

[51] Lee X, Yang Z, Shao Z, Rosenberg SS, Levesque M, Pepinsky RB, et al. NGF regulates the expression of axonal LINGO-1 to inhibit oligodendrocyte differentiation and myelination. J Neurosci. 2007 Jan 3; 27(1):220–5.

[52] Karnezis T, Mandemakers W, McQualter JL, Zheng B, Ho PP, Jordan KA, et al. The neurite outgrowth inhibitor Nogo A is involved in autoimmune-mediated demyelination. Nat Neurosci. 2004 Jul; 7(7):736–44.

[53] Mi S, Pepinsky RB, Cadavid D. Blocking LINGO-1 as a therapy to promote CNS repair: from concept to the clinic. CNS Drugs. 2013 Jul; 27(7):493–503.

[54] Mak JCW. Potential role of green tea catechins in various disease therapies: progress and promise. Clin Exp Pharmacol Physiol. 2012 Mar; 39(3):265–73.

[55] Balentine DA, Wiseman SA, Bouwens LC. The chemistry of tea flavonoids. Crit Rev Food Sci Nutr. 1997 Dec; 37(8):693–704.

[56] Lu Y-P, Lou Y-R, Liao J, Xie J-G, Peng Q-Y, Yang CS, et al. Administration of green tea or caffeine enhances the disappearance of UVB-induced patches of mutant p53 positive epidermal cells in SKH-1 mice. Carcinogenesis. 2005 Aug; 26(8):1465–72.

[57] Lin YL, Lin JK. (-)-Epigallocatechin-3-gallate blocks the induction of nitric oxide synthase by down-regulating lipopolysaccharide-induced activity of transcription factor nuclear factor-kappaB. Mol Pharmacol. 1997 Sep; 52(3):465–72.

[58] Aktas O, Prozorovski T, Smorodchenko A, Savaskan NE, Lauster R, Kloetzel P-M, et al. Green tea epigallocatechin-3-gallate mediates T cellular NF-kappa B inhibition and

exerts neuroprotection in autoimmune encephalomyelitis. J Immunol. 2004 Nov 1; 173(9):5794–800.

[59] Mähler A, Mandel S, Lorenz M, Ruegg U, Wanker EE, Boschmann M, et al. Epigallocatechin-3-gallate: a useful, effective and safe clinical approach for targeted prevention and individualised treatment of neurological diseases? EPMA J. 2013 Jan; 4(1):5.

[60] Zini A, Del Rio D, Stewart AJ, Mandrioli J, Merelli E, Sola P, et al. Do flavan-3-ols from green tea reach the human brain? Nutr Neurosci. Jan; 9(1–2):57–61.

[61] Kline CF, Kurata HT, Hund TJ, Cunha SR, Koval OM, Wright PJ, et al. Dual role of KATP channel C-terminal motif in membrane targeting and metabolic regulation. Proc Natl Acad Sci U S A. 2009 Sep 29; 106(39):16669–74.

[62] Nichols CG, Lederer WJ. Adenosine triphosphate-sensitive potassium channels in the cardiovascular system. Am J Physiol. 1991 Dec; 261(6 Pt 2):H1675–86.

[63] Proks P, Ashcroft FM. Modeling K(ATP) channel gating and its regulation. Prog Biophys Mol Biol. 2009 Jan; 99(1):7–19.

[64] Ashcroft FM, Gribble FM. New windows on the mechanism of action of K(ATP) channel openers. Trends Pharmacol Sci. 2000 Nov; 21(11):439–45.

[65] Kowaltowski AJ, Seetharaman S, Paucek P, Garlid KD. Bioenergetic consequences of opening the ATP-sensitive K(+) channel of heart mitochondria. Am J Physiol Heart Circ Physiol. 2001 Feb; 280(2):H649–57.

[66] Petit P, Loubatières-Mariani MM. Potassium channels of the insulin-secreting B cell. Fundam Clin Pharmacol. 1992 Jan; 6(3):123–34.

[67] Koch-Weser J. Diazoxide. N Engl J Med. 1976 Jun 3; 294(23):1271–3.

[68] Ramonet D, Rodríguez MJ, Pugliese M, Mahy N. Putative glucosensing property in rat and human activated microglia. Neurobiol Dis. 2004 Oct; 17(1):1–9.

[69] Ortega FJ, Gimeno-Bayon J, Espinosa-Parrilla JF, Carrasco JL, Batlle M, Pugliese M, et al. ATP-dependent potassium channel blockade strengthens microglial neuroprotection after hypoxia-ischemia in rats. Exp Neurol. 2012 May; 235(1):282–96.

[70] Ortega FJ, Jolkkonen J, Rodríguez MJ. Microglia is an active player in how glibenclamide improves stroke outcome. J Cereb Blood Flow Metab. 2013 Jul; 33(7):1138–9.

[71] Zhou F, Yao H-H, Wu J-Y, Ding J-H, Sun T, Hu G. Opening of microglial K(ATP) channels inhibits rotenone-induced neuroinflammation. J Cell Mol Med. 2008 Jan; 12(5A):1559–70.

[72] Virgili N, Espinosa-Parrilla JF, Mancera P, Pastén-Zamorano A, Gimeno-Bayon J, Rodríguez MJ, et al. Oral administration of the KATP channel opener diazoxide ameliorates disease progression in a murine model of multiple sclerosis. J Neuroinflammation. BioMed Central Ltd; 2011 Jan; 8(1):149.

[73] Rodríguez MJ, Martínez-Moreno M, Ortega FJ, Mahy N. Targeting microglial K(ATP) channels to treat neurodegenerative diseases: a mitochondrial issue. Oxid Med Cell Longev. 2013 Jan; 2013:194546.

[74] Robin E, Simerabet M, Hassoun SM, Adamczyk S, Tavernier B, Vallet B, et al. Postconditioning in focal cerebral ischemia: role of the mitochondrial ATP-dependent potassium channel. Brain Res. 2011 Feb 23; 1375:137–46.

[75] Roseborough G, Gao D, Chen L, Trush MA, Zhou S, Williams GM, et al. The mitochondrial K-ATP channel opener, diazoxide, prevents ischemia-reperfusion injury in the rabbit spinal cord. Am J Pathol. 2006 May; 168(5):1443–51.

[76] Espinosa-Parrilla JF, Martínez-Moreno M, Gasull X, Mahy N, Rodríguez MJ. The L-type voltage-gated calcium channel modulates microglial pro-inflammatory activity. Mol Cell Neurosci. 2015 Jan; 64:104–15.

[77] Virgili N, Mancera P, Wappenhans B, Sorrosal G, Biber K, Pugliese M, et al. K(ATP) channel opener diazoxide prevents neurodegeneration: a new mechanism of action via antioxidative pathway activation. PLoS One. 2013 Jan; 8(9):e75189.

[78] Virgili N, Mancera P, Chanvillard C, Wegner A, Wappenhans B, Rodríguez MJ, et al. Diazoxide attenuates autoimmune encephalomyelitis and modulates lymphocyte proliferation and dendritic cell functionality. J Neuroimmune Pharmacol. 2014 Sep; 9(4):558–68.

[79] Polman CH, Reingold SC, Banwell B, Clanet M, Cohen JA, Filippi M, et al. Diagnostic criteria for multiple sclerosis: 2010 revisions to the McDonald criteria. Ann Neurol. 2011 Feb; 69(2):292–302.

[80] Villoslada P, Rovira A, Montalban X, Arroyo R, Paul F, Meca-Lallana V, et al. Effects of diazoxide in multiple sclerosis: a randomized, double-blind phase 2 clinical trial. Neurol Neuroimmunol neuroinflammation. 2015 Oct; 2(5):e147.

[81] van den Elskamp IJ, Boden B, Dattola V, Knol DL, Filippi M, Kappos L, et al. Cerebral atrophy as outcome measure in short-term phase 2 clinical trials in multiple sclerosis. Neuroradiology. 2010 Oct; 52(10):875–81.

2

The Gateway Reflex, a Novel Neuro-Immune Interaction, is Critical for the Development of Mouse Multiple Sclerosis (MS) Models

Daisuke Kamimura, Yasunobu Arima,
Andrea Stofkova, Naoki Nishikawa, Kotaro Higuchi,
Takuto Ohki and Masaaki Murakami

Abstract

The central nervous system (CNS) is an immune-privileged tissue protected by the brain–blood barrier (BBB), which limits the absorption of substances and cells from blood flow. In the case of inflammatory diseases in the CNS, such as multiple sclerosis (MS), however, autoreactive T cells that attack brain autoantigens, including myelin proteins, circumvent the BBB. Despite the wide distribution of brain autoantigens, demyelination often occurs as discrete foci. This fact suggests that there might be a certain cue that guides autoreactive T cells to particular site(s) in the CNS. In other words, there exists a mechanism that facilitates a site-specific accumulation of autoreactive T cells in the CNS. Using a murine model of MS, experimental autoimmune encephalomyelitis (EAE), we identified dorsal vessels of the fifth lumbar (L5) spinal cord as the initial entry site of immune cells. The formation of a gateway for immune cells is defined by local neural stimulations. For example, neural stimulation by gravity creates this gateway by increasing the expression of chemokines that attract autoreactive T cells. Regional neural activation by the other stimuli, such as electric pulses or pain sensation, also induces gateway formation, but at different blood vessels via chemokine expression. These neuro-immune interactions are examples of the gateway reflex and are extensively reviewed in this chapter.

Keywords: gateway reflex, inflammation amplifier, NF-κB, STAT, multiple sclerosis

1. Introduction

Multiple sclerosis (MS) is a common neurological disease that is estimated to inflict more than 2.5 million patients worldwide [1–4]. MS is associated with chronic inflammation of the central nervous system (CNS) with myelin antigens as the immune target during the inflammation processes. The clinical manifestations of MS are variable and often include both symptoms of upper motor neurons, such as hyperreflexia, ataxia, spasticity, and visual defects, and lower motor neuron symptoms, such as sensory neuron defects and paralysis [5]. Given the uniform presence of myelin antigens in the CNS, however, variable local, rather than systemic clinical symptoms raise the possibility that there exists specific sites in the CNS that are vulnerable to immune cells thus triggering auto-reactivity. As discussed below, we observed using a murine model of MS, experimental autoimmune encephalomyelitis (EAE), that regional neural stimulations permit entry of immune cells into the CNS, which may explain the variable MS symptoms among patients.

Genetic susceptibility of MS is well studied, and major histocompatibility complex (MHC) genes and genes associated with CD4+ helper T-cell activation and homeostasis are identified as susceptible genes. The strongest genetic linkage was found at certain alleles of MHC class II, which suggests a relationship between autoreactive CD4+ T cells and MS development in humans [6]. Consistently, autoreactive CD4+ T cells have important roles in the development and relapse of animal models of MS [4, 7–13]. In addition to MHC genes, several genome-wide association studies (GWAS) of MS patients have identified additional genetic loci including interleukin (IL)-17, IL-2 receptor (CD25), and IL-7 receptor (CD127), which are important for CD4+ T-cell effector function, activation, and survival [14–16]. These lines of genetic evidence suggest that blocking CD4+ T-cell entry into the CNS, thereby blocking subsequent inflammation in the CNS, would be an effective way for the treatment of MS. Indeed, drugs that target T-cell migration such as fingolimod (FTY720) and natalizumab (anti-VLA4 antibody) have shown clinical success in the treatment of MS. Fingolimod is an orally available sphingosine-1-phosphate receptor modulator, which reduces CD4+ T-cell invasion to the CNS due to the inhibition of lymphocyte egress from lymph nodes [17]. Natalizumab, on the other hand, targets alpha4 integrin (a subunit of VLA4), which is required for the migration of CD4+ T cells to inflamed CNS [4, 18]. The prominent clinical effects of these drugs provide a proof of concept for therapeutic strategies to suppress the invasion of autoreactive CD4+ T cells into the CNS. Because side effects such as progressive multifocal leukoencephalopathy warrant caution for the use of fingolimod and natalizumab [19, 20], a novel strategy including a blockade of the entry site, or gateway, of immune cells to the CNS is desired.

It is widely known that the CNS is an immune-privileged site, protected by the blood–brain barrier (BBB), which restricts the exchange of substances and cell migration into and out of the organ. However, CNS invasion by immune cells occurs in not only neuropathologic conditions including MS, but also normal healthy conditions. We have been studying where and how immune cells can enter the CNS using EAE models. In this chapter, our recent findings about these gateways, a mechanism to operate them, and perspectives are discussed.

2. Blood–brain barrier and inflammation

The BBB is a specialized blood vessel formed by several cell types including vascular endothelial cells, pericytes, and astrocyte endfeet. In addition, tight junctions are critical for barrier development and are established through interactions of tight junction molecules, such as ZO-1, claudins, and occludins, between the vascular endothelial cells to cause a size exclusion of about 500 daltons [21, 22]. Despite this rigid barrier system, autoreactive T cells can enter to the CNS and cause autoimmune diseases such as MS. The breakdown of the BBB is also observed in neurodegenerative disorders such as Alzheimer's disease and Parkinson's disease [23]. Because neuroinflammation is associated with almost all diseases in the CNS [24], the relationship between a dysfunctional BBB and inflammatory cytokines has been well studied. For example, TNFαincreases BBB permeability during sepsis, and IL-1β regulates the BBB via reactivation of the HIF-VEGF axis in MS [25, 26]. IFNγ and TNFα decrease the expression of TWIK-related potassium channel-1 in human brain microvascular endothelial cells, which leads to increase the transmigration of various immune cells across the endothelial cells in vitro [27]. IL-17A, which is a signature cytokine of Th17 cells, also contributes to BBB leakage in vitro and in vivo. EAE was significantly suppressed in IL-17A-deficient mice [28], and IL-17A-deficient CD4+ T cells hardly invade the CNS through the fifth lumbar (L5) spinal cord unlike normal ones [12]. IL-17A-mediated BBB dysfunction involves the formation of reactive oxygen species by cellular oxidases, which down-regulate tight junction molecules and the activation of the endothelial contractile machinery in vitro [29, 30]. Seeing that GWAS and animal model data have revealed that autoreactive CD4+ T cells producing many cytokines play a central role in MS, understanding the in vivo behavior of disease-causing CD4+ T cells offers crucial insights about the pathophysiology of MS. Intravital two-photon imaging using a rat transfer EAE model showed that there are at least three stages for CNS invasion by autoreactive CD4+ T cells: intraluminal scanning, perivascular scanning, and CNS-surface scanning [31]. This study also suggested that the reactivation of CNS-invading CD4+ T cells by perivascular/ meningeal antigen-presenting cells is followed by parenchymal infiltration of pathogenic CD4+ T cells [31]. Chemokine guidance and cellular adhesion events of pathogenic CD4+ T cells are also critical for the CNS invasion [12, 31]. Myelin autoantigen candidates associated with MS including Myelin Basic Protein (MBP), myelin-oligodendrocyte protein (MOG) and proteolipid proteins (PLP) [32–35] are present throughout CNS white matter, while MS lesions are often observed by MRI as focal plaques [36]. These facts suggest that there exists an additional signal that directs pathogenic CD4+ T cells to initiate inflammatory reactions at particular region(s) of the CNS. We recently demonstrated that this signal is provided by several types of neural activations. We also defined a molecular mechanism of the resulting neuro-immune interactions for the development and relapse of murine models of MS, as discussed in the following sections.

3. Gravity-mediated gateway reflex

We first considered the initial site where the autoreactive CD4+ T cells invade the CNS. In EAE models, mice or rats are generally immunized with various CNS antigens such as myelin-oligodendrocyte protein (MOG) emulsified with complete Freund's adjuvant (CFA) in the presence of pertussis toxin administration, which are critical for the generation of autoreactive CD4+ T cells and the induction of MS-like symptoms, including a progressive paralysis that usually begins at the tip of the tail. EAE can also be induced in wild-type animals by the transfer of autoreactive CD4+ T cells isolated from other EAE mice. This transfer EAE model is induced without antigens, CFA, or pertussis toxin treatment, making this model suitable for investigating the behavior of the disease-causing CD4+ T cells in detail. Whole-mount sagittal sections of adult mice at a preclinical stage of the transfer EAE model (day 4 or 5 after MOG-reactive CD4+ T-cell transfer) revealed that MOG-reactive pathogenic CD4+ T cells preferentially accumulated at the L5 spinal cord, but not in the brain at this early stage. This observation suitably explains the first clinical symptom of typical EAE, a weakness of the tail tip. A closer analysis of the L5 spinal cord revealed that the accumulation of MOG-reactive CD4+ T cells occurred around the dorsal vessels. Various chemokines including Th17-attracting CCL20 were up-regulated at the L5 dorsal vessels during EAE compared with dorsal vessels from other spinal cords. Indeed, anti-CCL20 antibody treatment or transfer of MOG-reactive CD4+ T cells lacking its receptor, CCR6, compromised the L5 accumulation of these CD4+ T cells and subsequent development of EAE, which is consistent with a published study [37]. Interestingly, the selective up-regulation of chemokines at the L5 dorsal vessels was observed even at steady state, albeit to a lesser degree than in the EAE condition. These results suggested that the L5 dorsal vessels are the first gateway for pathogenic CD4+ T cells in this transfer EAE system (**Figure 1**), and some physiological effects under steady state that modulate chemokine levels at the L5 dorsal vessels are enhanced during EAE.

Further investigation revealed that the selective up-regulation of chemokines at the L5 dorsal vessels at steady state were the result of neuro-immune interactions. It is known that neurons in the dorsal root ganglion (DRG) beside the L5 spinal cord are connected to the soleus muscles, the main anti-gravity muscles [38]. Consistent with a constant stimulation of the soleus muscles by Earth's gravity, the L5 DRG is the largest among all DRGs in mice and humans [39]. We hypothesized that constant stimulation by gravity might mediate the uniqueness of the L5 spinal cord in establishing the gateway of immune cells including autoreactive CD4+ T cells. Consistent with this hypothesis, we found two peaks of CCL20 expression at the dorsal vessels of the cervical and lumbar cords, although CCL20 expression was higher at the latter. To examine the effect of gravity, mice were suspended by their tails so that their hind legs were released from gravity. This treatment resulted in a reduced accumulation of MOG-specific CD4+ T cells at the L5 cord. Instead, these CD4+ T cells invaded the cervical cords as if a new gateway was created by the additional gravitational burden on the forefeet muscles due to the tail suspension [12]. Consistently, the tail suspension downregulated CCL20 levels in the L5 dorsal blood vessels, but up-regulated CCL20 in the cervical cords. Moreover, electric stimulations to the soleus muscles in tail-suspended mice restored CCL20 levels and CD4+ T-cell accumulation at the L5 spinal cord [12]. These results suggest that a certain neural activation triggered by gravity contributes to the gateway at the L5 dorsal blood vessels for autoreactive CD4+ T cells to infiltrate the CNS (**Figure 1**).

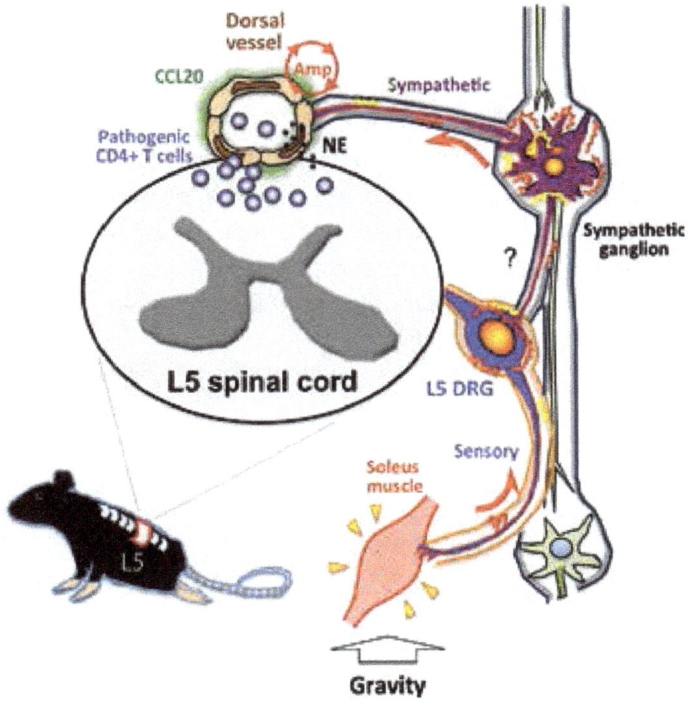

Figure 1. Gravity-mediated gateway reflex. Constant gravity-mediated stimulation of the soleus muscles induces the activation of sensory nerves, whose cell bodies are located at the dorsal root ganglion (DRG) of the fifth lumbar (L5) spinal cord. Signals via L5 DRG neurons travel to sympathetic neurons located nearby, resulting in norepinephrine (NE) secretion at the dorsal vessels there. NE enhances the inflammation amplifier (Amp) in the L5 dorsal vessel endothelium, causing an up-regulation of CCL20 and subsequent accumulation of pathogenic CD4+ T cells.

Sympathetic nerve activation was involved in the gravity-mediated chemokine expressions at the L5 dorsal vessels. c-Fos expression, which is a marker of neural activation, was higher in L5 sympathetic ganglions than in L1 sympathetic ganglions. Blood flow speeds at the L5 dorsal vessels, but not at other blood vessels including L1 dorsal vessels, femoral artery, and portal vein, became slower when mice were tail suspended, while electronic stimulation of the soleus muscles increased the flow speed, suggesting an involvement of autonomic nerves including sympathetic ones in this response [12]. Furthermore, pharmacological blockade of adrenergic receptors significantly inhibited CCL20 levels, NF-κB activation and MOG-reactive pathogenic CD4+ T-cell accumulation at the L5 dorsal vessels, and also suppressed clinical signs of EAE [12]. Thus, sensory nerve activation due to anti-gravity responses leads to a sympathetic nerve stimulation that creates a gateway for immune cells to pass through the CNS via the L5 dorsal vessels [12]. This neuro-immune response, which leads to change in the status of the vascular endothelium, is named the "gateway reflex" [40–42]. Other examples of the gateway reflex are described below.

4. Electric stimulation-mediated gateway reflex

Neural activations can be artificially induced by various methods including electric stimulations and treatment with reagents. We wondered if electric stimulation of different muscles could create gateways in blood vessels at distinct positions via regional neural activations. As discussed earlier, weak electric stimulation to the soleus muscles restored chemokine expression at the L5 dorsal vessels of tail-suspended mice, because the cell body of sensory neurons in the soleus muscles is mainly located in the L5 DRG. We applied this methodology to other muscles. As expected, electric stimulations to thigh muscles including the quadriceps, which are known to be regulated by L3 DRG neurons, led to an increased expression of chemokines in L3 dorsal vessels in mice, while electric stimulations of upper regions, such as forefoot muscles including the epitrochlearis and triceps brachii, resulted in an up-regulation of chemokines in the fifth cervical to fifth thoracic cord dorsal vessels, which is where the DRG

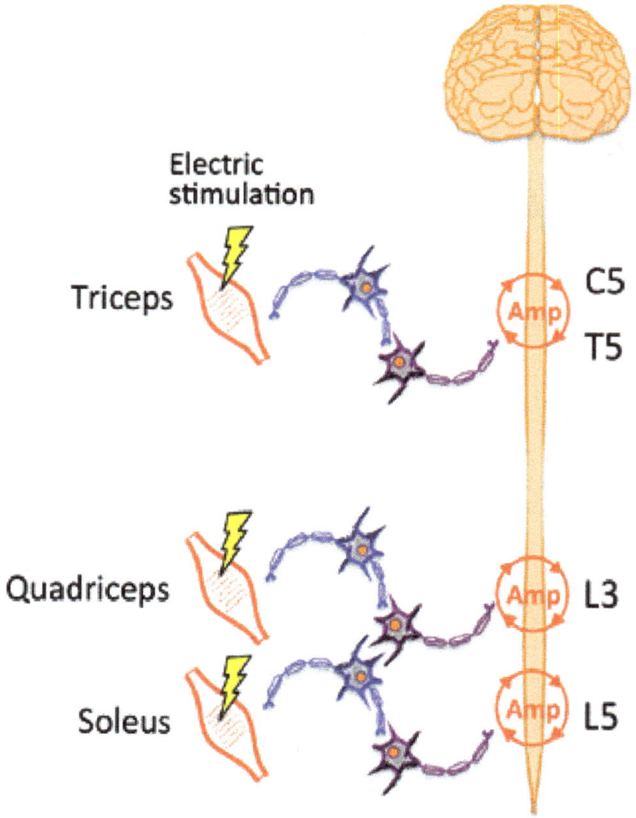

Figure 2. Electric stimulation-mediated gateway reflex. Artificially induced neural activation by weak electric stimulation followed by sensory-sympathetic cross talk can trigger the gateway reflex. Electric pulses to the triceps induce chemokine up-regulation at the dorsal vessels of the fifth cervical (C5) to fifth thoracic (T5) spinal cord through activation of the inflammation amplifier (Amp). Similarly, stimulation of the quadriceps induces a gateway at the dorsal vessels of the third lumbar (L3) cord, whereas the gateway dorsal vessels of the L5 cord are created by electric pulses to the soleus muscles.

neurons of the C5-T5 spinal cords project to/from these muscles. These results established the electric stimulation-mediated gateway as another example of the gateway reflex (**Figure 2**). In addition, they offer an important implication that the gateway reflex can be controlled by artificially stimulating specific neurons, providing a promising opportunity for a novel therapeutic strategy against inflammatory diseases in the CNS.

5. Pain-mediated gateway reflex

It is reported that many MS patients experience pain, and some patients take pain relief medication to improve their quality of life [43]. Pain is a common symptom in many diseases and disorders, but it is often considered a symptomatic effect that arises from tissue damage caused by the disease. However, it is known that pain triggers neural inputs via sensory neurons expressing nociceptors such as TRPV1 [44, 45]. Therefore, we assumed that a pain-mediated gateway reflex might exist, which would affect the disease status of MS and EAE. In EAE, modulations of nociception (pain sensation) are reported during the disease development [46]. Adoptive transfer of MOG reactive, pathogenic CD4+ T cells induces a transient EAE within a week after transfer, followed by a remission phase. Mice that experienced the first episode of EAE and are in the remission phase, which we termed EAE-recovered mice, never develop EAE symptoms again under normal conditions. We experimentally induced pain sensation in these EAE-recovered mice by ligating the middle branch of the trigeminal nerves, which has been reported as being composed of only sensory neurons [47]. Pain induction at the time of pathogenic T-cell transfer resulted in a persistence of EAE symptoms and caused considerable delay of the remission phase. On the contrary, suppressing pain by medication inhibited EAE development in several mouse models including an active immunization model in SJL mice. Because a majority of MS progresses with relapse and it is reported that pain is more intense in MS patients with higher disease scores [48], we examined whether pain induction triggers EAE relapse in mice. EAE-recovered mice were subjected to trigeminal nerve ligation to induce pain sensation. In separate experiments, pain-processing nerves were also chemically activated by the injection of capsaicin and substance P at the cheek or forefeet of EAE-recovered mice. All these treatments induced relapse of EAE, indicating that pain is not a simple by-product of the disease, but significantly contributes to the development and EAE relapse [13]. Similar to the gravity-mediated gateway reflex, a sensory-sympathetic pathway is involved in the pain-mediated EAE relapse, because pharmacological or genetic inhibition of pain-processing molecules such as TRPV1 and Nav1.8, and chemical ablation of sympathetic neurons by 6-hydroxydopamine (6-OHDA) suppressed EAE relapse induced by trigeminal nerve ligation. Interestingly, stress-mediated events, including immobilization stress and forced swimming stress (about 20 minutes/day), did not trigger EAE relapse although serum corticosterone, norepinephrine, and epinephrine were induced at a similar level to pain induction, suggesting that specific sensory-sympathetic nerve pathways, rather than systemic hormonal stress responses, mediate the relapse of EAE (**Figure 3**).

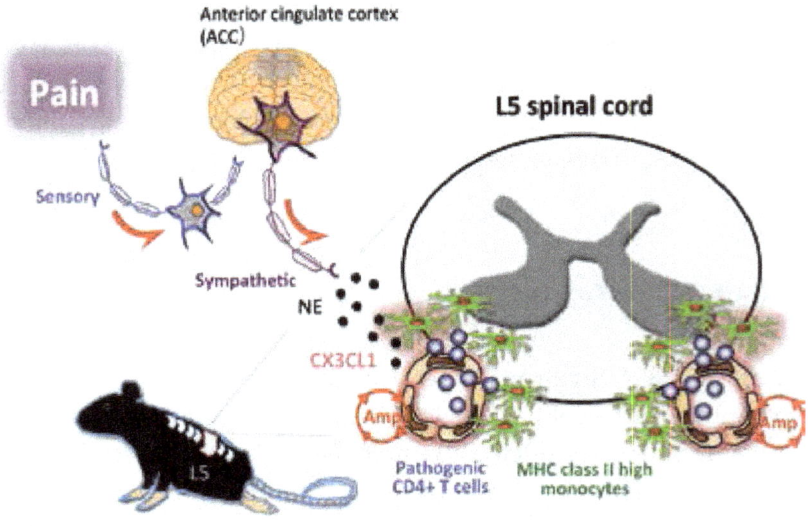

Figure 3. Pain-mediated gateway reflex. Pain-induced sensory neuron activation results in the activation of specific sympathetic neurons that control norepinephrine (NE) expression around the ventral vessels of every level of the spinal cords. This system is regulated by the anterior cinculate cortex (ACC) in the brain. Because the fifth lumbar (L5) spinal cord abundantly contains MHC class II high activated monocytes, this region is affected significantly during pain sensation. NE from pain-specific sympathetic neurons at the ventral vessels induces the production of CX3CL1 from the activated monocytes, further recruiting these cells in an auto/paracrine manner. The MHC class II high activated monocytes are able to present MOG antigens to pathogenic CD4+ T cells, which in turn activate the inflammation amplifier (Amp) in regional endothelial cells and subsequently cause a relapse in the disease.

During the first episode of EAE, MOG-reactive CD4+ T cells enter the CNS from the dorsal vessels of the L5 spinal cord [12]. The transferred CD4+ T cells are then found at the upper levels of the spinal cord and brain, which matches typical clinical manifestations of EAE including the initial tail tip weakness and subsequent ascending paralysis. Intriguingly, after pain induction in apparently normal EAE-recovered mice, the relapse also starts from the loss of tonicity of the tail tip, suggesting that the L5 cord could again be a gateway for relapse. However, an immunohistochemical examination of the L5 spinal cord from EAE-recovered mice showed differences with naïve mice, with many MHC class II high monocytes around the meningeal region. After pain induction, these cells accumulated at the L5 ventral vessels, but not dorsal vessels within a day. This accumulation is dependent on a chemokine CX3CL1, which is secreted from the MHC class II high monocytes themselves and astrocytes after norepinephrine stimulation. Therefore, the pain-mediated gateway reflex induces norepinephrine secretion from sympathetic neurons around the L5 ventral vessels and subsequent auto/paracrine induction of CX3CL1 followed by MHC class II high monocyte accumulations. Because these monocytes are able to present MOG peptides, circulating MOG-reactive pathogenic CD4+ T cells can recognize the L5 ventral vessels as an entry site to the CNS. Indeed, a depletion of CD4+ T cells including pathogenic ones from EAE-recovered mice abrogated the clinical symptoms of EAE relapse (i.e. paralysis), but the accumulation of MHC class II high monocytes around the L5 ventral vessels remained intact. These results suggested that the activated monocyte accumulation is an upstream event relative to pathogenic CD4+ T-cell invasion and required for EAE relapse induced by pain sensation [13].

The sympathetic nerve activation caused by pain appeared to be relatively systemic compared with that via the sensory pathway, since the expression levels of neural activation marker c-Fos increased in certain nerve cells in sympathetic ganglions at all spinal levels investigated, which is in contrast to the gravity-mediated gateway reflex in which the L5 sympathetic ganglion alone showed the highest expression of c-Fos. However, the pain-mediated gateway reflex affects blood vessels at the ventral sides of the L5 spinal cord. Why does the pain-mediated gateway reflex influence the L5 level alone, similar to the gravity-mediated gateway reflex? We assume that this property is related to the fact that the L5 cord is the first lesion in the transfer EAE model. Even at the remission phase of transfer EAE, MHC class II high monocytes that have infiltrated in the CNS during the initial episode remained mostly in the L5 spinal cord despite the disappearance of clinical symptoms [13]. Otherwise, gravity-mediated neural inputs might make the L5 environment different from other CNS regions. Whichever the explanation, we found that pain induction similarly triggers sympathetic neural activation to some neuron cells of every spinal level, but the L5 spinal cord responded strongest, most likely due to an abundance of activated monocytes.

It is known that pain-sensing neurons activate sympathetic neurons at least partially via the anterior cingulate cortex (ACC) in the somatosensory area of the brain [49, 50]. Blockade of this sensory-sympathetic connection by the injection of an N-methyl-D-aspartate (NMDA) receptor antagonist at the ACC suppressed the accumulation of MHC class II high monocytes at the L5 ventral vessels even after pain induction, and conversely, injection of an NMDA agonist at the ACC induced the accumulation of these cells without pain stimulation in EAE-recovered mice. These results clearly suggest that the sensory-sympathetic connection at the ACC is involved in pain-mediated EAE relapse. Thus, we showed a third pain-mediated gateway reflex where neural signals travel from a TRPV1 and Nav1.8-dependent sensory circuit to sympathetic neurons via the ACC, reaching the dorsal vessels of the spinal cords [13] (**Figure 3**).

The study of the pain-mediated gateway reflex also highlights the importance of MHC class II high monocytes for EAE relapse. Parabiosis experiments, in which two different congenically marked mice are joined together surgically to share blood circulation, revealed that MHC class II high monocytes that accumulated at the L5 ventral vessels were derived from the peripheral blood stream during the first EAE development and stayed in the CNS, but not from resident microglia in the CNS [13]. These infiltrated MHC class II high monocytes survive in the CNS during the remission phase and play a pathogenic role upon relapse when the mice have a pain sensation. Therefore, in addition to controlling neural pathways and/or molecular machinery of the gateway reflexes, MHC class II high monocytes could also be a potential cellular target for treatment of relapse-remitting MS and progressive-relapsing MS.

6. Other gateway reflexes

In addition to the sensory perceptions described above, including gravity-, electric stimulation-, and pain-mediated stimuli, neural excitations occur in response to emotional alterations and physical/mental stresses. These physiological events too are often associated with MS symptoms [51]. Worsening of the clinical symptoms of neurological diseases including MS when the body is exposed to high ambient temperatures, called Uhthoff's phenomenon, is another well-known example [52]. It is also known that stress burdens are associated with activation of the sympathetic nervous system, such as increased noradrenaline levels in the peripheral blood. Despite these correlations, a mechanical link between stress and disease development remains elusive. Neuronal activations, noradrenaline surge, and disease development are fundamental of the gateway reflex. Stress-induced neural signals traveling to the CNS might modulate specific blood vessels depending on stress type, opening or closing a gateway for immune cells in the CNS. To examine this possibility, we have been testing the effects of various stresses on the pathogenesis of EAE. Although restraint stress and forced swim stress did not provoke EAE relapse [13], some stresses were found to worsen the clinical symptoms, whereas another stress prevented EAE development. These phenomena represent the fourth and fifth examples of the gateway reflex. The effects of good stress, or eustress, have also been reported in cancer models, in which tumor growth is delayed when mice are reared under an enriched environment with running wheels, tunnels, etc. in a larger cage [53, 54]. We suggest it may be possible to prevent diseases if stimulating the appropriate neurons can trigger a good gateway reflex.

Kevin Tracey and his colleagues have reported that activation of the vagus nerves, which mainly consist of parasympathetic nerves, leads to the suppression of systemic inflammation during septic shock in mice. This neural reflex is specifically called the "inflammatory reflex." In this context, lipopolysaccharide treatment in mice leads to norepinephrine release in the spleen via vagus and splenic nerves. A subset of T cells that receive norepinephrine signaling produces acetylcholine, which acts on macrophages to suppress the lipopolysaccharide-induced expression of inflammatory mediators such as TNFα [55], thus acting as a negative feedback system for excessive inflammatory reactions such as septic shock. It is also reported that electro-acupuncture in mice at the ST36 Zusanli acupoint, which is located close to the common peroneal and tibial branches of the sciatic nerve, or directly to the sciatic nerve prevents a sepsis model through vagal activation and dopamine production [56]. A similar strategy may generate the gateway reflex in humans.

7. Inflammation amplifier

As described above, regional sensory neural activations transmit neural signals to sympathetic neurons, which then secrete norepinephrine at the target blood vessels to establish a gateway and recruit immune cells. Because chemokines have a critical role in immune cell recruitment, we hypothesized that machinery responsible for the production of chemokines could act as an interface between neural signals and immune reactions. Indeed, we discovered the inflammation amplifier, which is a local chemokine inducer. In this section, we describe the inflammation amplifier as a molecular mechanism for neuro-immune interactions in blood vessels.

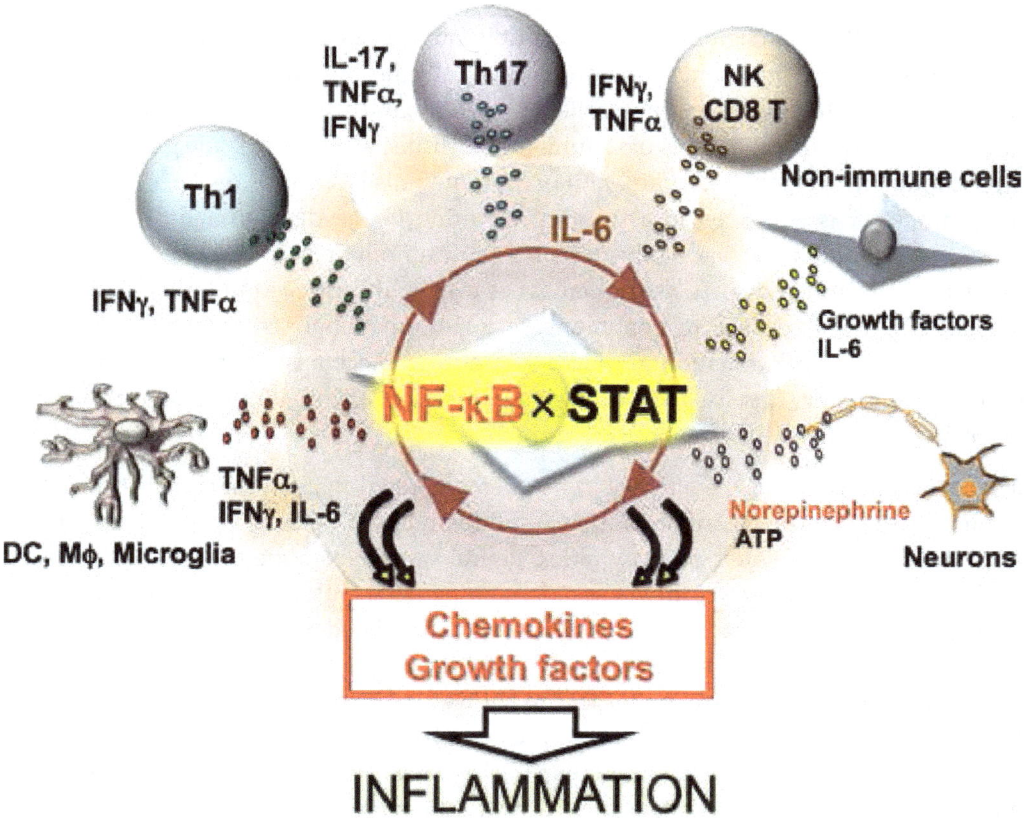

Figure 4. Inflammation amplifier. Simultaneous activation of the transcription factors NF-κB and STATs creates a synergistic effect on the production of inflammation mediators, such as chemokines, growth factors, and IL-6, in nonimmune cells, such as vascular endothelial cells and fibroblasts. Factors activating NF-κB and STATs are various and include IL-6, TNFα, and IL-17. IL-6 is expected to act on nonimmune cells to form a positive feedback loop that amplifies this synergistic effect. Massive chemokine and growth factor production by this mechanism, called the inflammation amplifier, plays a central role in the pathogenesis of many inflammatory diseases and disorders.

To establish an IL-6-dependent autoimmune mouse model, we previously generated a knock-in mouse strain called F759 mice, which lacks the SOCS3 binding site of the IL-6 signal transducer, gp130, thereby inhibiting SOCS3-dependent negative signaling and excessive STAT3 activation [57]. Accordingly, F759 mice developed spontaneous rheumatoid arthritis-like joint disease and autoantibody production [58], which is consistent with the high levels of IL-6 and clinical success of its signaling blockade in rheumatoid arthritis patients [59, 60]. Using these autoimmune-prone F759 mice, we performed mechanistic analyses for the pathogenesis of their autoimmunity and found that IL-6 signaling in nonimmune cells, such as vascular endothelial cells and fibroblasts, rather than immune cells, is important for the exaggerated inflammation [61, 62]. Mechanistically, coactivation of the transcription factors NF-κB and STATs in nonimmune cells led to a synergistic production of inflammatory agents, including chemokines and growth factors, compared with NF-κB or STAT activation alone (**Figure 4**). Factors that activate NF-κB and STATs and therefore trigger the inflammation amplifier include IL-17A, TNFα, IL-22, IL-6, and IFNγ. Furthermore, neurotransmitters, including norepinephrine and several growth factors, augment the amplifier by enhancing NF-κB activation [12, 63]. Since chemokines can recruit immune cells and promote inflammation, we named this synergistic mechanism in nonimmune cells the "inflammation amplifier" [64, 65]. Mice lacking gp130 or STAT3 in type 1 collagen+ cells including various nonimmune cells were highly resistant to animal models of rheumatoid arthritis, MS, and chronic graft rejection via suppression of the regional accumulation of immune cells [12, 13, 62, 63, 66, 67]. The inflammation amplifier is also seen in astrocytes, resulting in the development of EAE [68]. In addition, we found evidence of the inflammation amplifier activation in human clinical specimens, and human disease-associated genes are highly enriched in inflammation amplifier-related genes according to genome-wide RNA functional screening [67]. These data suggested that the inflammation amplifier is a critical mechanism for the development of various inflammatory diseases via excessive expression of inflammatory chemokines and growth factors from nonimmune cells (**Figure 4**).

Subsequent studies about the gateway reflex demonstrated that neural signals translate into inflammatory signals by the inflammation amplifier in target vascular endothelial cells. In the case of the gravity-mediated gateway reflex, neural signals from the soleus muscles reached the L5 dorsal vessel endothelium via sensory-sympathetic cross talk, where norepinephrine from the activated sympathetic neurons excessively stimulated the inflammation amplifier by increasing NF-κB activity to secrete various NF-κB-targets including chemokines. Moreover, the L5 but not L1 dorsal vessel endothelium showed activation of STAT3. Pharmacological inhibition of beta-adrenergic receptors suppressed NF-κB activation, chemokine production, and pathogenic CD4+ T-cell accumulation in the L5 dorsal vessels and EAE development [12]. Similarly, during the pain-mediated gateway reflex, treatment with a beta-adrenergic receptor antagonist resulted in no accumulation of activated monocytes or pathogenic CD4+ T cells around the target dorsal vessels of the L5 spinal cord. Neutralization of cytokines that activate the inflammation amplifier such as IL-6 and IL-17A also suppressed the pain-induced EAE relapse and pathogenic CD4+ T-cell accumulation [13]. These results indicate that the inflammation amplifier is a foundation of the immunological response induced by the gateway reflex.

8. Future directions

The CNS is an immune-privileged site protected by the BBB, but the gateway reflex, which can be triggered by various neural stimulations, can induce gateways for immune cells to circumvent the BBB. So far, three kinds of gateway reflex have been identified: gravity, electric stimulation, and pain-induced, all of which involve sensory-sympathetic communication. Further study of the mechanisms driving the gateway reflex should consider the neural network involved and whether it is present in other organs and tissues. Newly developed imaging techniques and tools including a tissue decolorization reagent, CUBIC [69, 70], will help elucidate the former. For the latter, it is recently reported there exists barrier architecture with similar components to the BBB in the gut endothelium, the so-called gut-vascular barrier [22]. A similar system may explain how immune cells breach this barrier. Because neuronal circuits run throughout the body, the gateway reflex could have a tremendous clinical benefit, as closing a specific gateway would dampen autoimmune inflammation in a target organ without massive systemic immune suppression, while opening it in tumors could enhance cancer immunotherapy.

Acknowledgements

We thank the excellent assistance by Ms. Chiemi Nakayama, Ms. Mitsue Ezawa and Ms. Satomi Fukumoto (Hokkaido University, Sapporo, Japan), and Dr. Peter Karagiannis for reading the manuscript. This work was supported by KAKENHI (D. K., Y. A., T. A., and M. M.), Takeda Science Foundation (M. M. and D. K.), Institute for Fermentation Osaka (M. M.), Mitsubishi Foundation (M. M.), Uehara Memorial Foundation (M. M.), Mochida Memorial Foundation for Medical and Pharmaceutical Research (D. K.), Suzuken Memorial Foundation (D. K. and Y. A.), Japan Prize Foundation (Y. A.), Ono Medical Research Foundation (Y. A.), Kanzawa Medical Research Foundation (Y. A.), Kishimoto Foundation (Y. A.), Nagao Takeshi Research Foundation (Y. A.), Tokyo Medical Research Foundation (M. M. and Y. A.), JSPS Postdoctoral Fellowship for Foreign Researchers (A.S.), JST-CREST program (M. M.), and the Osaka Foundation for the Promotion of Clinical Immunology (M. M.). The authors declare they have no conflicting financial interests.

Author details

Daisuke Kamimura*, Yasunobu Arima, Andrea Stofkova, Naoki Nishikawa, Kotaro Higuchi, Takuto Ohki and Masaaki Murakami

*Address all correspondence to: murakami@igm.hokudai.ac.jp

Molecular Neuroimmunology, Graduate School of Medicine, Institute for Genetic Medicine, Hokkaido University, Sapporo, Hokkaido ,Japan

References

[1] Noseworthy JH, Lucchinetti C, Rodriguez M, Weinshenker BG. Multiple sclerosis. N Engl J Med 2000;343(13):938–952. DOI: 10.1056/NEJM200009283431307

[2] Hafler DA, Slavik JM, Anderson DE, O'Connor KC, De Jager P, Baecher-Allan C. Multiple sclerosis. Immunol Rev 2005;204:208–231. DOI: 10.1111/j.0105-2896.2005.00240.x

[3] McFarland HF, Martin R. Multiple sclerosis: a complicated picture of autoimmunity. Nat Immunol 2007;8(9):913–919. DOI: 10.1038/ni1507

[4] Steinman L. Immunology of relapse and remission in multiple sclerosis. Annu Rev Immunol 2014;32:257–281. DOI: 10.1146/annurev-immunol-032713-120227

[5] Keegan BM, Noseworthy JH. Multiple sclerosis. Ann Rev Med 2002;53:285–302. DOI: 10.1146/annurev.med.53.082901.103909

[6] International Multiple Sclerosis Genetics C, Wellcome Trust Case Control C, Sawcer S, Hellenthal G, Pirinen M, Spencer CC, et al.: Genetic risk and a primary role for cell-mediated immune mechanisms in multiple sclerosis. Nature 2011;476(7359):214–219. DOI: 10.1038/nature10251

[7] Kuchroo VK, Anderson AC, Waldner H, Munder M, Bettelli E, Nicholson LB. T cell response in experimental autoimmune encephalomyelitis (EAE): role of self and cross-reactive antigens in shaping, tuning, and regulating the autopathogenic T cell repertoire. Annu Rev Immunol 2002;20:101–123. DOI: 10.1146/annurev.immunol.20.081701.141316

[8] Sospedra M, Martin R. Immunology of multiple sclerosis. Annu Rev Immunol 2005;23:683–747. DOI: 10.1146/annurev.immunol.23.021704.115707

[9] Steinman L, Zamvil SS. Virtues and pitfalls of EAE for the development of therapies for multiple sclerosis. Trends Immunol 2005;26(11):565–571. DOI: 10.1016/j.it.2005.08.014

[10] Goverman J. Autoimmune T cell responses in the central nervous system. Nat Rev Immunol 2009;9(6):393–407. DOI: 10.1038/nri2550

[11] Rangachari M, Kuchroo VK. Using EAE to better understand principles of immune function and autoimmune pathology. J Autoimmun 2013;45:31–39. DOI: 10.1016/j.jaut.2013.06.008

[12] Arima Y, Harada M, Kamimura D, Park JH, Kawano F, Yull FE, et al.: Regional neural activation defines a gateway for autoreactive T cells to cross the blood–brain barrier. Cell 2012;148(3):447–457. DOI: 10.1016/j.cell.2012.01.022

[13] Arima Y, Kamimura D, Atsumi T, Harada M, Kawamoto T, Nishikawa N, et al.: A pain-mediated neural signal induces relapse in murine autoimmune encephalomyelitis, a multiple sclerosis model. eLife 2015;4. DOI: 10.7554/eLife.08733

[14] Gregory SG, Schmidt S, Seth P, Oksenberg JR, Hart J, Prokop A, et al.: Interleukin 7 receptor alpha chain (IL7R) shows allelic and functional association with multiple sclerosis. Nat Genet 2007;39(9):1083–1091. DOI: 10.1038/ng2103

[15] Lundmark F, Duvefelt K, Iacobaeus E, Kockum I, Wallstrom E, Khademi M, et al.: Variation in interleukin 7 receptor alpha chain (IL7R) influences risk of multiple sclerosis. Nat Genet 2007;39(9):1108–1113. DOI: 10.1038/ng2106

[16] Australia, New Zealand Multiple Sclerosis Genetics C. Genome-wide association study identifies new multiple sclerosis susceptibility loci on chromosomes 12 and 20. Nat Genet 2009;41(7):824–828. 10.1038/ng.396

[17] Cohen JA, Barkhof F, Comi G, Hartung HP, Khatri BO, Montalban X, et al.: Oral fingolimod or intramuscular interferon for relapsing multiple sclerosis. N Engl J Med 2010;362(5):402–415. DOI: 10.1056/NEJMoa0907839

[18] Steinman L. Blocking adhesion molecules as therapy for multiple sclerosis: natalizumab. Nat Reviews Drug Discov 2005;4(6):510–518. DOI: 10.1038/nrd1752

[19] Bloomgren G, Richman S, Hotermans C, Subramanyam M, Goelz S, Natarajan A, et al.: Risk of natalizumab-associated progressive multifocal leukoencephalopathy. N Engl J Med 2012;366(20):1870–1880. DOI: 10.1056/NEJMoa1107829

[20] Van Schependom J, Gielen J, Laton J, Nagels G. Assessing PML risk under immunotherapy: if all you have is a hammer, everything looks like a nail. Mult Scler 2015. DOI: 10.1177/1352458515596458

[21] Steed E, Balda MS, Matter K. Dynamics and functions of tight junctions. Trends Cell Biol 2010;20(3):142–149. DOI: 10.1016/j.tcb.2009.12.002.

[22] Spadoni I, Zagato E, Bertocchi A, Paolinelli R, Hot E, Di Sabatino A, et al.: A gut-vascular barrier controls the systemic dissemination of bacteria. Science 2015;350(6262):830–834. DOI: 10.1126/science.aad0135

[23] Zlokovic BV. The blood–brain barrier in health and chronic neurodegenerative disorders. Neuron 2008;57(2):178–201. DOI: 10.1016/j.neuron.2008.01.003.

[24] Wyss-Coray T, Mucke L. Inflammation in neurodegenerative disease--a double-edged sword. Neuron 2002;35(3):419–432.

[25] Tsao N, Hsu HP, Wu CM, Liu CC, Lei HY. Tumour necrosis factor-alpha causes an increase in blood–brain barrier permeability during sepsis. J Med Microbiol 2001;50(9): 812–821.

[26] Argaw AT, Zhang Y, Snyder BJ, Zhao ML, Kopp N, Lee SC, et al.: IL-1beta regulates blood–brain barrier permeability via reactivation of the hypoxia-angiogenesis program. J Immunol 2006;177(8):5574–5584.

[27] Bittner S, Ruck T, Schuhmann MK, Herrmann AM, Moha ou Maati H, Bobak N, et al.: Endothelial TWIK-related potassium channel-1 (TREK1) regulates immune-cell trafficking into the CNS. Nat Med 2013;19(9):1161–1165. DOI: 10.1038/nm.3303

[28] Komiyama Y, Nakae S, Matsuki T, Nambu A, Ishigame H, Kakuta S, et al.: IL-17 plays an important role in the development of experimental autoimmune encephalomyelitis. J Immunol 2006;177(1):566–573.

[29] Huppert J, Closhen D, Croxford A, White R, Kulig P, Pietrowski E, et al.: Cellular mechanisms of IL-17-induced blood–brain barrier disruption. FASEB J 2010;24(4):1023–1034. DOI: 10.1096/fj.09-141978

[30] Kebir H, Kreymborg K, Ifergan I, Dodelet-Devillers A, Cayrol R, Bernard M, et al.: Human TH17 lymphocytes promote blood–brain barrier disruption and central nervous system inflammation. Nat Med 2007;13(10):1173–1175. nm1651 [pii] 10.1038/nm1651

[31] Bartholomaus I, Kawakami N, Odoardi F, Schlager C, Miljkovic D, Ellwart JW, et al.: Effector T cell interactions with meningeal vascular structures in nascent autoimmune CNS lesions. Nature 2009;462(7269):94–98. DOI: 10.1038/nature08478

[32] Ota K, Matsui M, Milford EL, Mackin GA, Weiner HL, Hafler DA. T-cell recognition of an immunodominant myelin basic protein epitope in multiple sclerosis. Nature 1990;346(6280):183–187. DOI: 10.1038/346183a0

[33] Allegretta M, Nicklas JA, Sriram S, Albertini RJ. T cells responsive to myelin basic protein in patients with multiple sclerosis. Science 1990;247(4943):718–721.

[34] Zhang J, Markovic-Plese S, Lacet B, Raus J, Weiner HL, Hafler DA. Increased frequency of interleukin 2-responsive T cells specific for myelin basic protein and proteolipid protein in peripheral blood and cerebrospinal fluid of patients with multiple sclerosis. J Exp Med 1994;179(3):973–984.

[35] Reindl M, Di Pauli F, Rostasy K, Berger T. The spectrum of MOG autoantibody-associated demyelinating diseases. Nat Reviews Neurol 2013;9(8):455–461. DOI: 10.1038/nrneurol.2013.118

[36] Polman CH, Reingold SC, Banwell B, Clanet M, Cohen JA, Filippi M, et al.: Diagnostic criteria for multiple sclerosis: 2010 revisions to the McDonald criteria. Ann Neurol 2011;69(2):292–302. DOI: 10.1002/ana.22366

[37] Reboldi A, Coisne C, Baumjohann D, Benvenuto F, Bottinelli D, Lira S, et al.: C-C chemokine receptor 6-regulated entry of TH-17 cells into the CNS through the choroid plexus is required for the initiation of EAE. Nat Immunol 2009;10(5):514–523. DOI: 10.1038/ni.1716

[38] Ohira Y, Kawano F, Stevens JL, Wang XD, Ishihara A. Load-dependent regulation of neuromuscular system. J Gravit Physiol 2004;11(2):P127-128.

[39] Shen J, Wang HY, Chen JY, Liang BL. Morphologic analysis of normal human lumbar dorsal root ganglion by 3D MR imaging. AJNR Am J neuroradiol 2006;27(10):2098–2103.

[40] Tracey KJ. Immune cells exploit a neural circuit to enter the CNS. Cell 2012;148(3):392–394. DOI: 10.1016/j.cell.2012.01.025

[41] Andersson U, Tracey KJ. Neural reflexes in inflammation and immunity. J Exp Med 2012;209(6):1057–1068. DOI: 10.1084/jem.20120571

[42] Sabharwal L, Kamimura D, Meng J, Bando H, Ogura H, Nakayama C, et al.: The Gateway Reflex, which is mediated by the inflammation amplifier, directs pathogenic immune cells into the CNS. J Biochem 2014;156(6):299–304. DOI: 10.1093/jb/mvu057

[43] Feinstein A, Magalhaes S, Richard JF, Audet B, Moore C. The link between multiple sclerosis and depression. Nat Rev Neurol 2014;10(9):507–517. DOI: 10.1038/nrneurol.2014.139

[44] Morales-Lazaro SL, Simon SA, Rosenbaum T. The role of endogenous molecules in modulating pain through transient receptor potential vanilloid 1 (TRPV1). J Physiol 2013;591(Pt 13):3109–3121. DOI: 10.1113/jphysiol.2013.251751

[45] Bennett DL, Woods CG. Painful and painless channelopathies. Lancet Neurol 2014;13(6):587–599. DOI: 10.1016/S1474-4422(14)70024-9

[46] Khan N, Smith MT. Multiple sclerosis-induced neuropathic pain: pharmacological management and pathophysiological insights from rodent EAE models. Inflammopharmacology 2014;22(1):1–22. DOI: 10.1007/s10787-013-0195-3

[47] Thygesen TH, Baad-Hansen L, Svensson P. Sensory action potentials of the maxillary nerve: a methodologic study with clinical implications. J Oral Maxillofac Surg : official journal of the American Association of Oral and Maxillofacial Surgeons 2009;67(3):537–542. DOI: 10.1016/j.joms.2008.02.015

[48] Ehde DM, Gibbons LE, Chwastiak L, Bombardier CH, Sullivan MD, Kraft GH. Chronic pain in a large community sample of persons with multiple sclerosis. Mult Scler 2003;9(6):605–611.

[49] Ikemoto K, Kitahama K, Nishimura A, Jouvet A, Nishi K, Arai R, et al.: Tyrosine hydroxylase and aromatic L-amino acid decarboxylase do not coexist in neurons in the human anterior cingulate cortex. Neurosci Letters 1999;269(1):37–40.

[50] Critchley HD. Neural mechanisms of autonomic, affective, and cognitive integration. J Comp Neurol 2005;493(1):154–166. 10.1002/cne.20749

[51] Karagkouni A, Alevizos M, Theoharides TC. Effect of stress on brain inflammation and multiple sclerosis. Autoimmun Rev 2013;12(10):947–953. DOI: 10.1016/j.autrev.2013.02.006

[52] Frohman TC, Davis SL, Beh S, Greenberg BM, Remington G, Frohman EM. Uhthoff's phenomena in MS--clinical features and pathophysiology. Nat Rev Neurol 2013;9(9):535–540. DOI: 10.1038/nrneurol.2013.98

[53] Cao L, Liu X, Lin EJ, Wang C, Choi EY, Riban V, et al.: Environmental and genetic activation of a brain-adipocyte BDNF/leptin axis causes cancer remission and inhibition. Cell 2010;142(1):52–64. DOI: 10.1016/j.cell.2010.05.029.

[54] Li G, Gan Y, Fan Y, Wu Y, Lin H, Song Y, et al.: Enriched environment inhibits mouse pancreatic cancer growth and down-regulates the expression of mitochondria-related genes in cancer cells. Sci Rep 2015;5:7856. DOI: 10.1038/srep07856

[55] Andersson U, Tracey KJ. Reflex principles of immunological homeostasis. Annu Rev Immunol 2012;30:313–335. DOI: 10.1146/annurev-immunol-020711-075015

[56] Torres-Rosas R, Yehia G, Pena G, Mishra P, del Rocio Thompson-Bonilla M, Moreno-Eutimio MA, et al.: Dopamine mediates vagal modulation of the immune system by electroacupuncture. Nat Med 2014;20(3):291–295. DOI: 10.1038/nm.3479

[57] Ohtani T, Ishihara K, Atsumi T, Nishida K, Kaneko Y, Miyata T, et al.: Dissection of signaling cascades through gp130 in vivo: reciprocal roles for STAT3- and SHP2-mediated signals in immune responses. Immunity 2000;12(1):95–105.

[58] Atsumi T, Ishihara K, Kamimura D, Ikushima H, Ohtani T, Hirota S, et al.: A point mutation of Tyr-759 in interleukin 6 family cytokine receptor subunit gp130 causes autoimmune arthritis. J Exp Med 2002;196(7):979–990.

[59] Nishimoto N, Kishimoto T, Yoshizaki K. Anti-interleukin 6 receptor antibody treatment in rheumatic disease. Ann Rheum Dis 2000;59 Suppl 1:i21-27.

[60] Nishimoto N, Kishimoto T. Inhibition of IL-6 for the treatment of inflammatory diseases. Curr Opin Pharmacol 2004;4(4):386–391. DOI: 10.1016/j.coph.2004.03.005

[61] Sawa S, Kamimura D, Jin GH, Morikawa H, Kamon H, Nishihara M, et al.: Autoimmune arthritis associated with mutated interleukin (IL)-6 receptor gp130 is driven by STAT3/IL-7-dependent homeostatic proliferation of CD4+ T cells. J Exp Med 2006;203(6):1459–1470. DOI: 10.1084/jem.20052187

[62] Ogura H, Murakami M, Okuyama Y, Tsuruoka M, Kitabayashi C, Kanamoto M, et al.: Interleukin-17 promotes autoimmunity by triggering a positive-feedback loop via interleukin-6 induction. Immunity 2008;29(4):628–636. DOI: 10.1016/j.immuni.2008.07.018

[63] Harada M, Kamimura D, Arima Y, Kohsaka H, Nakatsuji Y, Nishida M, et al.: Temporal expression of growth factors triggered by epiregulin regulates inflammation development. J Immunol 2015;194(3):1039–1046. DOI: 10.4049/jimmunol.1400562

[64] Murakami M, Hirano T. The pathological and physiological roles of IL-6 amplifier activation. Int J Biol Sci 2012;8(9):1267–1280. DOI: 10.7150/ijbs.4828

[65] Atsumi T, Singh R, Sabharwal L, Bando H, Meng J, Arima Y, et al.: Inflammation amplifier, a new paradigm in cancer biology. Cancer Res 2014;74(1):8–14. DOI: 10.1158/0008-5472.CAN-13-2322

[66] Lee J, Nakagiri T, Oto T, Harada M, Morii E, Shintani Y, et al.: IL-6 amplifier, NF-kappaB-triggered positive feedback for IL-6 signaling, in grafts is involved in allogeneic rejection responses. J Immunol 2012;189(4):1928–1936. DOI: 10.4049/jimmunol.1103613

[67] Murakami M, Harada M, Kamimura D, Ogura H, Okuyama Y, Kumai N, et al.: Disease-association analysis of an inflammation-related feedback loop. Cell Rep 2013;3(3):946–959. DOI: 10.1016/j.celrep.2013.01.028

[68] Ma X, Reynolds SL, Baker BJ, Li X, Benveniste EN, Qin H. IL-17 enhancement of the IL-6 signaling cascade in astrocytes. J Immunol 2010;184(9):4898–4906. DOI: 10.4049/jimmunol.1000142

[69] Susaki EA, Tainaka K, Perrin D, Kishino F, Tawara T, Watanabe TM, et al.: Whole-brain imaging with single-cell resolution using chemical cocktails and computational analysis. Cell 2014;157(3):726–739. DOI: 10.1016/j.cell.2014.03.042

[70] Tainaka K, Kubota SI, Suyama TQ, Susaki EA, Perrin D, Ukai-Tadenuma M, et al.: Whole-body imaging with single-cell resolution by tissue decolorization. Cell 2014;159(4):911–924. DOI: 10.1016/j.cell.2014.10.034

3

Social Cognition Impairments in Patients with Multiple Sclerosis and Comparison with Imaging Studies, Disease Duration and Grade of Disability

Valentina Ignatova, Lyudmila Todorova and Jivko Surchev

Abstract

Cognitive impairments in multiple sclerosis (MS) are heterogeneous and their rate varies between 43% and 70%. A less studied aspect of cognition is social cognition, which is not a uniform theoretical construct. It includes emotion perception, prosody, empathy, theory of mind (ToM) and assessment of mood. In addition to progressive physical disability, social cognitive impairments are a reason for job loss in 24–80% of patients with MS, increased divorce rate, dissolution of partnerships and social communication difficulties.

Social cognitive impairments are the result of disruptions in the mentalization network at the neuroanatomical, neurochemical and/or genetic level, which can lead to malfunctions in the dopaminergic–serotoninergic system and to compromising the development of neuroanatomical targets within the network. The wide dissemination of demyelinating lesions and cortical thinning typical of patients with MS often lead to anatomic and functional disorders of the above-mentioned specific brain structures. A correlation has been established among specific cortical areas involved in emotion identification from facial expression (right and left fusiform face area, frontal eye), emotion processing (right entorhinal cortex) and socially relevant information (left temporal pole). The most active brain region involved in social cognitive processing is the medal frontal cortex (MFC), which is described as the brain's social cognitive center. During performance of various sociocognitive tasks for mental state attribution, common areas of increased activation in the medial prefrontal gyrus and the temporoparietal junctions are registered bilaterally, while the area of the medial prefrontal cortex (the paracingulate cortex) is the only region uniquely activated by the performance of ToM.

Most MRI studies of patients with MS found a correlation between the cognitive and/or affective disorders, on the one hand, and lesion localization, total lesion load, or cerebral atrophy, on the other. A significant correlation was also reported between abnormal activities in specific cortical zones on fMRI, on the one hand, and clinical manifestation, conventional MRI findings and behavioral changes, on the other. Altered patterns of brain activity were found in all clinical phenotypes of MS, including when cognitive abilities were intact and/or restored, social cognitive dysfunction in MS actually affects all stages of the disease and all types of clinical course. The cortical plastic changes are a dynamic phenomenon that can be modulated by external factors. This phenomenon would facilitate the mapping of individual strategies for adequate treatment and rehabilitation of each patient.

Keywords: social cognition, multiple sclerosis, empathy, theory of mind, mentalization, emotional perception, faux pas, disability, social brain, imaging studies

1. Introduction

Multiple sclerosis (MS) is a chronic inflammatory autoimmune degenerative disease of the central nervous system (CNS) leading to both physical and neuropsychological disability. These two types of impairment may occur simultaneously or independently [1]. Until now the focus of scientific research has predominantly been on the physical disablement in patients with MS and its impact on their quality of life. Over the last few decades, researchers have shown an increasing interest in mood disorders, behavior and cognition in this disease.

Cognitive impairments in MS are heterogeneous [2] and their rate varies between 43% and 70% [3–5]. They are in an independent form of disability and make the performance of routine daily activities difficult, sometimes impossible. Up to now studies have mostly been conducted on impairments in the main cognitive domains such as memory, attention and executive functions. A less studied aspect of cognition is social cognition, which is not a uniform theoretical construct. It includes emotion perception, prosody, empathy, theory of mind (ToM) and assessment of mood [6, 7]. Findings in MS show disturbance not only in emotion recognition from facial expressions but in the whole area of general emotion processing. The connection between cognitive decline and impaired social cognitive skills in MS remains debatable.

Social cognitive dysfunction in MS actually affects all stages of the disease and all types of clinical course. Such disturbances are reported even in clinically isolated syndrome (CIS). Relatively, little is known about the evolution of cognitive deficits in MS, especially about those manifested in the early stages of the disease [8].

The frequency of social cognition impairments and the nature of pathological changes in the brain in patients with MS are reasonable grounds for seeking a relationship between deteriorated mentalization and findings from imaging/functional brain studies. Studies looking for a correlation between cognitive decline and MRI changes (lesion volume, lesion load, cortical thinning) are still at an early stage. This also applies to studies seeking to detect functional changes in specific brain areas responsible for the performance of relevant sociocognitive tasks. Additional data from future research in this field are needed for better understanding of social cognition impairments [9].

In addition to progressive physical disability, social cognitive impairments are a reason for job loss in 24–80% of patients with MS [10, 11], increased divorce rate, dissolution of partnerships [12] and social communication difficulties. Furthermore, these disturbances restrict the career development and social life of patients. This calls for a multidisciplinary approach in research and concurrent assessment of the physical, neuropsychological and social aspects of disability in MS.

The main objective is to evaluate the frequency and degree of social cognition impairments in patients with MS based on systematic analysis of advanced scientific research and to outline scientific trends in the field.

2. Methods

We conducted advanced search based on the following key words in different combinations: "social cognition", "multiple sclerosis", "empathy", "theory of mind (ToM)", "faux pas", "mentalization", "emotional perception", "disability", "social brain" and "imaging studies". The selection was made by two independent reviewers who retrieved relevant scientific works (original articles, book chapters, systematic reviews) published in English from electronic database (PubMed, MEDLINE). The search period was unrestricted. The following inclusion criteria were determined: (1) subjects, suffering from multiple sclerosis; (2) assessment of social cognition abilities; and (3) brain imaging findings and impaired social cognition. Case report articles were excluded. A relationship between social cognition skills, physical disability and duration of the disease was searched. We also checked up the bibliography of the related sources and included the relevant articles. We also checked up the bibliography of the related sources and included the relevant articles. We selected six books, seven book chapters, 43 scientific reviews, 86 original articles, one thesis, two conference papers and one manual regarding social cognition and/or MS. Finally, we retrieved two book chapters, 10 scientific reviews, 32 research studies, one thesis and two conference papers on the current topic "social cognition" in MS. Meta-analysis was not suitable for summarizing of the results due to methodological heterogeneity between reviewed studies. Quantitative assessment of the relevant data was conducted. Different points of views, as well as controversies within the scientific field, were presented. We highlighted key results, determined importance of social cognition impairments for quality of life in patients with MS and outlined a framework of research trends.

3. What is social cognition?

Numerous attempts to define social cognition have been made. In early 1994, Thomas M. Ostrom collected more than 100 definitions and accepted conceptual orientation in information processing in the context of cognitive psychology as the core of social cognition. According to him, the sociocognitive approach is based on the belief that constructs relevant to cognitive performance and processing are fundamental to understanding all human responses regardless of whether these responses are social or unsocial in nature. This basic definition has been supplemented and updated over time. Augoustinos et al. accept that social cognition is not a theory per se but an approach or perspective strongly influenced by the methods and concepts of cognitive psychology [13].

In 1980s, scientific research postulated that humans store and give meaning to complex social information by simplifying and organizing this information in understandable cognitive structures called schemata. The schemata theory implies that we use the same mental structures for the selection and processing of incoming information from the surrounding social environment. Schemata are based on the general expectations from experience (socialization) and allow the prediction and control of social interactions. This theory is applied to the following four key zones: person schemata, self-schemata, role schemata and event schemata [14]. The categorization process is borrowed from cognitive psychology. It includes the identification of stimuli, their grouping as part of a category similar to other parts in the same category and differentiating them from the components of other categories. It is fundamental to perception, thought, language and actions. In the 1990s, the concept was further developed with the assumption that categorization may present not only average abstraction but also a number of specific and concrete cases or samples found in this category. According to Mead and Vygotsky, intrapersonal processes originate and are modeled after interpersonal processes.

Social cognition is a level of mental capacity developed over the evolution process for successful adaptation to the social environment. The basic domains of social cognition are empathy and ToM.

Empathy is the natural ability to understand the emotions and feelings of others regardless of whether one is directly participating in a given situation, viewing photos, reading a book, listening to a story or just imagining. It refers to the phenomenological experience of compassion [15]. The term "empathy" comes from the German word Einfühlung translated by Titchener as "feeling into" [16, 17]. Empathy includes an intuitive feeling of having something in common with others which relies on socially shared emotional experience, cognitive mechanisms of perspective taking, the ability to maintain a self-other distinction during interpersonal interaction. The cognitive aspect of empathy is also defined as empathy accuracy [18].

ToM, also called mentalization, was described as a cognitive component of empathy by Baron-Cohen in 2003 [19, 20]. ToM is viewed as a specific capacity of the mind to understand ourselves and others in terms of mental states. It is based on "reading the thoughts and emotions" of others through analyzing their facial expressions and other behavioral signs [21, 22]. ToM provides the opportunity for establishing a connection between internal conditions manifested through expressions, gestures, signals and internal states of mind. The capacity to recognize the emotions, intentions and thoughts of others can be regarded as an important component of a broader set of skills called social competence or social intelligence.

More recent studies have explored ToM in two aspects—cognitive ToM (the ability to understand the intentions of others – 'cold') and affective ToM (the ability to infer others' emotional states – 'hot') [23]. The affective component of ToM requires empathy. According to Ickes, "everyday mind reading" [24] is not a skill that needs to be learned. However, one develops it in the course of life experience. In addition to personality traits, at least three types of mind-reading accuracy tests need to be examined, that is, the ability to assess someone in terms of the following: (1) mental state (both affective and nonaffective), (2) behavior, and (3) roles, identity and/or condition [25]. Emotion recognition is perhaps the most thoroughly investigated and best known of all mind-reading tasks.

The contemporary neurobiological ToM model includes both neuroanatomic and neurochemical levels of specificity. In this model, cortical and subcortical zones are functionally organized so as to ensure the expression of cognitive and affective mental states for both self and others. According to this model, the cognitive and affective aspects of ToM are based on dissociable but interacting prefrontal networks. The cognitive ToM network includes primarily the dorsomedial prefrontal cortex, the dorsal anterior cingulate cortex (ACC) and the dorsal striatum, while the affective ToM network comprises mainly the ventromedial and orbitofrontal cortices, the ventral anterior cingulate cortex, the amygdala and the ventral striatum. The ability to distinguish the mental condition for self from that for others is based on different brain representations within the mentalizing network and is modulated by the functional interaction between the dorsal and ventral systems for attention and selection in the temporoparietal junction and the anterior cingulate cortex.

The functioning of ToM depends on the integrity of the dopaminergic and serotonergic systems, which are primarily involved in the process of comprehension of mental states. Social cognitive impairments are the result of disruptions in the mentalization network at the neuroanatomical, neurochemical and/or genetic level, which can lead to malfunctions in the dopaminergic–serotoninergic system and to compromising the development of neuroanatomical targets within the network [26]. ToM abilities are variably influenced, depending on the type of pathology in the functioning of the mentalization network.

It is presumed that there are two systems involved in belief processing in humans: implicit ToM (iToM) and explicit ToM (eToM). The iToM system builds a hypothesis empirically in the absence of awareness. It is supposedly available from birth [27]. The eToM system is associated with thinking, control and awareness of the approach in mental state recognition. It responds and develops in the first years of life. Little is known about the connection between implicit and explicit processing of social cognition [28]. It is assumed that they are largely independent.

Social cognition comprises two levels relating to all its domains. The first level includes quick, relatively routine cognitive processing which is largely automatic, implicit and can occur without awareness. At the higher level, these processes are slow, flexible and explicitly require exertion of mental effort [28].

4. Clinical assessment of social cognition in patients with MS

Research on social cognition is experimental and focuses on intra-individual mental processing. Studies on emotional and cognitive impairments in patients with MS are based on different test batteries. Mental schemata are used for focusing attention and facilitating information encoding and retrieval.

Empathy can be regarded as a set of interrelated constructs including social competence, self-assessment, emotion and sensitivity to others [29]. Therefore, there is no universal tool objectively assessing empathy in all its aspects. In a recent review of empathy measurement tools [30], 1147 citations were used to select 50 articles describing 36 empathy tests, eight of which demonstrated satisfactory reliability, internal consistency and validity.

The empathy quotient is most often determined through self-assessment questionnaires. Interpersonal empathy is usually studied by applying the Hogan Empathy Scale (HES) [31], the Toronto Empathy Questionnaire (TEQ) and the 50 Item Interpersonal Skills Questionnaire (50 IISQ). The affective component of empathy can be assessed through the Questionnaire Measure of Emotional Empathy (QMEE), while the cognitive component is more precisely determined through HES. The Balanced Emotional Empathy Scale (BEES), developed by Mehrabian, evaluates responders' reaction to the mental state of others [32].

The instrument most often used for determining the level of self-empathy is Neff's self-compassion scale, which assesses self-kindness, common humanity and mindfulness [33]. The measurement of compassionate or altruistic love toward different targets through the Compassionate Love Scale (CLS) provides additional information about the perception of close others and all of humankind [34]. The Empathy Construct Rating Scale (ECRS) can test the ability to understand accurately the feelings of others through careful listening, thus checking whether the subject properly understands what others experience.

More complex information regarding compassion to self and others is provided by Baron-Cohen and Wheelwright in The Empathy Quotient, which measures cognitive empathy, emotional reactivity and social skills [35] and most of all in the Interpersonal Reactivity Index (IRI), which allows measuring of multidimensional individual empathy differences [36].

Recently, tests with nonverbal stimuli have also been applied to the evaluation of empathy. They are commonly used in patients with autism and aphasia but are also an important complement to self-assessment questionnaires, because they contribute to the greater objectivity of overall empathy assessment. Nonverbal tests provide additional information on the empathy quotient through analyzing what feelings and thoughts are inferred from facial expressions in pictures. Most often they are based on a series of photographs which depict people with different mental and emotional charge, thus measuring the cognitive and affective components of empathy. The most frequently used ones are the multifaceted empathy test (MET) [37], the visual recognition test, the Florida Affect Battery (FAB) and Ekman and Friesen's black and white stimulus set. The results of these tests minimize subjectivity in the patient's self-assessment [38].

ToM, as a key aspect of social cognition, requires greater cognitive effort for slower and more explicit processing. In general, ToM tests are classified into three groups: attribution of epistemic mental states, attribution of intention and attribution of affective mental states [39]. They are based on verbally or visually delivered information, and in recent years, ToM movies have been developed for increasing test sensitivity and approximating the demands of everyday life social cognition [40]. Verbal tests, such as "Strange Stories" and "Faux Pas Recognition", require interpretation of auditory information for grasping false belief and deception based on short stories with social context similar to real situations. Such tasks could be accompanied by pictures. Decoding complex emotions from voice is measured by "Reading the Mind in the Voice" [41] and the "Voice Emotion Identification Test" [42] and prediction of intentions and emotions—by "Reading the Mind in the Eyes" [43] and the "Facial Symbol Test", [44] which are sensitive indicators of the socioperceptual component involved in the immediate recognition of mental states [45]. Even more informative is the "Cambridge Mind-reading Face Voice Battery", [46] which combines verbal and dynamic visual stimuli.

ToM cartoons assess the ability to understand emotions and intentions by interpreting graphic design images and/or cartoon strips. Some of these use jokes involving false beliefs [47], and others combine representations of mental and physical states [48]. The following are some video tasks appropriate for ToM assessment in patients with MS: conversations and insinuations (C&I) [49], the social inference-enriched subtest of the TASIT, containing video-taped social interactions in which lies and sarcasm are presented [50], the Face Puzzle—for measuring the explicit and implicit aspects of facial emotion recognition, the social cue recognition test [51] and the videotape emotion identification test [52].

In the comprehensive evaluation of social cognitive skills in patients with MS, it is necessary to take into account the level of general cognition, personal characteristics, such as individual perspective, idiosyncrasies, purpose and attitudes [53], as well as a possible genetic modulation of individual empathic ability [54].

So far ToM research has used small groups of patients with MS and a narrow range of cognitive tasks. The fact that there is no unified neuropsychological battery for the assessment of social cognitive impairments should also be taken into account. For the reasons outlined earlier, it is difficult to generalize on their results for the entire MS population, numbering about 1.3 million worldwide, as well as to reach definitive conclusions

5. Impairment of social cognitive abilities in patients with MS

Social cognition is considered a main determinant of the functional outcome in many psychiatric and neurologic degenerative diseases, including MS. Social cognitive impairments have been registered even in the first clinical episode prior to conversion to MS.

Decreased empathy was reported in patients with MS (cohort of 34 MS subjects) compared to healthy controls of the same age and education level ($p < 0.01$) [55]. These results were obtained from a study by Benedict et al., which is the first of its kind. It matched self-reports of patients with MS on their level of empathy against external evaluation by informants. The authors found large discrepancies between the responses from the two groups—the scores obtained from patients were significantly higher ($p < 0.01$) than those of the informants. Personal abnormalities, such as elevated neuroticism, agreeableness and conscientiousness, were also registered in the patients. The authors emphasize the predictive role of executive control over the manifestation of these anomalies and suggest frontal lobe syndrome [55]. Ten years later,

Kraemer et al. also revealed a significantly lower level of empathy in patients with MS assessed by self-rating questionnaire ($p < 0.02$). A study of Banati et al. registered a higher level of empathy, attributed by ambulatory MS subjects to themselves by using self-assessment questionnaire. The patients ($n = 40$) showed 14 times better empathizing abilities to themselves compared to control individuals ($p < 0.05$) [56]. Ot self-compassion mechanisms suppress anxiety and negative thinking [57]. When self-compassion is lowered, mild symptoms of depression and anxiety could escalate into more severe ones.

A systematic review of 72 studies provides evidence of worse adjustment in MS, which is associated with emotional stress and specific emotionally focused coping strategies in these patients. The authors stress the need for further research in this direction because of insufficient evidence on the relation between adjustment outcomes and level of cognition, interaction with others, disease symptoms, social support obtained [58].

Significantly reduced self-perception in different subcategories was established in patients with MS as compared to healthy controls with similar demographic characteristics. Perception of emotional and social functioning (including global health perception) is impaired but mental characteristics are preserved [59].

Incorrect recognition of emotional information during the daily activities of patients with MS hinders the performance of social cognitive skills [60]. Alexithymia, the impaired ability to verbalize emotions due to violation of their processing, might have a significant impact on self-perception, emotion regulation, behavior control and interaction with others in these patients [61]. Alexithymia is a personal construct, characterized by subclinical inability to identify and describe the emotions in the self [62]. It is a common finding in patients with MS and further hinders social cognition [63], making them nonempathic and ineffective in emotional responding [64]. For example, in a study comparing 40 MS patients with the same number of normal volunteers, Montreuil and Petropoulo registered alexithymia in 50% of the patients and only in 9% of controls [65]. No correlation was found between alexithymia, on the one hand, and cognitive impairment, mood disorders and disease duration in MS patients, on the other. However, MRI studies established a significant connection between alexithymia and atrophy of the posterior part of corpus callosum [66]. This result supports the hypothesis of interhemispheric transfer dysfunction in patients with alexithymic MS [67].

One of the most sensitive indications of social cognition impairment, in particular in MS, is the difficulty in facial expression recognition [68, 69]. Most MS research detects a deficiency in emotional facial expression recognition. Beatty studied patients with MS and established impaired identification not only of facial affect, but also of neutral facial expressions [60]. Testing this ability in patients with MS again (cohort of 22 patients with MS and 11 healthy controls), Krause et al. detected unequivocal emotion recognition deficits in patients with MS who had shown no difficulties in face identification. In line with current findings, these impairments were most common in the recognition of unpleasant facial emotions, while deficits in the recognition of happy expression were not observed. Furthermore, the reaction times to happy facial expressions were significantly faster ($p < 0.001$) compared to that to negative emotional expressions. One reason may be that it is usually easier to recognize a happier facial expression, and consequently, these impairments can be better compensated for

[70]. Based on specific tests for perception from facial photographs, Philips expanded and supplemented the currently available data with the conclusion that MS leads to an impaired ability for processing emotional information from both static and dynamic images [71]. However, differences in emotion recognition are discreet and subtle, and according to some researchers, correlate significantly with cognitive functioning, suggesting a global deficiency in the speed of information processing [50]. Despite some variability in findings, several contemporary studies support the thesis that ToM impairments are independent from neuropsychological functioning in adult patients with MS [49, 56]. A correlation between impaired emotional perception and the physiological and social aspects of quality of life was found in MS [71]. Some studies have shown a correlation between the inability to recognize facial emotions from presented photographs and alexithymia [72–74].

In a study of patients with MS in 2003, which was the first of its kind, Beatty revealed affective prosody comprehension deficits not due to a hearing loss, cognitive decline, aphasia or depression (47 patients, 19 demographic controls). MRI studies of these patients did not detect a connection between affective prosody violations and the size of the corpus callosum or lesion load [75].

Empathy reflects the ability to infer and share the emotional state of others, therefore it is strongly related to ToM [76]. ToM (mentalization) refers to the perception of the mental condition of ourselves and others, which may serve for understanding and predicting their behavior [77].

ToM disorders are often detected in patients with MS. Their ability to read thoughts is reduced due to their impaired decoding of nonverbal signs such as facial expressions, gestures, gaze fixation and comprehensive processing of abstract verbal information.

The first study assessing ToM abilities in patients with MS was conducted in 2009 by Henry et al. [45], who applied both a test for basic recognition of emotional facial expressions and ToM tests (27 patients with MS and 30 controls). The "Reading the Mind in the Eyes" test (belonging to ToM tests) allowed the differentiation of more complex emotional states often associated with social relationships (e.g., attraction or repulsion, friendly or hostile attitude, noticing or ignoring the tested). The authors found impaired recognition of anger and fear in patients with MS but did not establish intergroup differences between subjects and controls in the recognition of surprise, sadness, disgust and happiness. A significant correlation was registered between dealing successfully with facial emotion recognition and ToM tasks. For both groups, a statistical correlation was discovered between the level of coping and executive control.

In the same year, Ouellet arrived at the conclusion that patients with MS suffering from cognitive deficits tend not to recognize the mental state of others unlike MS patients with preserved cognition (15 cognitively intact and 26 cognitively impaired patients) [49], while Henry (64 patients with relapsing-remitting MS (RRMS), 30 controls) [78] and Pöttgen (45 patients with MS, 45 healthy controls) [21] found that ToM deficits in MS appear independently of the well-known cognitive deficits. Emotion recognition impairments were more pronounced in patients with MS than impairments in thought and intention recognition [21, 79].

More errors of interpretation and lower total scores were reported in patients with MS when using nonverbal tests [56]. Subjects performed worse than controls ($p < 0.05$) at the facial symbol test (FST) [80].

In their pilot study, Genova et al. used a dynamic sociocognitive task—The Awareness of Social Inference Test (TASIT)—and established an impaired ability in patients with MS to interpret and understand lies and sarcasm. These impairments correlated with severe cognitive disorders in information processing speed, working memory, learning and memory and with premorbid IQ [50].

Charvet et al. devoted their scientific work on social cognition in patients with MS, which has debuted in childhood. The authors reported significantly worse results of the pediatric onset MS patients ($n = 28$) compared to those of healthy peers ($n = 32$) in the following three domains of social cognition: facial affect recognition ($p = 0.008$), detection of social faux pas ($p = 0.009$), perspective taking ($p = 0.06$) [81].

5.1. Social cognition impairments in different clinical subtypes of MS

Studies exploring the relatedness of social cognition impairments to clinical subtypes of MS are still insufficient. The available data indicate significant variation in the degree of cognitive impairment among individual phenotypes of the disease.

5.1.1. Clinically isolated syndrome (CIS)

In 2010, Jehna et al. conducted a study in which they established significant slower speed of emotional facial expression processing in patients with CIS compared to healthy persons ($p <$ 0.01). They suggested storage of facial emotion recognition based on the lack of significant differences in the number of correct answers. Since response time is an indicator of cognitive processing speed, the authors interpreted these results as evidence of general delay in information processing in MS [80].

5.1.2. Relapsing-remitting multiple sclerosis (RRMS)

Patients with RRMS demonstrated significantly lower levels of empathy toward others and fantasy compared to healthy subjects [82]. An earlier study by Beatty conducted in 1989 with MS patients assessed their ability to identify facial affect by viewing photographs depicting basic emotional states. Patients with RRMS fulfilled these tasks properly [60]. The findings of a new study, conducted by Kraemer et al. in 2013, with a homogeneous cohort of 25 patients with RRMS in the early stages of the disease (less than two years' duration) and with low levels of disability Expanded Disability Status Scale- <2 (EDSS <2) showed significantly worse results in affective prosody comprehension in MS subjects compared to the same number healthy controls. Patients gave less accurate solutions to "discrimination of affective prosody" and more incorrect responses in the subtest "matching of affective prosody to facial expression" for the emotion "anger". Paradoxically, regarding the emotion "fear" they showed better results than controls [6]. Gleichgerrcht et al found that MS subjects (patients $n = 38$; controls n

= 38) had significantly higher self-oriented personal distress ($p < 0.01$) and higher levels of alexithymia compared to controls [82].

So far the only available study in patients with MS examining the cognitive and affective components of ToM separately is that of Roca et al. from 2014. Using faux pas and executive function tests in 18 RRMS patients with low grade of disability, Roca et al. found deficits in the cognitive component of ToM in the presence of a stored affective component. Such dissociation between the cognitive and affective components of ToM has also been reported in other neurological and psychiatric disorders [83].

5.1.3. Primary progressive MS (PPMS)

Patients with primary progressive MS (PPMS) have experienced considerable difficulties in identifying the emotions of others, as well as their own emotions. Patients from this subgroup gave lower results in faux pas tasks compared to RRMS patients [84].

5.1.4. Secondary progressive multiple sclerosis (SPMS)

Patients with secondary progressive MS (SPMS) are significantly more alexithymic compared to healthy controls [61]. Beatty's study in 1989 revealed that the patients with chronic progradient MS experienced difficulties in the discrimination of facial affect and neutral faces, unlike those with RRMS. Error analysis demonstrated that patients had the same difficulties in depicting each of the represented seven emotional states without serious errors in indicating their polar opposites [60]. Current studies have not shown abnormal identification of neutral faces by subjects with SPMS. In patients with this subtype, lower accuracy has been reported in performing tasks for perception of fear, surprise, anger and sadness [61], while difficulties in identifying disgust and happiness were not reported. Compared to healthy controls, patients took less time in recognizing fear and surprise, while detecting anger and sadness took them longer.

A retrospective longitudinal review with 1845 MS patients, 351 of whom with chronic progradient multiple sclerosis (CPMS), 636 — with RRMS and 858 — with mixed or nonspecific MS, compared to 265 healthy individuals registered worse results in patients with CPMS than in RRMS patients at the Benton Facial Recognition Test (BFRT) [85].

5.2. Social cognition impairments depending on MS duration

A positive correlation was detected between duration of MS and level of empathy, that is, the greater the duration of the disease, the lower the empathy quotient [55, 56, 86]. Banati et al. found profoundly increasing of the empathizing quotient (p 0.03) among patients with short-term MS ($n = 40$) compared to controls ($n = 35$). In addition, Pakenham and Cox in longitudinal study of 388 persons with MS and 232 caregivers registered positive correlation between the time since diagnosis and compassion/empathy ($p < 0.01$), mindfulness ($p < 0.01$) and personal growth ($p < 0.01$). Contrarily, other studies found a significant decrease in the empathy level in patients with MS who are still in the early stages of the disease and with a low degree of disability compared to healthy subjects. The authors explain the unrealistic self-assessment results of most subjects with the greater impairment of ToM skills and partly with the higher emotional stress they were experiencing [22, 86].

In 2010, Banati et al. found more prominent ToM deficits in patients with longer disease duration ($p = 0.05$) [56]. In some research, the duration of the disease did not correlate with the emotional and cognitive scores from nonverbal tests [80], while Kraemer reported positive correlation between impaired social cognitive skills and executive function deficits in the early stages of the disease in fully ambulatory patients [6].

5.3. Social cognition impairments in MS depending on the grade of physical disability

Paradoxically, patients with more severe physical disorders relatively often show a higher level of empathy compared to controls and patients with mild neurological deficits. A positive correlation was found between the difficulty in emotional facial expression recognition and the degree of disability [44]. Patients with a higher grade of disability demonstrated greater difficulties in affective prosody recognition [75]. More interpretation errors and lower scores were reported for patients with MS when nonverbal tests were used [56]. With deterioration of the disability the results from ToM verbal tests also get worse [87]. In a study of Jehna, EDSS scores did not correlate significantly with scores from emotion recognition tests or with results from FST in MS subjects (sample of 20 patients: CIS $n = 12$, RRMS = 7, SPMS = 1) [80]. Results from other recent studies indicate that the severity of the disease (respectively the degree of physical disability) does not correlate with the degree of impaired emotion recognition or with the psychological and social aspects of the quality of life [71, 88]. Therefore, some researchers consider social cognition as a separate domain of cognition which could independently affect the quality of life of the individual, in particular, that of patients with MS. Based on the extensive review of the literature available, we can conclude that social cognition impairments in these patients require further in-depth research.

6. Social brain

Leslie Brothers was one of the first scientists talking about the social brain, using proof from studies in nonhuman animals [89]. Later Prinz created the common coding theory, according to which perception and actions rely on common codes [90]. The discovery of the so-called "mirror neurons" within the premotor and parietal cortices [91], activated while an action directed to the object is performed and while an action is perceived by the object [92, 93], became a basis for extensive research on the so-called social brain [91].

The discovery of social cognitive impairments in patients with MS presupposes brain damage. The difficulty in facial expression identification is among the most sensitive indicators for social cognition impairments. It is supposed that a disconnection mechanism due to white matter lesions and cortical thinning of specific brain zones causes a cognitive decline. This worsens the processing of emotions and the decoding of mental states from facial expressions. Functional MRI study, conducted by Jehna et al., provides evidence of altered functional brain processing in the posterior cingulate cortex and precuneus during emotion recognition in subjects with MS (sample of 15 patients and 15 healthy individuals) [88]. Abnormalities in face encoding and recognition vary in different stages of MS. Patients with CIS experience increased recruitment of the posterior visual areas. In patients with RRMS, the thalamus, parahippocampal gyrus and right anterior cingulum are more activated than in patients with CIS and SPMS. In SPMS, an increased recruitment in the frontal areas is also registered. Significant correlation has been described between the above-mentioned abnormal activations, on the one hand, and clinical symptoms, conventional MRI findings and behavioral disorders, on the other [94].

It is considered that mentalization is carried out by a large network of functionally related neurons [26]. A correlation has been established among specific cortical areas involved in emotion identification from facial expression (right and left fusiform face area, frontal eye), emotion processing (right entorhinal cortex) and socially relevant information (left temporal pole) [95]. According to a model of Ross and Mesulam, affective prosody comprehension could be related to the right-sided perisylvian region, whose structure is similar to the language areas in the left hemisphere [96]. Later studies have suggested an involvement of the basal ganglia and prefrontal cortex (PFC) [97, 98]. Alexithymia may be associated with deactivation and activation of the anterior cingulate cortex (ACC) in response to highly negative and respectively highly positive emotional stimuli [72].

The most active brain region involved in social cognitive processing is the medal frontal cortex (MFC) [99, 100], which is described as the brain's social cognitive center. This region is activated during tasks requiring self-knowledge and reflection, person perception and attribution of intentions. It is supposed that von Economo neurons [101] serve as a relay tract from the frontoinsular and anterior cingulate cortices (responsible for fast intuitive processes) to parts of the frontal and temporal cortices (associated with making slower conscious decisions), thus playing an important role in ToM [102]. It was discovered that damage to the VM frontal lobe plays a crucial role in the existence of a higher level of social cognition: social reasoning [69].

Individuals with bilateral damage of the orbitofrontal cortex show a decline in their ability to attribute higher-order mental states to other people from stories. In particular, they fail to detect faux pas during functional imaging study. Emotion recognition tasks establish priority activation of Brodman Area 47 (orbital area) compared to activation of the medial orbitofrontal region [103]. Tissue loss in BA47 correlates with the inability to recognize negative emotions [104].

It is reported that sections of the left medial prefrontal cortex also contribute significantly to understand the mental state of others [105] or to reasoning about the beliefs and intentions of others [106]. Functional MRI studies demonstrate activation of the amydgala during attribution of mental states and intentions to other people by viewing pictures of their eyes [107].

The wide dissemination of demyelinating lesions and cortical thinning typical of patients with MS often lead to anatomic and functional disorders of the above-mentioned specific brain structures. A subsequent disconnection mechanism leads to a cognitive decline [108]. Single-photon emission computed tomography (SPECT) studies in cognitively impaired patients with MS registered a deficiency of brain perfusion, mainly in the frontal and temporal lobe of the left hemisphere [109]. Positron emission tomography (PET) in these patients registered both global and regional reduction of cerebral glucose metabolism [110, 111]. An increase in the white matter lesion load, especially in the insula, precentral gyrus, prefrontal and temporal cortices, reduces the effectiveness of large-scale brain structural networks in patients with MS, which leads to cognitive deficits [108]. Functional MRI studies point to a positive correlation between the degree of activation of certain cerebral zones during performance of specific cognitive tasks and lesion load. These findings support the notion that increased cortical activity in patients with MS occurs as a result of axonal damage related to MS activity and aims to limit the clinical impact of structural damage [112].

According to Krause et al., the orbitoinsular cluster, which includes the ventral lateral prefrontal cortex (VLPF) and parts of the anterior insula, is crucial to deficits in emotional perception in patients with MS [70], which is one of the most sensitive indications of impaired social cognition. Functional MRI studies have indicated that after initial activation of the early visual fields visual stimuli are selectively processed in a specific region of the fusiform gyrus, the fusiform face area (FFA) and the facial part of the superior temporal sulcus (fSTS) [113]. FFA is activated mostly with invariable traits, which is possibly related to person identification [70, 113], while fSTS activation is more often associated with variable aspects related to the eyes, spoken speech and expression of emotions and intentions [114–116]. The high-level visual temporal cortex projects to a small proportion of amygdala neurons whose answers are relatively selectively modulated by viewing faces compared to other visual stimuli. Functional MRI research has proved that the amygdala is critical for emotion recognition from facial expression, especially with negative emotions, such as fear [117, 118]. The amygdala is involved in the automatic focusing of attention for detecting emotional stimuli and filtering emotionally relevant information through the signs perceived [119, 120]. Thus, it participates in making more complex social decisions in humans [121]. There is evidence that bilateral amygdala damage leads to severely impaired ability for the recognition of fear through facial expression [118, 122]. A study by Jehna et al. provided proof for functional differences between patients with MS and healthy controls concerning the perception of neutral and emotional facial expressions of anger and disgust. These differences were found relatively early in the course of the disease, even in the absence of behavioral differences between subjects and controls. Since the functional changes registered in the occipital areas of patients with MS during recognition of nonemotional faces are usually associated with face processing, the authors explain the excessive activation of the posterior cingulate and precuneus during emotion processing as an additional attentive requirement [88].

As regards the ability to simulate the emotional state of others, the anterior insula, functionally connected to the ventrolateral prefrontal cortex (VLPFC), shows reduced activation in subjects experiencing problems in facial emotion recognition [123]. More difficult cognitive tasks lead to higher activation of the more lateral regions of ventrolateral prefrontal cortex (VLPFC) [70, 124].

During performance of various sociocognitive tasks for mental state attribution, common areas of increased activation in the medial prefrontal gyrus and the temporoparietal junctions are registered bilaterally, while the area of the medial prefrontal cortex (the paracingulate cortex) is the only region uniquely activated by the performance of ToM tasks [47].

A hypothesis has been developed for explaining social cognition via three related but distinct dimensions of anatomical and functional brain organization [124]. It states that the medial-lateral dimension connects the medial prefrontal cortex (MPFC) (emotional aspects of mental state attribution and emotions) to the lateral prefrontal cortex (LPFC), associated with visuospatial centers supporting externally generated representations (cognitive aspects of mental state attribution and emotions) [125, 126]. The midline posterior-anterior dimension links the "first-order" perceptual substratum for the flow of socioemotional processing (superior temporal sulcus), the posterior insula and the middle ACC to the anterior insula and MPFC, where it is presented again with increased complexity [99, 127] and results in awareness and explicit judgments of affective mental states. The third dimension is the projection from ventral regions of the frontal midline involved mainly in stimulus-driven processes (amygdala, striatum and OFC) to dorsal regions supporting monitoring and reflective processes (dorso-medial and lateral prefrontal cortex) [124, 126]. This means that mental state attributions are supported by various neural structures depending on the type of sociocognitive task and processing demands.

Most MRI studies of patients with MS found a correlation between the cognitive and/or affective disorders, on the one hand, and lesion localization [128], total lesion load [129] or cerebral atrophy, on the other [129, 130]. A significant correlation was also reported between abnormal activities in specific cortical zones on fMRI, on the one hand, and clinical manifestation, conventional MRI findings and behavioral changes, on the other [94]. However, a study of voxel-based lesion symptom mapping did not reveal a significant connection of the total lesion volume to the degree of emotional recognition or to the activation of specific cortical areas during task performance. A statistically significant relationship was discovered between lesions in the left temporal periventricular white matter and decreased accuracy in dealing with cognitive tests, which points to a disturbance in information transmission from the temporal visual processing areas to the frontal regulation areas [70, 131].

Altered patterns of brain activity were found in all clinical phenotypes of MS, including when cognitive abilities were intact and/or restored [112, 132, 133]. However, such research is still insufficient. A recent fMRI study of different forms and stages of MS reported results from performance of face encoding and recognition [94]. In patients with CIS an increased recruitment of the posterior visual area, where face perception and encoding is processed, was revealed. The result was interpreted as an adaptive response of cerebral reorganization for compensating sociocognitive functioning in the early stages of the demyelinating disease. In patients with RRMS, an increased activation of the thalamus, parahippocampal gyrus and right anterior cingulum was reported. In patients with SPMS, an increased recruitment of the frontal fields, associated with higher cognitive functions, was registered. The findings suggest disadaptation and inadequate coping with cognitive tasks in a social context as the disease progresses. MRI findings show that in different clinical subtypes of MS the decreased cortical recruitment often correlates with increased T2 lesion load [112, 134].

Functional MRI studies in patients with MS prove that cortical plastic changes are a dynamic phenomenon that can be modulated by external factors. Unfortunately, fMRI studies of social cognitive abilities are still scarce, especially in patients with MS. Accumulation of data from future studies will allow early registering of the specifics of morphological and functional brain changes. This would facilitate the mapping of individual strategies for adequate treatment and rehabilitation of each patient.

7. Discussion

People are profoundly social creatures, and therefore, successful social communication is crucial to their satisfactory lifestyle. The quality of this communication depends on their ability to detect emotional and cognitive processes in others and to understand their own internal state. These two features of social cognition—affective and mental—are the basis for empathy and ToM (mentalization). During social interactions, these different levels of social cognitive response are highly intertwined and each is influenced by the other.

Between 40% and 70% of patients with MS are affected by cognitive impairments [5], which are linked to a significant decline in activities of daily living. Despite the rapidly growing amount of research establishing frequent social cognitive deficits in such patients, there is still no statistics on the frequency of this type of disturbances. We set ourselves the goal of providing an overview of studies in this scientific area and contributing, through summarizing the results, to a better understanding of the specifics of social cognitive disorders and the way they determine the functional outcome and quality of life of patients with MS. We also made attempts at discussing controversies, discovering outstanding issues and outlining a framework for future research.

A wide range of literary sources report that the pathology of white matter in MS has the potential not only to disrupt the basic parameters of cognitive functions but also to hinder important social perception skills. The accumulated data suggest that the neuronal processes of ToM and empathy are performed in different brain networks which partially overlap [56]. No significant controversies exist concerning the pathophysiological significance of altered brain activation patterns in MS [112]. Rather, various studies complement the knowledge on functional processing in specific brain areas responsible for the different aspects of social cognition. Common activation areas include the medial prefrontal cortex, the temporoparietal junction and the temporal poles. ToM stimuli lead to increased activation of the lateral orbitofrontal cortex, the middle frontal gyrus, the cuneus and the superior temporal gyrus, while empathy is associated with enhanced activations of the paracingulate, the anterior and posterior cingulate and the amygdale [135]. A more pronounced global and regional cortical atrophy in the left hemisphere, which is a frequent finding in MS [136], suggests more severe ToM deterioration. However, no studies have been conducted yet of the functional relation between empathy and ToM in MS.

Pathways composed of white matter, which have a key role in coordinating the information flow between different regions of gray matter of the brain, are particularly vulnerable in MS

[108]. Patients with lesions located in the ventromedial prefrontal cortex demonstrate selective deficits in affective ToM. Lesions in the inferior frontal gyrus are associated with extremely impaired empathy and emotion recognition [137].

ToM tests based on verbal and nonverbal stimuli not only serve for clinical evaluation of social cognitive impairments, but are also at the core of studying the functional anatomy of ToM in fMRI research [47]. The MPFC, associated with mentalizing tasks, activates whenever the person is attending to certain states of the self or others. The MPFC is equally active when the person is engaged in true beliefs, knowledge of the world based on past experience applied to the current situation, and partially in personal observations and behavioural predictions (STS) [48] There is increasing evidence of functional cortical changes in the early stages of MS, even after a single clinical episode [138, 139], when expansion and recruitment of additional cortical fields as common compensation of brain damage are registered [112].

The ability to decode specific facial emotions and ToM skills, which largely determines social communication in the real world, was first studied in MS patients in 2009 by Henry et al. For the first time, researchers presented clear evidence of increased difficulties in both aspects of emotion understanding, as well as in mental state attribution. Although the authors realized that their research was limited due to the lack of study of structural brain changes, their data were the first to establish a correlation between cognitive capacities and important aspects of emotion perception [45].

The diffuse demyelination and atrophy of both gray and white matter typical of MS lead to pronounced deficits in empathy and ToM. While white matter lesion load accounts only for some cognitive deficits in MS, this type of disorders can be better explained through pathological processes affecting gray matter, which are revealed in very early stages of the disease [140–142]. A significant positive correlation was established between neocortical volume and cognitive damage in patients with RRMS [143], as the gray matter atrophy occurring faster than white matter atrophy and, as recent research indicates, probably playing a central role in the emerging and deepening of cognitive deficits [144].

New technologies can help maximize our ability to assess cerebral integrity in MS. Regardless of the rapid development of imaging technology for detecting the earliest possible morphological abnormalities in MS, the focus of research has primarily been on the physical disability and/or general cognition. Unfortunately, the study of social cognition still remains outside the scope of such type of research. We strive to contribute to a better understanding of the neurobiological correlates of social cognitive deficits, hoping in this way to provide opportunities for future research to develop medicinal and therapeutic strategies for modifying the pathological brain processes involved in these deficits. This would increase the level of empathy and ToM skills in patients with MS and could also facilitate their successful social adaptation.

On the other hand, morphological damage in MS is highly variable both with regard to the load, location and size of demyelinating lesions and in relation to individual global and regional cortical thinning. The particular phenotype of MS introduces additional specific features of brain damage. This explains the heterogeneity of social cognition impairments in terms of their severity and regarding the predominant disturbance of certain social cognitive domains. According to Henry, while testing empathy and ToM skills, it is also recommended to perform in parallel direct mapping of underlying MS-related neuropathology for detecting a link between structural brain pathology and social cognitive impairments. Pöttgen established a deficient ability to reason about the mental state of others (ToM) and to have insight into the emotional stages and feelings of others (empathy) in the early stages of RRMS [21, 22], even in patients who have no substantial neuropsychological deficits. Emotional prosody comprehension may also be disrupted in the early stages of RRMS [6]. It is argued that this is the earliest social cognitive impairment in patients with MS. Deteriorated emotional perception at this early stage can create a difficulty in perceiving nuances, such as sarcasm, irony and sincerity, which may lead to interpersonal problems. To confirm these observations, international research with larger groups of patients is required. Data from this study indicate that one year after diagnosing a patient with CIS and RRMS, they experience diminished power of attention and memory speed, which is related to a capacity for fewer working hours, fatigue, depression and may have a negative impact, as opposed to self-efficacy, which affects working hours positively. The level of ToM abilities and their relation to the above-mentioned consequences have not been followed up.

Information on social cognition impairments and different forms of MS is still scarce. The main controversies that we encountered in the course of reviewing the material on the topic are about how the grade of disturbance of social cognition skills relates to the state of general cognition, on the one hand, and to the grade of physical disability and/or the duration of the disease, on the other. These issues remain disputable due to the small size of patient cohorts and the lack of homogeneity within the groups of conducted studies. Moreover, the majority of studies on social cognition skills in MS assess the patients' social cognitive skills at a given point without following up on their development over time. This prevents us from making conclusions about their dynamics during the course of the disease or taking into account the effect of a therapeutic and/or rehabilitation approach. Extensive long-term follow-up studies with well-defined inclusion criteria, consistent sample characteristics and a wide range of clinical and imaging measurements could establish which domains of ToM change in the course of the disease, in what way and at to what extent.

We devoted a lot of time to reviewing studies on social cognition also in other neurodegenerative and mental diseases. We were impressed with the extensive research in skills for interpersonal problem solving, for recognizing social cues, for detecting situational characteristics and for solving situation connection tasks. Our opinion is that a similar approach towards social cognitive impairments in MS would throw additional light on the objective evaluation of the patient's dealing with real situations in a social context. Even studies on the relation between social cognition disturbances and functional outcome define this relation in general terms, without specifying which domains of social cognition should refer to which functional outcome domains. Resolving these issues in the MS field is a challenge for scientists requiring uniform strategies, long-term follow-up, creativity and interdisciplinary cooperation among researchers.

Two longitudinal studies in schizophrenia provide evidence for the predictive role of emotional perception in the functional outcome at a later point in time [145, 146]. Their findings support the causal relationship between social cognition and functional outcome, which gives us good grounds for drawing attention to the opportunity for similar long-term studies in patients with MS. Surprisingly, despite the chronic nature of MS, which affects young people and inevitably disables them both physically and neuropsychologically, psychotherapeutic or psychoeducational programs are still widely lacking for MS, while being successfully implemented for other neuropsychiatric diseases associated with social cognition deficiency, such as alcoholism, schizophrenia, autism, Parkinson's disease and depression [22].

Irrespective of the limitations of most studies, they share the unanimous opinion that social cognition impairments in MS are a common finding in the early stages of the disease and are characterized by clinical significance. Functional MRI often objectifies deteriorations within the mentalizing network before structural brain disorders are detected. The cortical reorganization reported in these studies may serve as an objective marker for follow-up over time. Unfortunately, fMRI is not yet a routine method of examination due to the high cost, study complexity and lack of unified standards of interpretation.

8. Conclusion

Social cognitive impairments are a common finding in patients with MS and are often manifested at the initial stages of the disease. Both empathy and ToM deficits, regardless of physical disability, lead to psychosocial consequences such as failure to achieve life goals, limitations to employment and leisure activities, inadequacy in social relationships and daily activities [58, 61]. The preservation of a better quality of life in patients with MS requires special attention to the above mentioned aspects of the disease. Timely recognition of the deficit and adequate rehabilitation of social cognition would help patients enjoy a fulfilling social life for a longer time.

Author details

Valentina Ignatova[1*], Lyudmila Todorova[2] and Jivko Surchev[3]

*Address all correspondence to: valyaig@abv.bg

1 National Heart Hospital-MHAT, Clinic of neurology, Sofia, Bulgaria

2 Institute of Biophysics and Biomedical Engineering, Bulgarian Academy of Sciences, Sofia, Bulgaria

3 Medical University of Sofia, Department of Neurosurgery, St Ivan Rilski University Hospital, Clinic of Neurosurgery, Sofia, Bulgaria

References

[1] Chiaravalloti N, DeLuca J. Cognitive impairment in multiple sclerosis. Lancet Neurol. 2008;7:1139–1151.

[2] Langdon DW. Cognition in multiple sclerosis. Curr Opin Neurol. 2011;24:244–249.

[3] Pelosi L, Geesken JM, Holly M, Hayward M, Blumhardt LD. Working memory impairment in early multiple-sclerosis. Evidence from an event-related potential study of patients with clinically isolated myelopathy. Brain. 1997;120:2039–2058.

[4] Piras MR, Magnano I, Canu ED, et al. Longitudinal study of cognitive dysfunction in multiple sclerosis: neuropsychological, neuroradiological, and neurophysiological findings. J Neurol Neurosurg Psychiatry. 2003;74:878–885.

[5] DeLuca G, Yates R, Beale H, Morrow S. Cognitive impairment in multiple sclerosis: clinical, radiologic and pathologic insights. Brain Pathol. 2015;25:79–98.

[6] Kraemer M, Herold M, Uekermann J, et al. Perception of affective prosody in patients at an early stage of relapsing-remitting multiple sclerosis. J Neuropsychol. 2013;7(1): 91–106.

[7] Santiesteban I, White S, Cook J, Gilbert SJ, Heyes C, et al. Training social cognition: from imitation to theory of mind. Cognition. 2012;122:228–235.

[8] Amato MP, Zipoli V, Portaccio E. Multiple sclerosis-related cognitive changes: a review of cross-sectional and longitudinal studies. J Neurol Sci. 2006;245(1–2):41–46.

[9] Dulau C. Social cognition and multiple sclerosis. In: Brochet B, editor. Neuropsychiatric symptoms of inflammatory demyelinating diseases. Switzerland: Springer International Publishing; 2015. p. 213–226. DOI: 10.1007/978-3-319-18464-7-15

[10] Julian LJ, Vella L, Vollmer T, Hadjimichael O, Mohr DC. Employment in multiple sclerosis. J Neurol. 2008;255(9):1354–1360.

[11] Rao SM, Ellington L, Nauertz T, et al. Cognitive dysfunction I n multiple sclerosis. II. Impact of employment and social functioning. Neurology. 1991;41:692–696.

[12] Burgess M, editor. Multiple sclerosis: theory and practice for nurses. London: Whurr; 2002.

[13] Augoustinos M, Walker I, Donaghue N, editors. Social cognition: an integrated introduction. 3rd ed. Thousand Oaks, Calif: Sage; 2014.

[14] Fiske ST, Taylor SE, editors. Social cognition. 2nd ed. New York: McGraw-Hill; 1991.

[15] Decety J, Jackson PL. The functional architecture of human empathy. Behav Cogn Neurosci Rev. 2004;3(2):71–100.

[16] Titchener E, editor. Experimental psychology of the thought process. New York: Macmillan; 1909.

[17] Wispé L. History of the concept of empathy. In: Eisenberg N, Strayer J, editors. Empathy and its development. Cambridge: Cambridge University Press; 1987.

[18] Ickes W, editor. Empathic accuracy. New York: Guilford; 1997.

[19] Samson AC. The influence of empathizing and systemizing on humor processing: theory of mind and humor. Humor. 2012;25(1):75–98.

[20] Baron-Cohen S, Richler J, Bisarya D, Gurunathan N, Wheelwright S. The systemizing quotient: an investigation of adults with Asperger Syndrome or high-functioning autism, and normal sex differences. In: Frith U, Hill E, editors. Autism: mind and brain. Oxford: Oxford University Press; 2003. p. 161–186.

[21] Pöttgen J, Dziobek I, Reh S, Heesen C, Gold SM. Impaired social cognition in multiples clerosis. J Neurol Neurosurg Psychiatry. 2013;84(5):523–528.

[22] Kraemer M, Herold M, Uekermann J, Kis B, Wiltfang J, Daum I, Dziobek I, Berlit P, Diehl R, Abdel-Hamid M. Theory of mind and empathy in patients at an early stage of relapsing remitting multiple sclerosis. Clin Neurol Neurosurg. 2013;115:1016–1022.

[23] Brothers L, Ring B. A neuroethological framework for the representation of minds. J Cogn Neurosci 1992;4:107–118.

[24] Ickes W, editor. Everyday mind reading: understanding what other people think and feel. Amherst, NY: Prometheus Books; 2003.

[25] Davis MH, Kraus LA. Personality and empathic accuracy. In: Ickes W, editor. Empathic accuracy. New York: The Guilford Press; 1997. p. 144–168.

[26] Abu-Akel A, Shamay-Tsoory S. Neuroanatomical and neurochemical bases of theory of mind. Neuropsychologia. 2011;49(11):2971–2984.

[27] Apperly IA, Butterfill S. Do humans have two systems to track beliefs and belief like states? Psychol Rev. 2009;116:953–970.

[28] Frith CD, Frith U. Implicit and explicit processes in social cognition. Neuron. 2008;603(3):503–510.

[29] Davis MH. Measuring individual differences in empathy: evidence for a multidimensional approach. J Personal Soc Psychol. 1983;44:113–126.

[30] Hemmerdinger JM, Stoddart S, Lilford R. A systematic review of tests of empathy in medicine. BMC Med Educ. 2007;7:1–8.

[31] Hogan R. Development of an empathy scale. J Consult Clin Psychol. 1969;33:307–316.

[32] Mehrabian A, editor. Manual for the balanced emotional empathy scale (BEES). Available from Albert Mehrabian ed. 1130, Alta Mesa Road, Monterey, CA 93940; 2000.

[33] Neff KD. Development and validation of a scale to measure self-compassion. Self Identity. 2003;2:223–250.

[34] Sprecher S. Compassionate love for close others and humanity. J Soc Pers Relationsh. 2005;22(5):629–651.

[35] Lawrence EJ, Shaw P, Baker D, Baron-Cohen S, David A. Measuring empathy: reliability and validity of the Empathy Quotient. Psychol Med. 2004;34(05):911–920.

[36] Davis MH. A multidimensional approach to individual differences in empathy. JSAS Cat Sel Doc Psychol. 1980;10:85.

[37] Dziobek I, Rogers K, Fleck S, Bahnemann M, Heekeren HR, Wolf OT, et al. Dissociation of cognitive and emotional empathy in adults with Asperger syndrome using the Multifaceted Empathy Test (MET). J Autism Dev Disord. 2008;38:464–473.

[38] Feinstein AJ, DeLuca, Baune BT, Filippi M, Lassman H. Cognitive and neuropsychiatric disease manifestations in MS. Mult Scler Relat Disord. 2013;2(1):4–12.

[39] Stone VE, Baron-Cohen S, Calder A, Keane J, Young A. Acquired theory of mind impairments in individuals with bilateral amygdala lesions. Neuropsychologia. 2003;41:209–220.

[40] Dziobek I, Fleck S, Kalbe E, Rogers K, Hassenstab J, Brand M, Kessler J, Woike JK, Wolf OT, Convit A. Introducing MASC: a movie for the assessment of social cognition. J Autism Dev Disord. 2006;36:623–636.

[41] Rutherford MD, Baron-Cohen S, Wheelwright S. Reading the mind in the voice: a study with normal adults and adults with Asperger syndrome and high functioning autism. J Autism Developmental Disord. 2002;32:189–194.

[42] Kerr SL, Neale JM. Emotion perception in schizophrenia: specific deficit or further evidence of generalized poor performance? J Abnorm Psychol. 1993;102:312–318.

[43] Vellante M, Baron-Cohen S, Melis M, et al. The "Reading the Mind in the Eyes" test: systematic review of psychometric properties and a validation study in Italy. Cogn Neuropsychiatr. 2013; 18(4):326-354

[44] Scherer P, Penner IK, Rohr A, et al. The faces symbol test, a newly developed screening instrument to assess cognitive decline related to multiple sclerosis: first results of the Berlin Multi-Centre FST Validation Study. Mult Scler. 2007;13:402–411.

[45] Henry JD, Phillips LH, Beatty WW, McDonald S, Longley WA, Joscelyne A, et al. Evidence for deficits in facial affect recognition and theory of mind in multiple sclerosis. J Int Neuropsychol Soc. 2009;15(2):277–285.

[46] Golan O, Baron-Cohen S. Systemizing empathy: teaching adults with Asperger syndrome or high-functioning autism to recognize complex emotions using interactive multimedia. Dev Psychopathol. 2006;18:591–617.

[47] Gallagher HL, Happe F, Brunswick N, Fletcher PC, Frith U, Frith CD. Reading the mind in cartoons and stories: an fMRI study of 'theory of mind' in verbal and nonverbal tasks. Neuropsychologia. 2000;38:11–21.

[48] Frith U, Frith CD. Development and neurophysiology of mentalizing. Phil Trans R Soc Lond B. 2003;358:459–473.

[49] Ouellet J, Scherzer PB, Rouleau I, Me'tras P, Bertrand-Gauvin C, Djerroud N, et al. Assessment of social cognition in patients with multiple sclerosis. J Int Neuropsychol Soc. 2010;1:287–296.

[50] Genova H, Cagna C, Chiaravalloti N, DeLuca J, Lengenfelder J. Dynamic assessment of social cognition in individuals with multiple sclerosis: a pilot study. J Int Neuropsychol Soc. 2016;22(1):83–88.

[51] Ihnen GH, Penn, DL, Corrigan PW, Martin J. Social perception and social skill in schizophrenia. Psychiatry Res. 1998;80:275–286.

[52] Kee KS, Kern, RS, Green MF. Perception of emotion and neurocognitive functioning in schizophrenia: what's the link? Psychiatry Res. 1998;81:57–65.

[53] Taselli S, et al. The microfoundations of organizational social networks: a review and an agenda for future research. J Manag. 2015;41(5):1361–1387.

[54] Gong P, Liu J, Li S, Zhou X. Dopamine beta-hydroxylase gene modulates individuals' empathic ability. Soc Cogn Affect Neurosci. 2014;9:1341–1345.

[55] Benedict RHB, Priore RL, Miller C, et al. Personality disorder in MS correlates with cognitive impairment. J Neuropsychiatry Clin Neurosci. 2001;13:70–76.

[56] Banati M, Sandor J, Mike A, et al. Social cognition and theory of mind in patients with relapsing-remitting multiple sclerosis. Eur J Neurol. 2010;17:426–433.

[57] Raes F. Rumination and worry as mediators of the relationship between self-compassion and depression and anxiety. Personal Individ Differ. 2010;48:757–761.

[58] Dennison L, Moss-Morris R, Chalder T. A review of psychological correlates of adjustment in patients with multiple sclerosis. Clin Psychol Rev. 2009;29:141–153.

[59] Mostert S, Kesselring J. Effects of a short-term exercise training program on aerobic fitness, fatigue, health perception and activity level of subjects with multiple sclerosis. Mult Scler. 2002;8:161–168.

[60] Beatty WW, Goodkin DE, Weir WS, Staton RD, Monson N, Beatty PA. Affective judgements by patients with Parkinson's disease or chronic progressive multiple sclerosis. Bull Psychon Soc. 1989;27:361–364.

[61] Prochnow D, Donell J, Schafer R, Jorgens S, Hartung HP, et al. Alexithymia and impaired facial affect recognition in multiple sclerosis. J Neurol. 2011;258:1683–1688.

[62] Sifneos PE. The prevalence of 'alexithymic' characteristics in psychosomatic patients. Psychother Psychosom. 1973;22(2):255–262.

[63] Petropoulo H, Montreuil M, Truelle Jl, Lyon-Caen O, et al. Étude émotionnelle et cognitive de 40 patients attaints de sclérose en plaques récente. In: Atelier de conjoncture: développement, fonctionnement: perspective historico-culturelle. Société Française de Psychologie; 13–14 octobre; Paris. 2002.

[64] FeldmanHall O, Dalgleish T, Mobbs D. Alexithymia decreases altruism in real social decisions. Cortex. 2012;49:899–904.

[65] Montreuil M, Petropoulo H. Humeur et émotions dans la sclérose en plaques. Neuropsy News. 2003;2:91–96.

[66] Pelletier J, Montreuil M, Habib M, Ali Cherif A, et al. Alexithymia and multiple sclerosis: alteration of interhemispheric transfer. Eur J Neurol. 1996;3:63.

[67] Montel S, Bungener C. Les troubles de l'humeur et des émotions dans la sclérose en plaques: une revue de la littérature. Rev Neurol Mood and emotional disorders in Multiple Sclerosis: a literature review(Paris). 2007;163:27–37.

[68] Said CP, Haxby JV, Todorov A. Brain systems for assessing the affective value of faces. Philos Trans R Soc Lond B Biol Sci. 2011;366(1571):1660–1670.

[69] Adolphs R. Social cognition and the human brain. Trends Cogn Sci. 1999;3:469–479.

[70] Krause M, Wendt J, Dressel A, Berneiser J, Kessler C, Hamm AO, Lotze M. Prefrontal function associated with impaired emotion recognition in patients with multiple sclerosis. Behav Brain Res. 2009;205(1):280–285.

[71] Phillips LH, Henry JD, Scott C, Summers F, Whyte M, Cook M. Specific impairments of emotion perception in multiple sclerosis. Neuropsychology. 2011;25(1):131–136.

[72] Kano M, Fukudo S, Gyoba J. Specific brain processing of facial expressions in people with alexithymia: an H215O-PET study. Brain. 2003;126:1474–1484.

[73] Parker JDA, Taylor GJ, Bagby RM. Alexithymia and the recognition of facial expressions of emotion. Psychother Psychosom. 1993;59:197–202.

[74] Lane RD, Sechrest L, Riedel R, Shapiro DE, Kaszniak AW. Pervasive emotion recognition deficit common to alexithymia and the repressive coping style. Psychosom Med. 2000;62:492–501.

[75] Beatty WW, Orbelo DM, Sorocco KH, Ross ED. Comprehension of affective prosody in multiple sclerosis. Mult Scler. 2003;9:148–153.

[76] Chakrabarti B, Baron-Cohen S. Empathizing: neurocognitive developmental mechanisms and individual differences. Prog Brain Res. 2006;156:403–417.

[77] Premack D, Woodruff G. Does the chimpanzee have a theory of mind? Behav Brain Sci. 1978;4:515–526.

[78] Henry A, Tourbah A, Chaunu MP, et al. Social cognition impairments in relapsing–remitting multiple sclerosis. J Int Neuropsychol Soc. 2011;17:1122–1131.

[79] Phillips LH, Beatty WW, et al. Evidence for deficits in facial affect recognition and theory of mind in multiple sclerosis. J Int Neuropsychol Soc. 2009;15:277–285.

[80] Jehna M, Neuper C, Petrovic K, Wallner-Blazek M, Schmidt R, Fuchs S. An exploratory study on emotion recognition in patients with a clinically isolated syndrome and multiple sclerosis. Clin Neurol Neurosurg. 2010;112(6):482–484.

[81] Charvet LE, Cleary RE, Vazquez K, et al. Social cognition in pediatric-onset multiple sclerosis (MS). Mult Sclr J. 2014;20:1478–1484.

[82] Gleichgerrcht E, Tomashitis B, Sinay V. The relationship between alexithymia, empathy and moral judgment in patients with multiple sclerosis. Eur J Neurol. 2015;22(9):1295–1303.

[83] Roca M, Manes F, Gleichgerrcht E, Ibáñez A, González de Toledo ME, Marenco V, Bruno D, Torralva T, Sinay V. Cognitive but not affective theory of mind deficits in mild relapsing-remitting multiple sclerosis. Cogn Behav Neurol. 2014;27(1):25–30.

[84] Dulau C. Existe-t-il vraiment une atteinte de la cognition sociale dans la sclerose en plaques? [thesis]. Hum Health Pathol. 2014. Available from: <dumas-01089147>

[85] Zakzanis KK. Distinct neurocognitive profiles in multiple sclerosis subtypes. Arch Clin Neuropsychol. 2000;15:115–136.

[86] Pakenham KI, Cox S. The dimensional structure of benefit finding in multiple sclerosis and relations with positive and negative adjustment: a longitudinal study. Psychol Health. 2009;24:373–393.

[87] Berneiser J, Wendt J, Grothe M, et al. Impaired recognition of emotional facial expressions in patients with multiple sclerosis. Mult Scler Relat Disord. 2014;3(4):482–488.

[88] Jehna M, Langkammer C, Wallner-Blazek M, et al. Cognitively preserved MS patients demonstrate functional differences in processing neutral and emotional faces. Brain Imaging Behav. 2011;5(4):241–251.

[89] Brothers L. The social brain: a project for integrating primate behaviour and neurophysiology in a new domain. Concepts Neurosci. 1990;1:27–51.

[90] Prinz W. Perception and action planning. Eur J Cogn Psychol. 1997;9:129–154.

[91] Rizzolatti G, Craighero L. The mirror neuron system. Annu Rev Neurosci. 2004;27:169–172.

[92] Gallesse V, Metzinger T. Motor ontology: the representational reality of goals, actions and selves. Philos Psychol. 2003;13(3):365–388.

[93] Gallesse V, Fadiga L, Fogassi L, Rizzolatti G. Action recognition in the premotor cortex. Brain. 1996;119:593–609.

[94] Vacchi L, Rocca M, Riccitelli GC, Rodegher M. Processing face encoding in multiple sclerosis: a fMRI investigation (P6. 134). Neurology. 2015 April 6;84(14 Supplement):P6.134.

[95] Mike A, Strammer E, Aradi M, Orsi G, Perlaki G, Hajnal A, et al. Disconnection mechanism and regional cortical atrophy contribute to impaired processing of facial expressions and theory of mind in multiple sclerosis: a structural MRI study. PloS One. 2013 Dec 13;8(12):e82422.

[96] Ross ED, Mesulam MM. Dominant language functions of the right hemisphere? Prosody and emotional gesturing. Arch Neurol. 1979;36:144–148.

[97] Buchanan TW, Lutz K, Mirzazade S, Specht K, Shah NJ, Zilles K, Jancke L. Recognition of emotional prosody and verbal components of spoken language: an fMRI study. Cogn Brain Res. 2000;9:227–238.

[98] Abdel-Hamid M, Lehmkamper C, Sonntag C, Juckel G, Daum I, Brune M. Theory of Mind in schizophrenia: the role of clinical symptomatology and neurocognition in understanding other people's thoughts and intentions. Psychiatry Res. 2009;165:19–26.

[99] Amodio DM, Frith CD. Meeting of minds: the medial frontal cortex and social cognition. Nat Rev Neurosci. 2006;7(4):268–277.

[100] Fiske ST, Markus HR. Facing social class: how societal rank influences interaction. New York, NY: Russell Sage Foundation, 2012.

[101] Von Economo C, Koskinas G, editors. Die Cytoarchitectonik der Hirnrinde des erwachsenen Menschen.Berlin, Springer: 1925.

[102] Allman JM, Watson KK, Tetreault NA, Hakeem AY. Intuition and autism: a possible role for Von Economo neurons. Trends Cogn Sci. 2005;9:367–373.

[103] Steele JD, Lawrie SM. Segregation of cognitive and emotional function in the prefrontal cortex: a stereotactic meta-analysis. Neuroimage. 2004;21:868–875.

[104] Rosen HJ, Wilson MR, Schauer GF, et al. Neuroanatomical correlates of impaired recognition of emotion in dementia. Neuropsychologia. 2006;44:365–373.

[105] Stone VE, Baron-Cohen S, Knight RT. Frontal lobe contributions to theory of mind. J Cogn Neurosci. 1998;10:640–656.

[106] Goel V, et al. Modeling other minds. Neuro Report. 1995;6:1741–1746.

[107] Baron-Cohen S, et al. Social intelligence in the normal and autistic brain: an fMRI study. Eur J Neurosci. 1999;11:1891–1898.

[108] He Y, Dagher A, Chen Z, Charil A, Zijdenbos A, Worsley K, Evans A. Impaired small-world efficiency in structural cortical networks in multiple sclerosis associated with white matter lesion load. Brain. 2009;132(12):3366–3379.

[109] Paulesu E, Perani D, Fazio F, et al. Functional basis of memory impairment in multiple sclerosis: a [18F]FDG PET study. NeuroImage. 1996;4:87–96.

[110] Blinkenberg M, Rune K, Jensen CV, et al. Cortical cerebral metabolism correlates with MRI lesion load and cognitive dysfunction in MS. Neurology. 2000;54:558–564.

[111] Penner IK, Opwis, Kappos L . Relation between functional brain imaging, cognitive impairment and cognitive rehabilitation in patients with multiple sclerosis. J Neurol. 2007;254(2):II53–II57.

[112] Pantano P, Mainero C, Caramia F. Functional brain reorganization in multiple sclerosis: evidence from fMRI studies. J Neuroimaging. 2006;16:104–114.

[113] Kanwisher N, Yovel G. The fusiform face area: a cortical region specialized for the perception of faces. Philos Trans R Soc Lond B Biol Sci. 2006;361:2109–28.

[114] Allison T, Puce A, McCarthy G. Social perception from visual cues: role of the STS region. Trends Cogn Sci. 2000;4:267–278.

[115] Thompson JC, Hardee JE, Panayiotou A, Crewther D, Puce A. Common and distinct brain activation to viewing dynamic sequences of face and hand movements. Neuro-image. 2007;37(3):966–973.

[116] Esterman M, Yantis S. Perceptual expectation evokes category-selective cortical activity. Cereb Cortex. 2010;20(5):1245–1253.

[117] Morris JS, et al. A differential neural response in the human amygdala to fearful and happy facial expressions. Nature. 1996;383:812–815.

[118] Adolphs R, et al. Impaired recognition of emotion in facial expressions following bilateral damage to the human amygdala. Nature. 1994;372:669–672.

[119] Vuilleumier P, Pourtois G. Distributed and interactive brain mechanisms during emotion face perception: evidence from functional neuroimaging. Neuropsychologia. 2007;45:174–194.

[120] Adolphs R, Spezio M. Role of the amygdala in processing visual social stimuli. Prog Brain Res. 2006;156:363–378.

[121] Buchel C, Morris J Dolan RJ, Friston KJ. Brain systems mediating aversive conditioning: an event-related fMRI study. Neuron. 1998;20:947–957.

[122] Young AW, Aggleton JP, Hellawell DJ, Johnson M, Broks P, Hanley JR. Face processing impairments after amygdalotomy. Brain. 1995;118(Pt 1):15–24.

[123] Singer T, Seymour B, O'Doherty J, Kaube H, Dolan RJ, Frith CD. Empathy for pain involves the affective but not sensory components of pain. Science. 2004;303:1157–1162.

[124] Olsson A, Ochsner KN. The role of social cognition in emotion. Trends Cogn Sci. 2008;12:65–71.

[125] Lieberman MD. Social cognitive neuroscience: a review of core processes. Annu Rev Psychol. 2007;58:259–289.

[126] Ochsner KN et al. Reflecting upon feelings: an fMRI study of neural systems supporting the attribution of emotion to self and other. J Cogn Neurosci. 2004;16:1746–1772.

[127] Burgess PW, et al.. The gateway hypothesis of rostral prefrontal cortex (area 10) function. Trends Cogn Sci. 2007;11:290–298.

[128] Reischies FM, Baum K, Nehrig C, Schorner W. Psychopathological symptoms and magnetic resonance imaging findings in multiple sclerosis. Biol Psychiatry. 1993;33:676–678.

[129] Bobholz JA, Rao SM, Lobeck L, et al. fMRI study of episodic memory in relapsingremitting MS: correlation with T2 lesion volume. Neurology. 2006;67:1640–1645.

[130] Lazeron RH, Boringa JB, Schouten M, et al. Brain atrophy and lesion load as explaining parameters for cognitive impairment in multiple sclerosis. Mult Scler. 2005;11:524–531.

[131] Cavada C, Company T, Tejedor J, Cruz-Rizzolo RJ, Reinoso-Suarez F. The anatomical connections of the macaque monkey orbitofrontal cortex. A review. Cereb Cortex. 2000;10:220–242.

[132] Audoin B, Ibarrola D, Ranjeva JP, et al. Compensatory cortical activation observed by fMRI during a cognitive task at the earliest stage of MS. Hum Brain Mapp. 2003;20:51–58.

[133] Staffen W, Mair A, Zauner H, et al. Cognitive function and fMRI in patients with multiple sclerosis: evidence for compensatory cortical activation during an attention task. Brain. 2002;125:1275–1282.

[134] Lee M, Reddy H, Johansen-Berg H, et al. The motor cortex shows adaptive functional changes to brain injury from multiple sclerosis. Ann Neurol. 2000;47:606–613.

[135] Völlm BA, Taylor AN, Richardson P, Corcoran R, Stirling J, McKie S, et al. Neuronal correlates of theory of mind and empathy: a functional magnetic resonance imaging study in a nonverbal task. Neuroimage. 2006;29(1):90–98.

[136] Narayana PA, Govindarajan KA, Goel P, et al. Regional cortical thickness in relapsing remitting multiple sclerosis: a multi-center study. NeuroImage Clin. 2012;2:120–131.

[137] Shamay-Tsoory SG, Aharon-Peret J, Perry D. Two systems for empathy: a double dissociation between emotional and cognitive empathy in inferior frontal gyrus versus ventromedial prefrontal lesions. Brain. 2009;132:617–627.

[138] Pantano P, Iannetti GD, Caramia F, et al. Cortical motor reorganization after a single clinical attack of multiple sclerosis. Brain. 2002;125:1607–1615.

[139] Rocca MA, Mezzapesa DM, Falini A, et al. Evidence for axonal pathology and adaptive cortical reorganization in patients at presentation with clinically isolated syndromes suggestive of multiple sclerosis. Neuroimage. 2003;18:847–855.

[140] Amato MP, Bartolozzi ML, Zipoli V, Portaccio E, Mortilla M, Guidi L, Siracusa G, Sorbi S, Federico A, De Stefano N. Neocortical volume decrease in relapsing-remitting MS patients with mild cognitive impairment. Neurology. 2004;63(1):89–93.

[141] Lazeron RH, Langdon DW, Filippi M, van Waesberghe JH, Stevenson VL, Boringa JB, Origgi D, Thompson AJ, Falautano M, Polman CH, et al. Neuropsychological impairment in multiple sclerosis patients: the role of (juxta)cortical lesion on FLAIR. Mult Scler. 2000;6(4):280–285.

[142] Rovaris M, Filippi M, Minicucci L, Iannucci G, Santuccio G, Possa F, Comi G. Cortical/subcortical disease burden and cognitive impairment in patients with multiple sclerosis. AJNR Am J Neuroradiol. 2000;21(2):402–408.

[143] Amato MP, Ponziani G, Siracusa G, Scorbi S. Cognitive dysfunction in early-onset multiple sclerosis: a reappraisal after 10 years. Arch Neurol. 2001;58:1602–1606.

[144] Pirko I, Lucchinetti CF, Sriram S, Bakshi R. Gray matter involvement in multiple sclerosis. Neurology. 2007;68:634–642.

[145] Brekke JS, Kay DD, Kee KS, Green MF. Biosocial pathways to functional outcome in schizophrenia. Schizophr Res. 2005;80:213–225.

[146] Kee KS, Green MF, Mintz J, Brekke JS. Is emotion processing a predictor of functional outcome in schizophrenia? Schizophr Bull. 2003;29:487–497.

4

Pediatric Multiple Sclerosis

Ozgul Ekmekci

Abstract

Multiple sclerosis (MS) is an autoimmune inflammatory demyelinating disorder of the central nervous system. Although pediatric and adult-onset MS have similar neurologic symptoms, there are some differences from adults in radiologic findings, cognitive features, clinical course, and diagnostic criteria of pediatric MS. Diagnostic criteria and radiologic features of pediatric MS have been defined in recent years. There are no large, randomized, controlled therapeutic trials in pediatric MS. In this chapter, clinical characteristics, diagnostic criteria, laboratory findings, differential diagnosis, and treatment of pediatric MS are summarized.

Keywords: multiple sclerosis, pediatric multiple sclerosis, childhood multiple sclerosis, demyelinating disorders, demyelination

1. Introduction

Multiple sclerosis (MS) is an autoimmune chronic inflammatory disease of the central nervous system; it is characterized by demyelination and axonal loss. MS primarily affects young adults. Recently, it has been increasingly recognized in children and adolescents. Approximately 2–5% of all MS patients have onset before age 18 [1, 2]. Onset before 10 years of age occurs in less than 1% of all patients. There are some differences, including clinical presentation, magnetic resonance imaging (MRI) findings, and neuroimmunologic features, between pediatric and adult MS patients. The first attack can be acute disseminated encephalomyelitis, particularly in young children. Relapses are more frequent in pediatric MS patients than in adults, though improvement is better. Cognitive impairment including linguistic dysfunction and reduction in IQ scores also differs from adults. T2 lesion burden is higher in pediatric patients in MRI as compared to adult MS patients. These differences are more marked in prepuberal children [3]. The still developing central nervous and immune systems may be responsible for these differences. However, studies on pathogenesis and pathology of pediatric MS are limited.

2. Epidemiology

The incidence of pediatric MS is unknown, but its estimated prevalence has been reported to be 1.35–2.5 per 100,000 children [4]. The gender ratio varies with the age of onset: in patients older than 10 years, the female-to-male ratio is similar to adults; there is female dominance. In children younger than 10 years old, the female-to-male ratio decreases. This difference may be due to hormonal influence or gender-specific genetic influence on immunological reactivity [5].

3. Etiology and risk factors

Pediatric MS has a complex etiology related to both genetic and environmental factors. Vitamin D deficiency has been implicated as a risk factor for MS in children, as it is in adults. Mowry et al. have demonstrated an association between relapse rate and vitamin D level in pediatric MS patients [6]. Smoking has been considered as a risk factor in adults, whereas passive smoke exposure has been recognized as a risk factor in children [7]. One of the most studied environmental risk factors is viral exposure and studies have found that viral exposure in childhood may predispose some individuals to the development of MS. Epstein-Barr seropositivity and serum anti-EBV antibody titers tend to be higher in MS patients than they are in normal individuals. The relationship between the Epstein-Barr virus and MS has also been shown in pediatric MS [8]. Another risk factor is obesity. Childhood and adolescent obesity has been suggested as a risk factor for the development of MS in both adults and children [9]. Genetic susceptibility is also a risk factor for MS. HLA-DRB1 locus has been associated with multiple sclerosis in children. Twin studies have demonstrated a concordance rate of 27% in monozygotic twins. The incidence for first-degree relatives of patients with MS is 2–5%, whereas the incidence for the general population is under 0.1% [10].

4. Pathogenesis

Multiple sclerosis is a neuroimmunologic disorder characterized pathologically by inflammation, demyelination, and axonal loss. Neuropathological findings and animal models such as experimental allergic encephalomyelitis support the immunopathogenesis in multiple sclerosis. HLA Class II genes which are associated with MS risk are also related to the immune system.

The first step in the immunopathogenesis of MS is peripheral activation of CD4+ T lymphocytes in response to an antigen. This antigen is unknown. It has been suggested that molecular mimicry between this antigen and central nervous system antigens causes cross reactivity. Subsequently, activated T lymphocytes migrate through the blood-brain barrier into the central nervous system [10, 11]. Lymphocyte migration represents an important step in MS pathogenesis. This multistep process includes adhesion, chemoattraction, and active infiltration into the central nervous system. Adhesion molecules, chemokines, and cytokines play an important role in these steps [10]. $\alpha 4\beta 1$ integrin (VLA-4, very late activating antigen) is an adhesion molecule which is expressed on the lymphocyte surface and binds to the vascular cell adhesion molecule-1 (VICAM-1) located on the endothelium. As a result of this interaction, lymphocytes adhere to the endothelium and transmigrate across the endothelial cell layer into the central nervous system [12]. Chemokines regulate migration of immune cells into the brain; they also manipulate the lymphocyte transendothelial migration and locomotion within the tissue along chemoattractant gradients. Reactivation of infiltrating immune cells within the central nervous system leads to perivascular inflammation and injury. This injury results in the release of additional central nervous system antigens such as myelin proteins and leads to immune responses to these self-antigens (antigen spreading/epitope spreading). T cells reactive to myelin proteins including myelin basic protein (MBP), myelin oligodendrocyte glycoprotein (MOG), and myelin proteolipid protein (PLP) are involved in the central nervous system inflammatory response of MS patients [10]. Myelin-reactive T cells have differences in MS patients as compared with healthy controls. In MS patients myelin-reactive T cells differ by having memory phenotype. Memory T cells play an important role in MS pathogenesis. Other immune cells including proinflammatory and anti-inflammatory/regulatory CD4+ T cells (helper T lymphocytes), CD8+ T cells (cytotoxic T lymphocytes), myeloid cell subsets, B cells, and natural killer cells contribute to the pathogenesis of MS in adults. After activation by antigen-presenting cells such as dendritic cells, naïve T cells differentiate into one of the several subsets with different effector functions. Th1 lymphocytes secrete proinflammatory cytokines such as interferon gamma, while Th2 lymphocytes produce anti-inflammatory cytokines such as interleukin 4, interleukin 10. The imbalance between proinflammatory and anti-inflammatory cytokines has been invoked in MS pathogenesis. Proinflammatory cytokines play crucial roles in MS pathogenesis including peripheral immune activation, enhancement of trafficking of activated immune cells into the CNS, and direct damage to oligodendrocytes, myelin, and axons [10, 12]. Th17 lymphocytes are also a subgroup of CD4+ T cells that produce the proinflammatory cytokines interleukin 17A and interleukin 17F. Th17 lymphocytes are developmentally distinct from Th1 and Th2 lineages. Interleukin 23 produced by macrophages and dendritic cells contributes to development of Th17. High Th17 to Th1 ratios are associated with T cell infiltration and inflammation in the brain parenchyma [13]. The presence of interleukin 17 in MS lesions and increased interleukin 17 expression in both blood and CSF of MS patients have been demonstrated [14, 15]. Other subgroups of T cells also have been implicated in the immunopathogenesis of MS. Regulatory T (Treg) cells control potentially pathogenic autoreactive T cells. Studies demonstrated that regulatory T cell functions are altered in MS. In a study, similar T cell responses to myelin basic protein and myelin oligodendrocyte glycoprotein epitopes have been found in both adult and pediatric MS patients [16]. Vargas Lowy demonstrated increased CD4+ T cell proliferation to myelin peptides in children with MS and also found an increased proportion of dividing CD4+ T cell to myelin peptides with a memory phenotype which produced interleukin 17 [10].

Humoral immunity has also been implicated in MS pathogenesis. B lymphocytes, plasma cells, immunoglobulins, and complement deposition have been shown in MS lesions. Anti-myelin oligodendrocyte glycoprotein antibodies (anti-MOG) have been reported in pediatric cases with inflammatory demyelinating diseases, predominantly in children with ADEM-like first episodes and in pediatric MS patients younger than 10 years of age at disease onset. Anti-MOG antibodies have also been observed in pediatric patients with recurrent optic neuritis and seronegative NMO [10, 17]. The presence of anti-MOG antibodies has been reported in a subgroup of adults with seronegative NMO but only rarely in adults with MS [18]. Moreover, antibody-independent functions of B lymphocytes such as cytokine production play a role in MS immunopathogenesis.

Neurodegeneration and axonal damage are other processes in the pathogenesis of MS. Mechanisms of axonal damage in multiple sclerosis include a specific immunologic attack on axons; the presence of soluble mediators such as proteases, cytokines, and free radicals released during the inflammatory process and lack of neurotrophic factors provided to the axon by oligodendrocytes as a result of chronic demyelination [10, 19].

5. Pathology

The cellular content of MS lesions includes primarily T lymphocytes (CD4+ and CD8+) and macrophages. Lucchinetti et al. have described four distinct pathological patterns of demyelination in autopsy and biopsy samples from adult MS patients. Patterns I and II showed T cell/macrophage inflammation and there was also T cell plus antibody-mediated autoimmune damage in pattern II. Patterns III and IV were suggestive of a primary oligodendrocyte dystrophy. Oligodendrocyte apoptosis or death and lesser macrophage-T cell inflammation were observed in patterns III and IV [20]. In another study, Trapp et al. demonstrated axonal damage in normal appearing white matter [21]. Additionally, subpial cortical, intracortical, and leukocortical lesions were found in adult-onset multiple sclerosis patients' biopsy specimens. Immune cells were also identified within the pia-arachnoid in adult-onset multiple sclerosis and ectopic B-cell follicles with germinal centers were detected in the meninges of patients with secondary progressive multiple sclerosis. All these pathological findings were identified in adult patients [10, 22, 23]. Neuropathological studies are limited in pediatric multiple sclerosis [10]. Tumefactive demyelinating lesions have been investigated in pediatric patients with MS [24]. The pathological characteristics of tumefactive demyelinating lesions include relative axonal preservation, perivascular and parenchymal lymphocyte and macrophage inflammation [25].

6. Diagnostic criteria

In 2007, the International Pediatric Multiple Sclerosis Study Group (IPMSSG) proposed a consensus on definitions for pediatric acquired demyelinating disorders of the central nervous system and pediatric MS. Pediatric MS referred to "children" (under the age of 10) and "adolescents" (aged 10 and above but younger than 18) in this definition. In 2012, the study group revised the criteria in consideration of studies that had applied 2007 pediatric MS criteria and the 2010 revised McDonald's criteria for adults [26–28].

According to the 2012 revised criteria, pediatric MS can be satisfied by any of the following:

- Two or more non-encephalopathic (e.g. not ADEM-like) clinical central nervous system (CNS) events with a presumed inflammatory cause, separated by more than 30 days and involving more than one area of the CNS.
- One non-encephalopathic episode typical of MS which is associated with MRI findings consistent with the 2010 revised McDonald criteria for DIS (dissemination in space) and in which a follow-up MRI shows at least one new enhancing or non-enhancing lesion consistent with DIT (dissemination in time) MS criteria.
- One ADEM attack followed by a non-encephalopathic clinical event, three or more months after the onset of symptoms, which is associated with new MRI lesions that fulfill the 2010 revised McDonald DIS criteria.
- A first single, acute event that does not meet ADEM criteria and whose MRI findings are consistent with the 2010 revised McDonald criteria for DIS and DIT (applies only to children ≥ 12 years old).

7. Clinical features

Most of the patients with pediatric MS have a relapsing remitting course. A primary progressive course is extremely rare in pediatric MS. The definition of an attack (relapse/exacerbation) in pediatric MS is similar to that in adults. An attack is defined as "the appearance of new symptoms and neurologic signs, or worsening of old symptoms and signs due to an acute inflammatory demyelinating event in the CNS, with duration of at least 24 hours in the absence of fever or infection," and the onset of the attack should be separated from the onset of a previous attack by at least 30 days [27].

Visual, sensory, motor, brainstem, cerebellar symptoms, sphincter, and cognitive dysfunctions may also occur in pediatric MS, as they do in adults. Polysymptomatic and ADEM-like onset are more common in prepuberal patients, particularly in very young children. Visual and sensory symptoms may go unnoticed in very young children. In adolescents, the presentation of monosymptomatic and sensorimotor symptoms is frequent, and optic neuritis is the most common initial presentation. The interval between the initial demyelinating event and the second attack varies, and this interval may be longer in very young children. Relapses are more frequent and may be more severe in pediatric patients but recovery is often better than it is in adults. The accumulation of disability takes a long time in pediatric MS; however, over the long term, patients can become disabled at a younger age. The transition to secondary progressive MS occurs at a younger age in pediatric-onset MS than in adult-onset MS. The risk of transition to secondary progressive MS in pediatric patients is associated with a higher frequency of relapses and shorter intervals between attacks in the first few years of the disease [2, 29–31].

Cognitive disturbance is an important feature in pediatric MS. Cognitive impairment can occur even in the first few years of the disease and does not correlate with physical disability, number of relapses, and disease duration. The onset of multiple sclerosis in very young children increases the risk of cognitive impairment [3]. In adult MS patients, the most commonly affected cognitive functions include processing speed, visual-spatial function, memory, and executive functions. The most commonly affected cognitive areas in pediatric MS are attention span, processing speed, and visual-motor skills as adults. Receptive language, verbal fluency, and intelligence also are affected in pediatric MS, and they are affected differently than they are in adult MS. Linguistic involvement (verbal fluency, naming, and comprehension) is an important neuropsychological difference between pediatric and adult-onset MS [32, 33]. Pediatric MS patients are also at risk for a lower IQ [3]. Differences in cognitive dysfunctions between pediatric MS and adult MS may be due to the effect of inflammatory demyelination on the developing central nervous system and neuronal networks. All patients with pediatric MS should be checked for cognitive dysfunction because it occurs in the early stages of the disease and is unrelated to physical disability [29, 30, 33].

Psychiatric disorders such as depression or anxiety are common in pediatric MS, as they are in adults. Fatigue is also reported in patients with pediatric MS. Cognitive impairment, depression, and fatigue disrupt the child's academic performance and quality of life [3].

8. Diagnostic evaluation

8.1. Magnetic resonance imaging features

MRI is the most important paraclinical tool for the diagnosis of MS, and it also provides information for differential diagnosis.

Demyelinating plaques are demonstrated as an increased signal on T2 and FLAIR sequences and are typically located in deep white matter, corpus callosum, periventricular zone, juxtacortical, and posterior fossa. Hypointense lesions occur on T1 sequences. These hypointense lesions are named "black holes." Black holes are a result of tissue loss due to previous inflammatory events. Acute MS plaques may appear to be T1 hypointense as a result of transient edema, but these are not true T1-black holes. T1 hypointensity may remain for months after an acute event with such lesions evolving to isointensity (loss of edema or repair) or persisting as chronic, permanent hypointensity [34]. Active demyelinating plaques may show gadolinium enhancement due to a blood-brain barrier breakdown and enhancement is often incomplete around the periphery (open ring sign) (**Figures 1** and **2**).

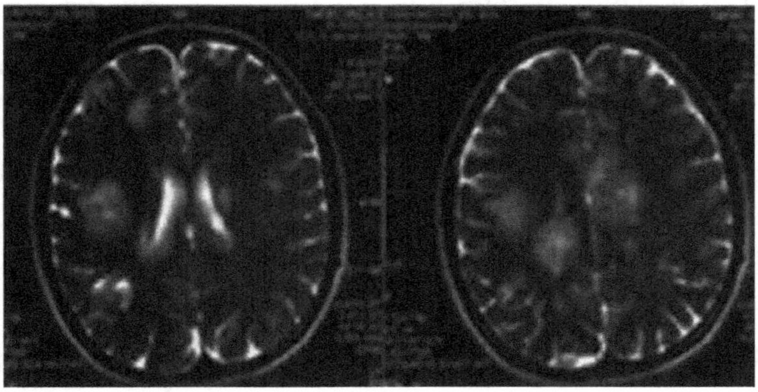

Figure 1. Large, hyperintense lesions on T2-weighted sequences.

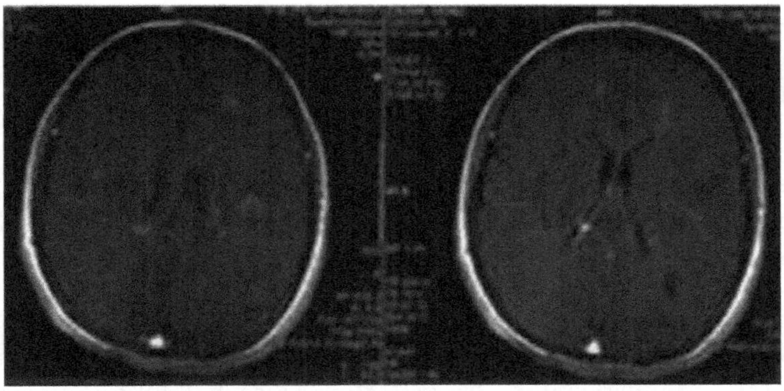

Figure 2. Gadolonium enhanced demyelinating plaques and black holes on T1-weighted sequences.

MRI findings in McDonald's diagnostic criteria are important and provide a diagnosis of MS at the first demyelinating event. According to McDonald's diagnostic criteria, dissemination in space (DIS) can be demonstrated by one or more T2 lesions in at least two of four areas of the CNS (periventricular, juxtacortical, infratentorial, spinal cord) and dissemination in time (DIT) can be demonstrated by a new T2 and/or gadolinium-enhancing lesion(s) on a follow-up MRI, with reference to a baseline scan, irrespective of the timing of the baseline MRI or the simultaneous presence of asymptomatic gadolinium-enhancing and non-enhancing lesions at any time [10]. These criteria have been found to be highly sensitive (100%) and highly specific (86%) for children older than 12 years with non-ADEM presentation, but they may not be appropriate for young children [35].

There are some differences in MRI findings between children and adults, particularly in prepuberal cases: T2-hyperintense lesion volume and lesion load in the infratentorial area are higher in children than they are in adults; first presentation may be as ADEM; there is an increased incidence of larger, tumefactive lesions in young children; spinal cord lesions may be longer than three vertebral segments in children with MS as in neuromyelitis optica [29, 36].

8.2. Cerebrospinal fluid (CSF) features

Analysis of CSF provides information about both the inflammatory process and differential diagnosis such as infection and malignancy. Cell count, presence of oligoclonal bands, and IgG index are examined in CSF analysis. A mild lymphocytic pleocystosis may be seen in children, but it has been shown that children younger than 11 years have more neutrophils in the CSF than older children. Oligoclonal band positivity has been found in 92% of patients with pediatric MS [37, 38]. An increased IgG index is more common in adolescents than in young children.

8.3. Evoked potentials

Evoked potentials help to demonstrate subclinical demyelination and to evaluate prior demyelination [39]. Visual evoked potentials are more informative than brainstem auditory and somatosensory evoked potentials.

9. Differential diagnosis

Other immune-mediated central nervous system demyelinating disorders (clinically isolated syndrome, acute disseminated encephalomyelitis, neuromyelitis optica) must be excluded in pediatric patients presenting a first demyelinating attack.

Clinically isolated syndrome (CIS) is a monofocal (optic neuritis, brainstem syndrome, transverse myelitis, cerebellar syndrome, or hemispheric syndrome) or polyfocal clinical CNS event with a presumed inflammatory demyelinating cause without a prior clinical history of a CNS demyelinating disease and encephalopathy. MRI features do not meet McDonald's criteria. Therefore, a follow-up check for the possibility of developing MS is necessary; however, the likelihood of developing MS is low in patients with a normal brain MRI [28].

Acute disseminated encephalomyelitis (ADEM) is an inflammatory demyelinating disease which is characterized by acute encephalopathy and polyfocal neurologic deficits. Encephalopathy is an important feature and diagnostic criterion. Encephalopathy is defined as an alteration in consciousness or behavioral change unexplained by fever, systemic illness, or postictal symptoms in IPMSSG criteria 2012. Encephalopathy is an unexpected finding in MS. MRI features are also defined for pediatric ADEM in the 2012 IPMSSG criteria [28]. Diffuse, large (>1–2 cm), poorly demarcated hyperintense lesions are detected in cerebral white matter on T2-weighted and fluid-attenuated inversion recovery (FLAIR) sequences; T1 hypointense lesions are rare and deep gray matter lesions can be present in the thalamus or basal ganglia. White matter lesions are multiple, bilateral, and asymmetrical in the cerebral hemispheres, cerebellum, brainstem, and spinal cord. Deep gray matter lesions are usually symmetrical and more characteristic of ADEM than of MS. The presence of T1 hypointense lesions in white matter leads to a diagnosis of MS. Periventricular lesions are less common. Cerebrospinal fluid (CSF) oligoclonal bands are rarely observed and usually transient in ADEM. Anti-MOG antibodies may be transiently present in the serum. ADEM is usually a monophasic disorder.

Clinical and radiologic findings may fluctuate in the first 3 months after the onset of disease. A second attack of ADEM may occur rarely, and it is named "multiphasic ADEM" [28]. This second ADEM event can involve either new neurologic symptoms and MRI findings or the re-emergence of prior neurologic symptoms and MRI findings. In the 2012 IPMSSG criteria, multiphasic ADEM is defined as two episodes consistent with ADEM separated by 3 months but not followed by any further events [28]. Sometimes pediatric ADEM may be the first manifestation of pediatric MS. Mikaeloff et al. showed that 18% of patients with pediatric ADEM had a second attack suggesting MS [40]. The second attack usually occurs within 2 years of the initial event.

Neuromyelitis optica (NMO) is an inflammatory disorder characterized by severe acute transverse myelitis and optic neuritis. Pediatric NMO can be monophasic or relapsing. Optic neuritis and myelitis are more severe in NMO and the prognosis is worse than it is for MS. Atypical presentations such as encephalopathy, persistent hiccups, nausea, and vomiting may occur. A brain MRI does not meet the criteria for MS and can show lesions in the supratentorial area, periaquaductal gray matter, hypothalamus, medial thalamus, dorsal pons, and medulla. The presence of longitudinally extensive spinal cord lesions (more than three vertebral segments) in a spinal MRI is an important finding and a supportive criterion. Anti-aquaporin-4 IgG seropositivity is another supportive criterion and it is 99% specific and 60–70% sensitive in children [41]. CSF oligoclonal bands are generally absent.

Other causes such as vasculitis, vascular, infectious, or neoplastic diseases must be excluded in pediatric patients with acute neurologic deficits. The presence of encephalopathy, persistent headaches, fever, polyneuropathy, and hearing loss, the involvement of other organs such as arthritis, skin rashes, oral/genital ulcers, lymphadenopathy, nephropathy, or hepatopathy with a progressive course should be suggestive of other causes. A progressive course and the involvement of the peripheral nervous system usually occur in mitochondrial diseases or neurometabolic disorders such as leukodystrophies. The diseases that should be kept in mind in the differential diagnosis are shown in **Table 1**. Markedly elevated pleocytosis, low glucose, and increased protein in CSF analysis should rouse suspicions. Persistent gadolinium enhancement and continued enlargement of lesions, leptomeningeal enhancement, T2 hyperintensities in the basal ganglia, thalamus, and hypothalamus, and calcifications in an MRI should also eliminate the diagnosis of MS.

Other demyelinating disorders
Clinically isolated syndrome
ADEM
Neuromyelitis optica
Vasculitis/inflammatory diseases
Primary CNS angiitis
Systemic lupus erythematosus
Sjögren syndrome
Behcet disease

- Neurosarcoidosis

Cerebrovascular disorders

İnfection

- Neurborreliosis
- Tuberculosis
- Viral encephalitis
- HIV
- Progressive multifocal leukoencephalopathy (PML)

Neurometabolic/genetic disorders

- Mitochondrial diseases
- Leukodystrophies

Neoplasm

- CNS lymphoma
- Other CNS tumors

Table 1. Differential diagnosis of pediatric MS.

10. Treatment

10.1. Treatment of the acute demyelinating attack

A mildly acute demyelinating attack that does not impair the patient's functions may not require treatment. The first option in the treatment of an acute demyelinating attack is a high-dose intravenous corticosteroid. Corticosteroids increase the speed of recovery and reduce the number of gadolinium-enhancing lesions on an MRI. The presumed mechanisms of action are modification of cytokine responses, reduction in T cell activation, and reduction in blood-brain barrier permeability. Intravenous corticosteroid is administered as 20–30 mg/kg (up to 1 g/day) methyl prednisolone over 3–5 days in children. There is no consensus on tapering oral corticosteroid. Oral prednisone may be administered to patients with incomplete recovery after intravenous treatment. Plasma exchange can be considered for patients with severe, life-threatening attacks or patients who were unresponsive to intravenous steroid treatment. The typical course is 5–7 exchanges over the course of 10–14 days. Plasma exchange therapy is an invasive treatment; its side effects include infection, blood clotting issues, and electrolyte disturbances. Another option is intravenous immunoglobulin (IVIG) if the steroids are contraindicated or the response is inadequate. There have been no controlled studies for the efficiency of this treatment in pediatric MS. IVIG influences cytokine production, T cell proliferation, and autoantibodies against myelin. It is given at a dose of 2 g/kg over 2–5 days. Side effects include fever, headache, aseptic meningitis, thromboembolism, and allergic reactions. Severe allergic reactions may develop in people with IgA deficiency; therefore, serum IgA levels should be examined before treatment [42, 43].

10.2. Disease-modifying therapy

The aims of treatment are to reduce disease activity, prevent disability, and preserve cognitive functions. Therefore, it is recommended to start treatment at an early stage.

First-line disease-modifying therapy includes interferon beta and glatiramer acetate. These drugs are used in adults for 15–20 years. Their efficacy, side effects, and safety are well known in adults. Both interferon beta and glatiramer acetate reduce relapse rates by approximately 30% and the accrual of new lesions on the MRI. There have been no randomized controlled trials in pediatric patients.

Glatiramer acetate is a synthetic amino acid polymer that resembles myelin basic protein. Its mechanism is not clear. It modulates T cells, shifts the population of T cells from proinflammatory Th1 cells to regulatory Th2 cells, and reduces antigen presentation. Standard dosage is 20 mg daily by subcutaneous injection. Its side effects include injection reactions, lipoatrophy at injection sites, chest pain, and a post-injection reaction (anxiety, flushing, palpitations, dyspnea, and chest pain) [42–44].

Interferon beta inhibits autoreactive T cells, increases production of anti-inflammatory cytokines, reduces proinflammatory cytokines, and decreases the migration of inflammatory cells into CNS. There are two subgroups: interferon beta 1a and 1b. Interferon beta 1a is given three times a week at a dose 22 or 44 μg via subcutaneous injection or intramuscularly at a dose of 30 μg a week. A pegylated form of interferon beta 1a is used in adults, but the safety and efficacy of this form in children and adolescents have not been established. The standard dose of interferon beta-1b is 0.25 mg (8 MIU), injected subcutaneously every other day. Dose titration is recommended at the start of treatment for interferons. Most pediatric patients tolerate the adult dose. The most frequent side effects are flu-like symptoms, injection site reaction, transient transaminase elevation, bone marrow suppression, thyroid dysfunction, and depression. Paracetamol and ibuprofen are effective in managing the flu-like symptoms. Liver transaminases, blood counts, and a thyroid function test should be carried out following the treatment.

The aim of disease-modifying therapy is to reduce clinical and radiological disease activity. Disease activity is defined as clinical relapses, new or enlarging lesions on an MRI, or gadolinium-enhancing lesions on an MRI. When the first-line disease-modifying therapy remains insufficient to reduce disease activity, second-line therapies can be used. The second-line therapies that have been used in pediatric MS include natalizumab, rituximab, and cyclophosphamide [42–44].

Natalizumab is a humanized monoclonal antibody. Natalizumab selectively binds to the 4-integrin component of adhesion molecules found in lymphocytes, monocytes, eosinophils and inhibits the α4-mediated adhesion of leukocytes to their counter-receptors. It decreases clinical relapse rate by about 70% and reduces the accumulation of new or enlarging T2 hyperintense lesions. Natalizumab is given at a dose of 300 mg intravenously every 4 weeks. Its side effects include hypersensitivity and headaches. The most serious risk is progressive multifocal leukoencephalopathy (PML) in adults. This fatal risk is higher in patients who have been exposed to the JC virus and have been treated with immunosuppressive drugs previously.

There is also a relationship between the duration of natalizumab therapy and an increased risk. There have been no controlled, randomized trials in pediatric MS to date.

Rituximab is a monoclonal antibody. It selectively depletes CD20+ B lymphocytes. There have been no controlled, randomized trials. Salzer et al. suggested that rituximab treatment is safe, effective, and well tolerated in their case series with pediatric MS [45].

Trials on the safety and efficacy of new oral therapies including fingolimod, dimethyl fumarate, and teriflunamide in pediatric MS patients have not been finalized.

10.3. Symptomatic treatment

Spasticity, fatigue, tremor, neuropathic pain, paroxysmal symptoms, epileptic seizures, bladder dysfunctions, and depression can be persistent symptoms in MS and affect patient's quality of life. Medical drugs can be effective in the treatment of these symptoms as in adult patients.

Baclofen, tizanidine, and benzodiazepines are effective for spasticity. Amantadine, modafinil, methylphenidate can be used for fatigue. Antiepileptic drugs such as carbamazepine, gabapentine are effective for both paroxysmal symptoms and neuropathic pain [42]. Anticholinergic agents (oxybutynin, tolterodine) can be used for detrusor hyperreflexia, and desmopressin may be beneficial for nocturia.

10.4. Rehabilitation

The aim of MS rehabilitation is to reduce symptoms including spasticity, gait disturbances, imbalance, bladder-bowel dysfunction, speech and swallowing disorders, fatigue, pain and improve quality of life. Rehabilitation interventions for MS symptoms include methods such as exercise (stretching/strengthening), gait training, endurance training, aerobic training, hydrotherapy, physiotherapy, exercise-pelvic floor training, occupational therapy, psychological training [46]. Rehabilitation interventions should be selected according to patient's characteristics such as age and functional deficits.

Cognitive rehabilitation is an important part of MS rehabilitation, but there is no specific cognitive rehabilitation intervention for pediatric MS. Rehabilitative strategies include rehabilitation of attention and language based on other disease such as trauma, stroke, and tumor [47].

11. Conclusion

Two to 5% of all MS patients have their first attack during childhood or adolescence. Pediatric MS has different clinical features from adult-onset MS, particularly in very young children. ADEM can occur as first attack in children, especially those under 10 years of age. The relapse rate in pediatric MS is higher than in adult MS, but recovery from relapse is better than in adults. However, the onset of secondary progression occurs at a younger age as compared with adult-onset MS. The primary progressive form of MS is extremely rare in pediatric patients. Primary progressive course should suggest other diagnoses in children. Cognitive impairment is one of the most important causes of disability and has different characteristics from adults. Linguistic dysfunction and decrease in IQ scores can occur during the first year of disease. Despite all these differences from adult MS, the therapeutic approach is based on information in adult MS. There are no randomized controlled trials on efficacy and safety of immunomodulatory and immunosuppressive drugs. Studies on pathogenesis are also limited in pediatric MS. One of the most important differences in the pathogenesis of pediatric-onset and adult-onset MS is the presence of anti-MOG antibodies in children. More studies on pathogenesis will provide insight into clinical differences and the development of more safe and effective treatment.

Author details

Ozgul Ekmekci

Address all correspondence to: ozgul.ekmekci@ege.edu.tr

Ege University, Faculty of Medicine, Department of Neurology, Izmir, Turkey

References

[1] Duquette P, Murray TJ, Pleines J, et al.: Multiple sclerosis in childhood: clinical profile in 125 patients. J Pediatr. 1987;111:359–363. DOI: 10.1016/S0022-3476(87)80454-7.

[2] Ghezzi A, Deplano V, Faroni J, et al.: Multiple sclerosis in childhood: clinical features of 149 cases. Mult Scler. 1997;3:43–46. DOI: 10.1177/135245859700300105.

[3] Bigi S, Banwell B: Pediatric multiple sclerosis. J Child Neurol. 2012;27(11):1378–1383. DOI: 10.1177/0883073812452784

[4] Gadoth N: Multiple sclerosis in children. Brain Dev. 2003;25:229. DOI: 10.1016/S0387-7604(03)00035-4.

[5] Banwell B, Ghezzi A, Bar-Or A, Mikaeloff Y, Tardieu M: Multiple sclerosis in children: clinical diagnosis, therapeutic strategies, and future directions. Lancet Neurol. 2007;6:887–902. DOI: 10.1016/S1474-4422(07)70242-9.

[6] Mowry EM, Krupp LB, Milazzo M, et al.: Vitamin D status is associated with relapse rate in pediatric onset multiple sclerosis. Ann Neurol. 2010;67(5):618–624. DOI: 10.1002/ana.21972.

[7] Mikaeloff Y, Cardidade C, Tardieu M, Suissa S: Parental smoking at home and risk of childhood onset multiple sclerosis in children. Brain. 2007;130:2589–2595. DOI: 10.1093/brain/awm198.

[8] Ascherio A, Munger KI: Environmental risk factors for multiple sclerosis: part 1: the role of infection. Ann Neurol. 2007;61(4):288–289. DOI: 10.1002/ana.21117.

[9] Langer-Loud A, Brara SM, Beaber BE, et al.: Childhood obesity and risk of pediatric multiple sclerosis and clinically isolated syndrome. Neurology. 2013;80(6):548–552. DOI: 10.1212/WNL.0b013e31828154f3.

[10] Vargas-Lowy D, Chitnis T: Pathogenesis of pediatric multiple sclerosis. J Child Neurol. 2012;27(11):1394–1407. DOI: 10.1177/0883073812456084.

[11] Chitnis T: The role of CD4 T cells in the pathogenesis of multiple sclerosis. Int Rev Neurobiol. 2007;79:43–72. DOI: 10.1016/S0074-7742(07)79003-7.

[12] Ciccarelli O, Barkhof F, Bodini B, et al.: Pathogenesis of multiple sclerosis: insights from molecular and metabolic imaging. Lancet Neurol. 2014;13:807–822. DOI: 10.1016/S1474-4422(14)70101-2.

[13] Stromnes IM, Cerretti LM, Liggitt D, et al.: Differential regulation of central nervous system autoimmunity by TH1 and TH17 cells. Nat Med. 2008;14:337–342. DOI: 10.1038/nm1715.

[14] Lock C, Hermans G, Pedotti R, et al.: Gene-microarray analysis of multiple sclerosis lesions yields new targets validated in autoimmune encephalomyelitis. Nat Med. 2002;8:500–508. DOI: 10.1038/nm0502-500.

[15] Graber JJ, Allie SR, Mullen KM, et al.: Interleukin-17 in transverse myelitis and multiple sclerosis. J Neuroimmunol. 2008;196:124–132. DOI: 10.1016/j.jneuroim.2008.02.008.

[16] Correale J, Tenembaum SN: Myelin basic protein and myelin oligodendrocyte glycoprotein T-cell repertoire in childhood and juvenile multiple sclerosis. Mult Scler. 2006;12:412–420. DOI: 10.1191/135248506ms1282oa.

[17] Fernandez-Carbonell C, Vargas-Lowy D, Musallam A, et al.: Clinical and MRI phenotype of children with MOG antibodies. Mult Scler J. 2016;22(2):174–184. DOI: 10.1177/1352458515587751.

[18] Kitley J, Woodhall M, Waters P, et al.: Myelinoligodendrocyte glycoprotein antibodies in adults with a neuromyelitis optica phenotype. Neurology. 2012;79:1273–1277. DOI: 10.1212/WNL.0b013e31826aac4e.

[19] Chitnis T, Imitola J, Khoury SJ.: Therapeutic strategies to prevent neurodegeneration and promote regeneration in multiple sclerosis. Curr Drug Targets Immune Endocr Metabol Disord. 2005;5:11–26.

[20] Lucchinetti C, Bruck W, Parisi J, et al.: Heterogeneity of multiple sclerosis lesions: implications for the pathogenesis of demyelination. Ann Neurol. 2000;47:707–717.

[21] Trapp BD, Peterson J, Ransohoff RM, et al.: Axonal transection in the lesions of multiple sclerosis. N Engl J Med. 1998;338:278–285. DOI: 10.1056/NEJM199801293380502.

[22] Kutzelnigg A, Lucchinetti CF, Stadelmann C, et al.: Cortical demyelination and diffuse white matter injury in multiple sclerosis. Brain. 2005;128(pt 11):2705–2712. DOI: 10.1093/brain/awh641.

[23] Kutzelnigg A, Faber-Rod JC, Bauer J, et al.: Widespread demyelination in the cerebellar cortex in multiple sclerosis. Brain Pathol. 2007;17:38–44. DOI: 10.1111/j.1750-3639.2006.00041.x.

[24] McAdam LC, Blaser SI, Banwell BL.: Pediatric tumefactive demyelination: case series and review of the literature. Pediatr Neurol. 2002;26:18–25. DOI: 10.1016/S0887-8994(01)00322-8.

[25] Lucchinetti CF, Gavrilova RH, Metz I.: Clinical and radiographic spectrum of pathologically confirmed tumefactive multiple sclerosis. Brain. 2008;131(7):1759–1775. DOI: 10.1093/brain/awn098.

[26] Krupp LB, Banwell B, Tenenbaum S: Consensus definitions proposed for pediatric multiple sclerosis and related disorders. Neurology. 2007;68:S7–S12. DOI: 10.1212/01.wnl.0000259422.44235.a8.

[27] Polman CH, Reingold SC, Banwell B, et al.: Diagnostic criteria for multiple sclerosis: 2010 revisions to the McDonald criteria. Ann Neurol. 2011;69:292–302. DOI: 10.1002/ana.22366.

[28] Krupp LB, Tardieu M, Amato MP et al.: International Pediatric Multiple Sclerosis Study Group criteria for pediatric multiple sclerosis and immune-mediated central nervous system demyelinating disorders: revisions to the 2007 definitions. Mult Scler. 2013;19(10):1261–1267. DOI: 10.1177/1352458513484547.

[29] Narula S: New perspectives in pediatric neurology-multiple sclerosis. Curr Probl Pediatr Adolesc Health Care. 2016:46(2):62–69. DOI: 10.1016/j.cppeds.2015.11.002.

[30] Pena JA, Lotze TE: Pediatric multiple sclerosis: current concepts and consensus definitions. Autoimmune Dis. 2013:2013, Article ID 673947:12 p. DOI: 10.1155/2013/673947.

[31] Huppke B, Ellenberger D, Rosewich H, Friede T, Gartner J, Huppke P: Clinical presentation of pediatric multiple sclerosis before puberty. Eur J Neurol. 2014;21(3):441–446. DOI: 10.1111/ene.12327.

[32] Cardoso M, Olmo NR, Fragoso YD: Systematic review of cognitive dysfunction in pediatric and juvenile multiple sclerosis. Pediatr Neurol. 2015;53:287–292. DOI: 10.1016/j.pediatrneurol.2015.06.007.

[33] Suppiej A, Cainelli E: Cognitive dysfunction in pediatric multiple sclerosis. Neuropsychiatr Dis Treat. 2014;10:1385–1392. DOI: 10.2147/NDT.S48495.

[34] Simon JH, Li D, Traboulsee A, et al.: Standardized MR imaging protocol for multiple sclerosis: consortium of MS centers consensus guidelines. Am J Neuroradiol. 2006;27:455–461.

[35] Sadaka Y, Verhey LH, Shroff MM, et al.: 2010 McDonald criteria for diagnosing pediatric multiple sclerosis. Ann Neurol. 2012;72(2):211–223. DOI: 10.1002/ana.23575.

[36] Waubant E, Chabas D, Okuda T, et al.: Difference in disease burden and activity in pediatric patients on brain magnetic resonance imaging at time of multiple sclerosis onset vs adults. Arch Neurol. 2009;66(8):967–971. DOI: 10.1001/archneurol.2009.135.

[37] Ghezzi A, Pozzilli C, Liguori M, et al.: Prospective study of multiple sclerosis with early onset. Mult Scler. 2002;8(2):115–118. DOI: 10.1191/1352458502ms786oa.

[38] Pohl D, Rostasy K, Reiber H, Hanefeld F: CSF characteristics in early-onset multiple sclerosis. Neurology. 2004;63(10):1966–1967. DOI: 10.1212/01.WNL.0000144352.67102.BC.

[39] Pohl D, Rostasy K, Treiber H et al.: Pediatric multiple sclerosis: detection of clinically silent lesions by multimodal evoked potentials. J Pediatr. 2006;149:125–127. DOI: 10.1016/j.jpeds.2006.01.003.

[40] Mikaeloff Y, Suissa S, Vallée L, Lubetzki C, et al.: First episode of acute CNS inflammatory demyelination in childhood: prognostic factors for multiple sclerosis and disability. J Pediatr. 2004;144(2):246–252. DOI:10.1016/j.jpeds.2003.10.056.

[41] Banwell B, Tenenbaum S, Lennon VA, et al.: Neuromyelitis optica-IgG in childhood inflammatory demyelinating CNS disorders. Neurology. 2008;70(5):344–352. DOI: 10.1212/01.wnl.0000284600.80782.d5.

[42] Narula S, Hopkins SE, Banwell B: Treatment of pediatric multiple sclerosis. Curr Treat Options Neurol. 2015;17:10. DOI: 10.1007/s11940-014-0336-z.

[43] Bernton JN, Banwell BL. Therapeutic approach to the management of pediatric demyelinating disease: multiple sclerosis and acute disseminated encephalomyelitis. Neurotherapeutics. 2016;13:84–95. DOI: 10.1007/s13311-015-0396-0.

[44] Kornek B. Treatment of pediatric multiple sclerosis. Neuropediatrics. 2013;44(06):309–313. DOI: 10.1055/s-0033-1359308.

[45] Salzer J, Lycke J, Wickstrom R, Naver H: Rituximab in paediatric onset multiple sclerosis: a case series. J Neurol. 2016;263(2):322–326. DOI: 10.1007/s00415-015-7979-x.

[46] Beer S, Khan F, Kesselring J. Rehabilitation interventions in multiple sclerosis: an overview. J Neurol. 2012;259(9):1994–2008. DOI: 10.1007/s00415-012-6577-4.

[47] Portaccio E, Goretti B, Zipoli V, et al.Cognitive rehabilitation in children and adolescents with multiple sclerosis. Neurol Sci. 2010;31(Suppl 2):S275–S278. DOI: 10.1007/s10072-010-0377-3.

5

Genetic and Biochemical Factors Related to the Risk and Disability Progression in Multiple Sclerosis

Daniel Čierny, Jozef Michalik, Ema Kantorová, Egon Kurča and Ján Lehotský

Abstract

Sclerosismultiplex(multiplesclerosis,MS)isachronicautoimmuneinflammatorydisease of the central nervous system. The immune regulatory defects lead to the process of inflammation and neurodegenerationthat results in the deterioration of neurological functions. It is still unclear as to why MS is so devastating and rapidly progressive in one patient and less so in another. It is known that the etiopathogenesis of MS is very complex, and many factors can be involved in the risk and character of the disease and its progression. In this chapter, we discuss the general molecular and cellular mechanisms of action of genetic and biochemical factors that are related to immune system regulation and thus can be connected to the individually varying risk and disability progression of MS. We found that gene variants of the gene polymorphism rs6897932 in interleukin 7 receptor α chain gene rs10735810 in vitamin D receptor gene and *HLA-DR* and *HLA-DQ* genes as well as the serum level of vitamin D are associated with MS risk or disability progression in Central European Slovak population.

Keywords: multiple sclerosis, risk, disability progression, gene polymorphism, biochemical marker

1. Introduction

In triggering an autoimmune response in multiple sclerosis (MS), environmental factors have a strong effect and interact with complex risk-conferring genetic variants [1–3]. In this process, the myelin reactive Tcells with altered functional characteristics are formed and activated [4]. The immune regulatory defects and increased migration of autoreactive lymphocytes within the brain, that are the typical traits in MS, lead to the process of inflammation, myelin sheath breakdown, demyelination, remyelination, neuronal and axonal degeneration, and subsequent deterioration of neurological functions [5]. Neurodegeneration, neuronal and axonal damage that correlate with the progression of the disease can be a process partly independent from inflammation and demyelination or even can be the cause of demyelination occurring from the disease onset. Axonal damage in MS is a result of many pathological processes [6, 7].

It is still unclear as to why MS is so devastating and rapidly progressive in one patient and less so in another. Because the etiopathogenesis of MS is very complex, disease development as well as the characteristics of disease progression is probably the consequence of multifactorial interaction. Our work is dedicated to genetic and biochemical markers that were chosen according to their possible role in the modulation of the immune response in MS patients and thus could be associated with MS risk and disability progression. In our work, we discuss the immune response-related genetic factors associated with MS that can be generally classified into *HLA* genes and *non-HLA* genes. Since vitamin D can have an important role in the pathogenesis of MS, great part of our work is dedicated to its metabolism, functions, mechanisms of action in MS and genetic factors that can modify these effects. In this work, we also present the results of our own analysis of genetic and biochemical markers that we found to be associated with MS risk or progression in the group consisting of MS patients with clinically diagnosed MS and healthy individuals from the region of Central Slovakia. To evaluate the disease progression rate, we used the widely accepted multiple sclerosis severity score (MSSS, score range 0.01–9.99) [8] that considers the neurological impairment of the functional systems (expanded disability status scale score) [9] together with disease duration. For the purpose of the association analysis of these markers with the rate of disease disability progression, we stratified MS patients by MSSS scores to three groups—slowly progressing MS (MSSS < 3), mid-rate progressing MS (MSSS 3–6) and rapidly progressing MS (MSSS > 6) [10].

2. Immune response-related genetic factors in the risk and progression of multiple sclerosis

MS is a typical gender-dependent disease; a higher risk of MS is observed in women than in men in all populations and races. A study conducted in Canada found female to male ratio in individuals affected by MS to be 3:1 [11]. The risk of MS development in siblings of an affected individual is estimated to be 5%, in children 2%, in monozygotic twins 25% [5]. However, it has been shown that genetic predisposition is not strong enough to induce disease development, and appropriate environmental triggers are necessary to start the disease process [1, 12]. In general, the MS-associated genes can be classified into genes of the HLA-complex and*non-HLA* genes [3].

3. Gene polymorphisms and haplotypes in the aetiology of multiple sclerosis

The single-nucleotide polymorphism (SNP) is a variation of a single nucleotide, which is present in the population in a frequency higher than 0.01. SNPs are the most common type of genetic variation and are usually caused by somatic or gametic mutations. Nucleotide change can cause the formation or loss of restriction sites for bacterial endonucleases that are able to cleave the specific DNA sequence. The identification of gene polymorphisms that are in correlation with other risk factors, including biochemical markers, can be useful in establishing the risk of MS development, prognosis, clinical course of the disease and response to therapy. Haplotype (haploid genotype) is a certain combination of alleles or SNPs in the sequence of the DNA, whichis localized on one chromosome and is inherited together. When two alleles are in linkage disequilibrium, they are inherited together in a higher frequency than expected randomly [13]. The combination of more alleles, known as tagging SNPs, enables us to identify the other associated alleles. For example, the allele A of gene polymorphism rs3135388 corresponds to the incidence of allele HLA-DRB1*1501, which is the most common genetic risk factor for MS development [14–16].

4. *HLA* genes and MS

Antigen expression that is inducible by cytokines is different on the various immune cells. Major histocompatibility complex II (MHCII) antigens are transmembrane proteins localized on the immune cells, thus having an important role in the process of exogenous antigen presentation to Tcells. MHCII molecules are coded by the gene of human leucocyte antigens D (*HLA-D* gene) that is localized on chromosome 6 and has three regions—HLA-DP, HLA-DQ and HLA-DR [17]. The susceptibility of the population to autoimmune diseases depends on the individual ability to express HLA-DQ and HLA-DR antigens. This expression can be induced by virus infection, most likely by EBV, influenza or paramyxovirus [18]. *MHCII* gene expression is regulated by vitamin D through its binding to the *vitamin D–responsive elements(VDREs)* that are localized in the promoter region of *HLA-DRB1* gene. This fact can explain the interaction between vitamin D, that is an important factor modifying MS development and disease course, and genetic predisposition to MS represented mainly by a highly conservative allele HLA-DRB1*1501. HLA-DRB1*1501 allele is in general considered to be the most important susceptibility allele of MS [19–24]. This allelewas found to be present in over 50% of MS cases [25, 26]. The increased frequencies of the DRB1*15 allele in MS patients have been described in Northern Europeans [23, 27], South and North Americans [20, 28], Mediterraneans [29, 30] and African Americans [21]. In Spanish cohorts, the DRB1*03 was the second most frequent allele associated with MS, but only after eliminating HLA-DRB1*15 [29]. The DRB1*03 allele has also been found to be significantly associated with the increased risk of MS in Scandinavians [27], Sardinians [31], and Australians [32]. Fernández et al. [33] found that the DRB1*13 allele is protective against MS development in Spaniards. A protective effect of the alleles DRB1*01, DRB1*07, DRB1*12 and DRB1*14 was confirmed in the recent meta-analysis in Caucasians [24]. The allele DRB1*07 was found to be protective against MS also in Scandinavians [34]. The DRB1*13.03 allele was found to be the primary risk allele in MS patients of European descent [23]. The protective effect against MS has also been shown for the HLA-DRB1*11 allele [24, 29].

The DQB1*06:02 allele was found to be linked to the increased risk of MS with a proved tight linkage disequilibrium between DRB1*15 and DQB1*06 in Caucasians [35]. As the risk factor of MS, DQB1*06:02 allele has also been identified in a cohort of Afro-Brazilians [36] and Spaniards [33]. Kaushansky et al. [37] suggested that the role of the DRB1*15:01 and DQB1*06:02 alleles in MS depends on the heterogeneous interaction of target antigen, genotype, and phenotype. On the contrary, Isobe et al. [38] found none of the HLA-DQB1 alleles to be associated with MS in African Americans. According to the combinations of HLA-alleles, the association of HLA-DRB1*15/*15 genotype with MS was identified by several studies [32, 34, 39]. In multi-case MS families, Barcellos et al. [39] identified a high risk DRB1*15/*08 genotype and protective DRB1*15/*14 genotype. The study of Sawcer et al. [23] indicates that in all populations of North-European ancestry, a predisposition to MS is linked with the DRB1*15:01-DQB1*06:02 haplotype. Furthermore, Link et al. [34] in a Scandinavian cohort showed that risk haplotypes for MS are almost all DRB1*15 bearing haplotypes, while protective effect against MS development are HLA class I A*02 allele-bearing haplotypes. In Sardinian MS patients, Cocco et al. [40] confirmed a positive association of the haplotype HLA DRB1*03:01-DQB1*02:01 with MS.

In the study from our laboratory, we analysed the association of the *HLA-DRB1/DQB1* genes, alleles and their combinations with susceptibility to MS in the population from central Slovakia. We found that the increased risk of MS is in individuals carrying alleles HLA-DRB1*15, DRB1*03 and DQB1*06, genotypes HLA-DRB1*15/*15 DQB1*06/*06 and haplotype DRB1*15-DQB1*06. In addition, we also found that HLA-DRB1/DQB1 class II alleles DRB1*07, DRB1*13, DQB1*03, genotypes DRB1*13/*11, DQB1*05/*03 and haplotypes DRB1*13-DQB1*06 and DRB1*11-DQB1*03 are associated with the protection against MS development. We cannot exclude that the proposed protective effects of the DRB1*11-DQB1*03 and DRB1*13-DQB1*06 haplotypes in our cohort could be, at least partially, due to the linkagedisequilibrium with alleles in the HLA class I region which is primarily associated with MS [41].

5. *Non-HLA* genes and MS

Gene products of *non-HLA* genes can contribute to the genetic risk of MS by modulation of different processes. These genes are involved in the regulation of functions of T- and Bcells, dendritic cells, NKcells, cytokine signalization, metabolism of interferons, vitamin D metabolism, neuronal regeneration and many others [3]. It has been found that these genes can contribute not only to the increased inherited risk of MS development but also to the risk of other autoimmune diseases [42, 43]. The examples of the SNPs involved in the etiopathogenesis of MS are summarised in **Table 1**.

Gene	*function*	*Localization*	*SNP*	*Alleles*
HLA-DRB1*1501*(human leucocyte antigen DRB1*1501)*	Antigen presentation	6p21	rs3135388	C/T
			rs3135005	C/T
IL-7Ra *(interleukin 7 receptor receptor alpha chain)*	Proliferation of memory Tcells, T- and B-cell development	5p13	rs6897932	C/T
IL-2Ra *(interleukin 2 receptor receptor alpha chain)*	Sensitization of Tcells to IL-2, proliferation of Tcells	10p15	rs2104286	A/G
			rs12722489	A/G
			rs11256369	C/G
			rs7076103	C/T
CD58 *(cluster of differentiation 58)*	Function of regulatory Tcells	1p13	rs2300747	A/G
			rs6677309	A/C
			rs12044852	A/C
CD6*(cluster of differentiation 6)*	Regulation, adhesion of T_{H17} and other Tcells	11q13	rs17824933	C/G
			rs12288280	G/T
CLEC16A *(C-type lectin domain family 16 member A)*	Cell receptor, induction of immune response	16p13	rs6498169	A/G
			rs12708716	A/G
VAV1 *(vav guanine nucleotide exchange factor 1)*	Lymphocyte survival, differentiation and proliferation	19p13	rs2546133	C/T
			rs2617822	A/G
PRKCA *(protein kinase C alpha)*	Regulation of IL-2 expression, receptor	17q22-q23	Allele variants in introns 3, 8	
EVI 5 *(ecotropic viral integration site 5 protein homolog)*	Nuclear protein, cell cycle regulation	1p22	rs6680578	A/T
			rs11808092	A/C
			rs11804321	C/T
IRF5 *(interferon regulatory factor 5)*	Regulation of cytokine activation	7q32	rs4728142	A/G
			rs3807306	A/C
IRF8 *(interferon regulatory factor8)*	Expression of interferon response genes, development of Bcells	16q24	rs17445836	A/G
TYK2 *(tyrosin kinase 2)*	Gene expression	19p13	rs34536443	C/G
			rs55762744	C/T
TNFRSF1A *(tumour necrosis factor receptor superfamily member 1A)*	Receptor for tumour necrosis factor	12p13	rs1800693	A/G
			rs4149584	A/C/G
			rs767455	C/T
			rs4149577	C/T
CD40 *(cluster of differentiation 40)*	Receptor for tumour necrosis factor	20q12-q13	rs1883832	C/T
CD226 *(cluster of differentiation 226)*	Activator of NKcells, lymphocyte adhesion, co-stimulator of Tcells	18q22	rs763361	C/T
KIF1B *(kinesin family member 1B) kinesin family member 1B)*	Neuronal regeneration	1p36	rs10492972	C/T
GPC 5 *(glypicane 5)*	Neuronal growth and reparation	13q32	rs9523762	A/G

Table 1. Gene polymorphisms involved in the etiopathogenesis of MS [3, 44–48].

6. Genetic variants in *interleukin 7 receptor α chain (IL-7Ra)* gene

IL7 is a type 1 short-chain cytokine of the haematopoietin family involved in the modulation of T- and B-cell development and T-cell homeostasis. To perform the immune system functions, IL7 binds to the transmembrane receptor that is formed by heterodimerisingthe common cytokine gamma chain and IL7 receptor alpha chain (IL7Ra or CD127). IL7Ra is a membrane glycoprotein folded to bind and mediate the action of IL7 and other alpha helical cytokines. IL7Ra consists of an extracellular domain, transmembrane region and cytoplasmic tail, which uses kinases for signal transduction [49]. The localization of the *IL7Ra* gene is chromosome 5p13.3. An increased expression of IL7Ra in peripheral blood mononuclear cells was found in MS patients when compared to controls [50, 51]. The IL7Ra and IL7 mRNA increased expression was found also in the cerebrospinal fluid of MS patients, possibly suggesting an altered balance between the isoforms of IL7Ra and a higher signal-inducing immune cell proliferation and survival [52]. According to the alternative splicing of exon 6 in *IL7Ra* gene, membrane-bound or soluble isoforms of IL-7Ra are produced [53]. A significantly increased ratio of the membrane-bound to soluble isoforms of IL7Ra in MS patients can facilitate the aberrant activation of potentially auto-reactive T cells [54].

Single-nucleotide polymorphisms in *IL7Ra* gene are involved in the dysregulation of immune homeostasis and thus can be associated with susceptibility to MS [55]. A genome-wide study in a large group of subjects from the UK and USA identified the strong association between SNP rs6897932 in *IL7Ra* gene and the risk of MS [2]. The non-conservative aminoacid change on position 244 (Ile→Thr) ofIL7Ra is a result of the SNP rs6897932 (ATC → ACC) in exon 6 of *IL7Ra* gene [56]. This aminoacid change has a functional effect on the product of expression of alternative spliced *IL7Ra* gene, which is manifested by changes in the proportion of the soluble versus membrane-bound isoforms of IL7Ra. The change of this ratio can be followed by a different regulation of the IL7 signal transduction pathway and directly associates the SNP rs6897932 with MS [57].

It has been found that allele C of SNP rs6897932 in *IL7Ra* gene contributes to the increased genetic risk of MS in groups of MS patients from the USA [57, 58], South Spain [59], Nordic countries—Denmark, Finland, Norway and Sweden [52], France [60], Netherlands [61] and Japan [62]. The homozygosity for C allele was identified as a risk genotype for MS susceptibility in Netherlands [61] and Spain [59]. A genotype association was also confirmed by the finding of increased counts of CC genotype of rs6897932 in MS patients compared to controls in the cohorts from the USA [58] and Japan [62]. Corresponding with the contribution of allele C to the risk of MS, the protective effect of allele T for MS risk in a Nordic case-control group has been reported by Lundmark et al. [52]. The protective effect of allele T has been reported also in Spain by Alcina et al. [59]. On the contrary, no association between SNP rs6897932 and MS was found in cohorts of MS patients from Northern Ireland [58], Germany [44] and Western Balkan countries—Serbia, Croatia and Slovenia [63].

Only a few studies addressed the question whether the rs6897932 in *IL7Ra* gene contributes only to the genetic risk of MS, or whether it can also affect the disease course and disability progression [44, 57, 61, 64]. Groups of patients with different forms of MS were compared in several studies. In Northern European primary-progressive MS cases (PP MS), the underexpression of *IL7Ra* gene as well as different allele frequencies of IL7Ra promoter SNP was confirmed. Moreover, *IL7Ra* gene expression was found to be up-regulated in secondary-progressive MS (SP MS) patients [64]. In a study by Akkad et al. [44] in German MS patients, it was found that the soluble IL7Ra reduced the expression and allelic and genotypic association between rs6897932 and SP or PP MS but not with RR MS. In their study, a significantly higher frequency of allele C and genotype CC of rs6897932 in SP and PP MS patients was found, but not in RR MS patients compared to controls. The assessment of the severity of MS by MSSS did not show any association between rs6897932 genotype and disease severity in the USA [57]. Differences in allele frequencies in SP MS patients compared to healthy controls were reported in Dutch MS patients by Sombekke et al. [61]. In spite of that, no association between rs6897932 genotype and disease severity (MSSS, EDSS, other clinical tests) and disease activity (relapse rate and MRI markers) was found.

Results of our own work suggest the relevance of rs6897932 allele and gene variants in MS pathogenesis in Slovaks [10]. Our results have revealed that allele C is present in a higher frequency in MS patients (77.4%) as compared to the control group (72.3%), which indicates an increased risk of MS development (OR=1.314, 95% CI=1.004–1.720, p=0.047). Interestingly, allele T was manifested in MS patients in a significantly lower frequency representing only 22.6% as compared to 27.7% in controls. This suggeststhat allele T seems to be protective against MS development (OR = 0.761, 95% CI= 0.582–0.996, p = 0.047). The additive model fitted the best to assess association between genotypes and MS risk. Logistic regression analysis adjusted for sex and age revealed that there is a significant associationbetween IL7Ra rs6897932 genotype and MS risk (OR = 0.764, 95% CI = 0.586–0.995, $p_{\log}$ = 0.045). The genotype analysis showed that MS patients manifested a lower frequency of genotype CT when compared to controls (34.8% vs. 36.3) and genotype TT (5.2% vs. 9.9%) and a higher frequency of genotype CC (60.0% vs. 54.1%). When we used the additive genetic model, we found a significantly decreased risk of MS development in carriers of allele T with genotype CT (OR = 0.865, 95% CI = 0.609–1.228, p = 0.05) as well as with genotype TT (OR = 0.565, 95% CI = 0.282–1.132, p = 0.05).

After stratification of MS patients according to the disease disability progression rate, we found a significantly lower frequency of allele T in the subgroup of rapidly progressing MS patients (18.1%) as compared to 27.7% in controls. These results suggest that allele T is associated with protection against rapid disability progression of MS (OR = 0.576, 95% CI = 0.348–0.955, p = 0.031). An additive genetic model adjusted for sex and age fitted the best to assess the association between genotypes and the rate of disease disability progression. Linear logistic regression with disease disability rate as the dependent variable—MSSS (1, 2, 3 and 0 for controls) revealed that there is a significant association between IL7Ra rs6897932 genotype and disability progression of MS ($p_{\log}$ = 0.034). Genotype analysis showed that the frequency of genotype TT is higher in controls (9.6%) and lower in MS patients with rapid disability progression (3.5%). Frequency of genotype CC was higher in rapidly progressing MS patients (67.2%) and lower in controls (54.1%). The data suggest that individuals carrying genotype TT are protected against rapid disease disability progression of MS.

We have shown for the first time in a Central European Slovak population that allele C of rs6897932 is associated with the risk of MS, and allele T has a protective additive effect against MS susceptibility. Moreover,we revealed that minor allele T and genotype TT of rs6897932 in the *IL7Ra* gene are protective against rapid disease disability progression in MS [65].

7. Vitamin D and its role in risk and progression of multiple sclerosis

In the past decades, much attention has been given to vitamin D and its role in MS and other autoimmune diseases. The following sectionsare dedicated to the metabolism and structure of vitamin D, its immunological effects, serum level and mechanisms of action of vitamin D in the prevention and treatment of MS. We also describe the genetic factors that can modulate the biological effects of vitamin D.

7.1. The structure and metabolism of vitamin D

Vitamin D in the human body undergoes a complex metabolism. Cholecalciferol (vitamin D_3), as a precursor of a hormonally active form, is produced in the skin from 7-dehydrocholesterol after sunlight exposure and can also be absorbed from the diet. Subsequently, cholecalciferol is hydroxylated in the liver forming 25-hydroxycholecalciferol, calcidiol. The hormonally active form of vitamin D, 1,25- dihydroxycholecalciferol, calcitriol, is produced by further hydroxylation especially in the kidneys and also in other tissues. The enzyme catalysing this hydroxylation is 25-hydroxyvitamin D-1α-hydroxylase, coded by *CYP27B1* (cytochrome P450 family 27 subfamily B member 1) gene [66, 67]. In various cells, the bioactive form of vitamin D binds to the vitamin D receptor (VDR) providing its physiological functions by modulation of the target gene's transcription [68]. The circulating serum level of vitamin D depends not only on environmental factors such as exposition to sunlight and vitamin D intake but also on genetic and epigenetic factors.The genetic factors can influence the effects of vitamin D through the variability of the genes participating in its activation and degradation, transport and receptor signalling [69].

7.2. The effect of vitamin D on the functions of immune cells

There is growing evidence that vitamin D not only regulates bone metabolism but also has large-scale immunomodulatory and anti-inflammatory effects. A linkage has been found between vitamin D deficiency and increased risk of autoimmune diseases [70]. The immunocompetent cells—macrophages, dendritic cells, Tcells and Bcells are able to produce calcitriol and express the VDR at the high rate. Through this, vitamin D modulates the synthesis of various cytokines and immunoglobulins and is involved in the regulation of innate and adaptive immune response. Autocrine and paracrine effects of vitamin D depend also on its serum level, and individuals with hypovitaminosis D are in a state of immune system dysfunction and are predisposed to the development of autoimmune diseases [71].

In Tcells, calcitriol inhibits the production of IL-12 and IFN-γ and subsequent differentiation of T_{H1} lymphocytes that are the key cells involved in the MS development. Calcitriol improves the immunosuppressive functions of T_{REG}cells and ameliorates the T_{H2}-cell development by the activation of the promotor region of *IL-4* gene [19, 72]. Vitamin D increases the expression of IL-4, IL-5 and IL-10 that are able to activate T_{H2} cells, decreases the production of IFN-γ, blocks the formation of T_{H1}cells after antigen stimulation and has positive effects on the T_{H1}-mediated autoimmune diseases [73, 74]. Bcells, which also participate in the demyelinating process and produce intrathecalimmunoglobulins, express VDR and vitamin D hydroxylases. In Bcells, calcitriol reduces the intracellular signal pathways of nuclear transcription factor NF-kappa B (NF-kB) and CD40 signalling [75]. Calcitriol inhibits the maturation and proliferation of Bcells, induces apoptosis of Bcells, inhibits the differentiation of plasma and memory cells and decreases the production of immunoglobulinsIgG and IgM [76]. Immature Bcells are more prone to regulation by calcitriol when compared to plasma cells. Calcitriol also decreases the expression of MHCII molecules and co-stimulatory molecules in Bcells [19].

Calcitriol formed in macrophages inhibits the immune response by suppressing proliferation of T_{H1}- and T_{H17}cells and promoting the functions of T_{H2}- and T_{REG}cells [71]. Calcitriol inhibits the secretion of IL-12 by antigen-presenting cells and monocytes [77]. Vitamin D blocks the differentiation of immature dendritic cells and the expression of co-stimulatory molecules CD40, CD80, CD86 and MHC II, thus decreasing the capacity of dendritic cells to activate autoreactive Tcells. Vitamin D also ameliorates the spontaneous apoptosis of mature dendritic cells [73]. In macrophages, calcitriolsuppresses intracellular oxidative burst and listericidal activity. It also suppresses the expression of Fc and TLR receptors induced by IFN-γ that are important for antigen recognition [78]. Vitamin D suppresses the proliferation of antigen-specific Tcells and chemotaxisof dendritic cells by decreasing the expression of differentiation antigens CD80, CD86 and HLA-DR molecules [79].

7.3. The murine model of MS and vitamin D

In mice that lack the *VDR* gene or the gene of the enzyme catalysing vitamin D activation, an abnormal development and function of T_{H1}-lymphocytes and deficiency of peripheral T-lymphocytes have been observed [80, 81]. Calcitriol treatment can prevent the induction and progression of autoimmune diseases including experimental autoimmune encephalomyelitis (EAE), a murine model of MS [82, 83]. Calcitriol can also decrease the severity of EAE symptoms, and its deficiency causes an increased susceptibility of animals to EAE induction [77, 82]. In mice with chronic EAE, vitamin D administration suppresses the proliferation of specific T_{H1} cells, inhibits IL-12 dependent production of IFN-γ, prevents relapses and reduces perivascular infiltration, demyelination plaque formation and axonal degeneration in the brain and spinal cord [84].

7.4. Serum level of vitamin D and dose management

To reflect vitamin D status in the human body, calcidiol plasma level measurement is usually used. Calcidiol is the main circulating form of vitamin D in plasma, and its biological half-time is 19 days [85]. The recommended daily dose of vitamin D is approximately 10times higher than in the past. The optimal serum level of vitamin D is 75–250 nmol/l (30–100 ng/ml). In countries with less sunny climate, the necessary daily dose of vitamin D is 1000–4000 IU/day (1 μg = 40 IU) [86].

The risk of vitamin D overdosing is hypercalcaemia and subsequent organ and tissue damage. Whole body exposure to sunlight results in the production of around 10,000 IU of vitamin D, so it is not simple to cause vitamin D intoxication by its short-term peroral supplementation. The results of several studies suggest that even high-dose vitamin D_3 supplementation in MS patients is safe and clinically useful. Burton et al. [87] administered high peroral doses of vitamin D to healthy individuals and MS patients. The initial dose was 40,000 IU/dayduring 28 weeks, followed by 10,000 IU/day during 12 weeks; later it was gradually decreased to 0 IU/day, combined with 1.2 grams of calcium per day. During the period of 40,000 IU of vitamin D per day, the serum levels reached 413 nmol/l, which was higher than the conventional limit established for vitamin D toxicity (250 nmol/l). Calcidiol serum levels remained around this limit for 18 weeks without any observed negative effects. The serum level of calcium was in the physiological reference range during the whole study duration. Moreover, no cardiac rhythm abnormalities or impairment of hepatic or renal functions was observed. Kimball et al. [88] administered 4000–40,000 IU/day to patients in the active phase of MS together with 1.2 grams of calcium. Medium serum level of calcidiol was 78 ± 35 nmol/l and rose to 386 ± 157 nmol/l. Serum calcium level and urinary calcium to creatinine ratio did not exceed the physiological reference values. Vitamin D supplementation in this study did not cause any change in the serum level of hepatic enzymes, creatinine, electrolytes, proteins and parathormone. Although the serum level of calcidiol doubled the physiological upper range value, hypercalcaemia or hypercalciuria was not observed.

Although the significant toxicity of vitamin D_3 was not observed even in doses of 40,000 IU/day, its daily dose in healthy individuals should not exceed 2000 IU. The optimal daily dose of vitamin D_3 that should be routinely recommended to women during pregnancy and lactation is 1000 IU. Children born in families with MS history should be administered daily 200–400 IU of vitamin D_3 [66].

7.5. Vitamin D and the course, prevention and treatment of MS

The role of vitamin D in the prevention of MS development has been confirmed by many experimental, epidemiological, genetic and immunological studies. Vitamin D insufficiency during the whitematter development can alter the pathways of axonal differentiation and adhesion and increase the apoptosis of oligodendrocytes that express VDR. This results in local microenvironmental changes and altered regeneratory and remyelinating capacity [66]. In individuals with an increased genetic risk of MS, it is possible to prevent the demyelination process by preventive vitamin D administration. This preventive strategy would be better than reparation of already developed myelin and axonal damage [12, 66].

High-dose peroral vitamin D intake has been found to be inversely associated with the risk of MS in a cohort of more than 90,000 women. Peroral vitamin D supplementation in a dose higher than 400 IU/day leads to the reduction of MS risk when compared to the individuals with no vitamin D intake (RR = 0.59, 95% CI = 0.38–0.91,p = 0.006) [89]. Also,calcidiol plasma levels are inversely correlated with MS risk. This association is particularly obvious in whites, while among blacks and Hispanics with lower 25-hydroxyvitamin D levels than whites, there was no significant association between vitamin D and MS risk [90]. Vitamin D also has reparative effects for the nervous tissue, especially in patients in the early phases of the disease. In countries with low sun exposure, food supplementation of vitamin D could be a simple and cheap method of MS prevention [86]. The incidence of MS could be reduced by the administration of vitamin D to pregnant women, and all children living in mild climates should be more exposed to sunlight and should be on a vitamin D–rich diet [66].

Vitamin D is not only a factor modifying MS risk, but it can also have a role in the modulation of disease course. It has been observed that in relapsing remitting MS, calcidiol plasma levels are lower during relapses compared to the periods of remission [91]. In addition, there is evidence that lower calcidiol levels are associated with higher relapse rates and higher risk of exacerbation, as well as higher expanded disability status scale (EDSS) scores and progressive forms of MS [92–94]. Vitamin D can improve memory and cognitive impairments in patients with MS, Alzheimer disease and in patients after chemotherapeutical treatment [95]. High-dose peroral vitamin D supplementation has immunomodulatory effects and leads to reduction in the number of relapses and suppression of the inflammatory activity and proliferation of Tcells [87], as well as the decrease in the number of gadolinium-enhancing lesions in brain [88].

In our study, we examined the serum levels of calcidiol in a group of MS patients from the Central-Northern part of Slovakia. We found that hypovitaminosis D is more frequent in MS patients, when compared to healthy individuals. Serum levels of calcidiol were significantly lower in MS patients when compared to controls (15.0 ± 6.1 ng/ml vs. 18.2 ± 8.3 ng/ml, $p_{(K-W)}$= 0.001). Moreover, we found that there is an association of the serum level of vitamin D with the rate of MS disability progression ($p(K-W)$ = 0.000). We detected similar serum levels of calcidiol in slow progressing and mid-rate progressing MS patients (15.7 ± 5.0 ng/ml vs. 15.8 ± 6.6 ng/ml), but interestingly we noticed a marked decrease of calcidiol serum levels in rapidly progressing MS patients (12.8 ± 5.9 ng/ml). In addition, calcidiol levelwas significantly lower in all subgroups of MS patients when compared to controls (18.2 ± 8.3 ng/ml). Thus we can conclude that decreased serum level of calcidiol in MS patients can be one of the factors related to increased risk of MS development, as well as increased risk of rapid disease disability progression.

7.6. Genetic factors related to vitamin D effects in MS

Nucleotide exchange in DNA sequence can cause the production of protein products with different activities. Polymorphisms of the genes involved in the activation, transport, signalling and degradation of vitamin D can, together with other factors, modify the individual immune response and thus can be related to MS. Because of the beneficial effects of vitamin D, in individuals with genes predisposing to its higher serum levels, the risk of MS should be reduced [96]. The serum level of vitamin D can be modified by *VDR* gene polymorphisms [97–99]. The fact that serum levels of vitamin D are similar in twins, and especially when they are monozygotic twins, speaks in favour of a genetic regulation. Gene polymorphisms FokI in

VDR gene, rs4646536 and rs703842 in the *CYP27B1* gene and rs10741657 in the *CYP2R1* gene are the significant predictors of caldiciol serum level [99]. Hypovitaminosis D is common in higher latitudes because of the lack of sun exposure [100]. The fact that not all vitamin D–deficient individuals develop MS is probably the result of the complexity of the etiopathogeneis of MS and the interaction of many factors. The positive effects of vitamin D in MS can be dampened for example by the allele HLA-DRB1*15 [96]. In MS patients, it is necessary to find out the link between the genotype and the vitamin D serum level and also the genetic interactions among the genes *CYP27B1, VDR* and *HLA* [19]. The gene polymorphisms associated with vitamin D metabolism are summarized in **Table 2**.

Gene	*function*	*Localization*	*SNP*	*Allele*
CYP27B1 *(cytochrome P450 family 27 subfamily B member 1, 25-hydroxyvitamin D_3 1-alpha-hydroxylase)*	Hydroxylation	12q13	rs703842	C/T
			rs10877012	G/C
			rs4646536	C/T
			rs10877015	A/G
			rs118204009	A/G
			rs118204012	A/G
			rs118204011	C/T
CYP2R1 *(cytochrome P450 family 2 subfamily R member 1, vitamin $D_3$25-hydroxylase)*	Hydroxylation	11p15	rs10741657	A/G
			rs10500804	G/T
			rs12794714	A/G
DBP *(vitamin D binding protein)*	Transport in plasma	4q12	rs7041	G/T
			rs4588	A/C
VDR *(vitamin D receptor)*	Receptor	12q13	rs1544410 (BsmI)	A/G (B/b)
			rs7975232 (ApaI)	T/C (A/a)
			rs731236 (TaqI)	T/C (T/t)
			rs10735810 (FokI)	C/T (F/f)
			rs11568820 (Cdx2)	G/A
			rs2254210	A/G
			rs98784	C/T
CYP24A1 *(cytochrome P450 family 24 subfamily A polypeptide, vitamin D 24-hydroxylase)*	Deactivation	20q13	rs2296241	A/G

Table 2. The gene polymorphisms associated with vitamin D metabolism [19, 98, 99, 101].

7.6.1. Genetic variants in vitamin D receptor gene in MS

According to the effects of vitamin D in MS, the molecular mechanisms of vitamin D function should be considered. As mentioned earlier, vitamin D executes its physiological effect via binding and activation of VDR. Interestingly, the activation of VDR by calcitriol can suppress the induction of EAE, while animals that lack VDR are not protected against EAE [102]. The gene for VDR is located on the 12q13 chromosomal region and consists of 11 exons. Non-coding exons 1A, 1B and 1C are located in the 5′ end of the VDR gene, and exons 2–9 encode the structural portion of the VDR protein [103]. VDR sequence is similar to that of the receptors for steroid hormones and hormones of the thyroid gland. VDR is a regulatory transcription factor and consists of highly conservative DNA-binding and ligand-binding domains. The signal pathways associated with the VDR regulate the transcription of genes involved in the regulation of bone metabolism, immune response and cancer [83]. The polymorphisms in the initiation codon of the *VDR* gene can cause the formation of transcription variants coding different proteins [104]. In the *VDR* gene, SNPs ApaI (rs7975232), BsmI (rs1544410), FokI (rs10735810) and TaqI (rs731236) have functional biological effects and are mostly studied in MS as well as in other diseases. These gene polymorphisms can alter mRNA level, its stability and alternative splicingand also the stability of the final gene product, amount of protein isoforms and their interactions [105]. FokI gene polymorphism is located in exon 2 of the *VDR* gene, and its variants result in a change of protein structure. There are two possible allele variants, f (presence of a restriction site for FokI endonuclease) and F (absence of a restriction site for FokI endonuclease). It has been confirmed that the f (T) allele leads to the expression of a VDR protein, which is three amino acids longer (427 amino acids) than the F (C) allele (424 amino acids). The shorter isoform of the receptor is more transcriptionally potent through a more efficient interaction with transcription factor TFIIB [105, 106]. Near the 3′ end of the *VDR* gene, we can find the ApaI and BsmI polymorphism in the intron between exon 8 and 9 and TaqI gene polymorphism in exon 9 [107]. The allele variants of these gene polymorphisms and their combinations regulate the functions of VDR through the modulation of mRNA stability. In Caucasians, TaqI, ApaI and BsmI polymorphisms are in strong linkage disequilibrium and are present in five haplotype blocks. Haplotype2 (t-A-B) probably results in a lower number of 'A' in polyA variable number of tandem repeats (VNTR), while haplotype 1 (T-A-b) is connected to a large number of 'A', thus modulating mRNA stability [106]. Morrison et al. [108] found that allele b (G) of the BsmI polymorphism causes a decreased expression of VDR mRNA.

Interestingly, several studies have found an association between *VDR* gene polymorphisms and the risk of MS. Differences in allele frequency of the BsmI polymorphism in the *VDR* gene were found in Japan by Fukazawa et al. [109], who for the first time pointed out the involvement of *VDR* gene polymorphisms in the pathogenesis of MS. The association of *VDR* gene polymorphisms with MS has been confirmed in cohorts of MS patients from Japan [110], theUK [111, 112], Australia [107] and the USA [98]. On the contrary, no association of VDR gene polymorphisms with the risk of MS was found by studies in MS patients from Canada [113], Netherlands [114], Greece [115], Spain [116, 117], Tasmania [118] and Iran [119]. The presence of specific haplotypes of the *VDR* gene can increase the risk of MS development, especially its progressive forms. Tajouri et al. [107] in Australia found haplotype A-t (T-C) of ApaI and TaqI polymorphism to increase the risk of MS development, especially its progressive forms. The carriership of allele t (C) in their study increased MS risk twice. Fukazawa et al. [109] found allele b (G) and genotype bb (GG) of BsmI polymorphism to increase MS risk, but without any association with the form and severity of MS (EDSS, magnetic resonance imaging (MRI)). Allele b (G) of BsmI polymorphism of VDR has been found to be associated with MS risk in combination with allele A (T) of ApaI polymorphism by Niino et al. [110]. However, in their study, they did not find any association of ApaI gene polymorphism with clinical form and severity of MS evaluated by the EDSS score, disease duration and MRI findings. Agliardi et al. [120] in Italy found that allele T (T) and genotype TT (TT) are protective against MS development, supported by the finding that the expression of VDR mRNA is increased four times by genotype Tt (TC) and eight times by genotype TT (TT) when compared to genotype tt (CC). The observed effect is present especially when the protective allele Tis present in the combination with HLA-DRB1*15 allele.

The role of VDR gene polymorphisms is still not completely understood, and it seems to vary among different populations. For proper cell signalling to decrease the risk of MS, it is probably necessary to reach a certain level of the transcriptional activity of VDR that is also modified genetically. For proper immunoregulation, the individuals that have the genotype causing the decreased VDR protein activity can need a higher peroral vitamin D intake or higher level of sun exposure. Contrarily, in individuals with higher transcriptional activity of VDR, a lower sun exposure or vitamin D intake can be sufficient for proper immune system regulation.

The findings of our previous study in MS patients from the Central-Northern region of Slovakia have confirmed the association of FokI heterozygous genotype Ff with an increased risk of MS in women [10]. Although we found no statistically significant differences in the proportions of FokI genotypes or allele frequencies between total MS patient and the control group, we have observed significant differences in the FokI genotype distribution between women with MS and the female control group ($p = 0.042$). Our results have shown a significantly higher frequency of heterozygous Ff genotypes in FokI polymorphism in the female MS group (53.4%) as compared to 43.7% in the female control group (OR = 1.48, 95% CI = 1.01–2.16). In spite of this fact, when we compared the subgroup of rapidly progressing MS patients with the subgroup of slow progressing MS patients, allele and genotype counts were not significantly different between them (allele f: 34.5 vs. 43.3%, allele F: 65.5 vs. 56.7%, genotype ff: 10.3 vs. 13.4%, genotype Ff: 48.3 vs. 59.8%). Since we have not shown any significant association between FokI VDR gene polymorphism and the rate of disease disability progression in our cohort of Slovak MS patients, we observed a trend of higher frequency of homozygotes FF to be 41.4% in MS patients with rapid progression of disease as compared to 26.8% in slow progressing MS patients (OR = 1.93, 95% CI=0.94–3.94) with a marginal level of significance ($p = 0.071$). From the results of our study, it seems that contributions from genetic and allelic variants of FokI VDR gene polymorphism have only a small impact in a disease as complex as MS, andits role in the etiopathogenesis of MS still remains controversial.

8. Conclusions

In summary, we can conclude that many genetic and biochemical factors can be involved in the etiopathogenesis of MS. These markers could be used to evaluate the risk of MS development and the risk of rapid disease disability progression.

The proposed markers that have been found to be associated with MS risk or disability progression in Central European Slovak population are summarized in **Table 3**. In our studies, we identified decreased serum level of vitamin D, allele C and genotype CC of polymorphism rs6897932 in the *IL7Ra* gene, genotype Ff of rs10735810 in the *VDR* gene (only in women); HLA-alleles DRB1*15, DRB1*03, DQB1*06; HLA-genotypes DRB1*15/*15, DQB1*06/*06 and HLA-haplotype DRB1*15-DQB1*06 as the main risk factors for MS development. On the contrary, allele T of rs6897932 in the *IL7Ra* gene (in individuals with genotype CT and TT); HLA-alleles DRB1*07, DRB1*13, DQB1*03; HLA-genotypes DRB1*13/*11, DQB1*05/*03 and HLA-haplotypes DRB1*13-DQB1*06 and DRB1*11-DQB1*03 displayed a protective effect against MS development. Genotype CC of rs6897932 in the *IL7Ra* gene and decreased serum level of vitamin D were identified as negative prognostic factors for rapid disability progression in MS, while minor allele T of rs6897932 in the *IL7Ra* gene (especially in individuals with TT genotype) was identified as a protective factor disability progression.

	MS development	*Rapid disease disability progression*
Risk factors	Decreased serum vitamin D	Decreased serum vitamin D
	rs6897932 in *IL7Ra* gene—allele C, genotype CC	rs6897932 in *IL7Ra* gene—genotype CC
	HLA-alleles DRB1*15, DRB1*03, DQB1*06; HLA-genotypes DRB1*15/*15, DQB1*06/*06; HLA-haplotype DRB1*15-DQB1*06	
	rs10735810 in *VDR* gene —genotype Ff (only women)	
Protective factors	rs6897932 in *IL7Ra* gene—allele T, genotype CT and TT	rs6897932 in *IL7Ra* gene—allele T, genotype TT
	HLA-alleles DRB1*07, DRB1*13, DQB1*03; HLA-genotypes DRB1*13/*11, DQB1*05/*03; HLA-haplotypes DRB1*13-DQB1*06, DRB1*11- DQB1*03	

Table 3. The proposed markers associated with the MS risk or disability progression in Slovaks [10, 41, 65].

From the results of our study, we conclude that rs6897932 of the *IL7Ra*gene, rs10735810 in the *VDR* gene, HLA-DR and DQ genotypes, as well as serum level of vitamin D may be the important markers that could be used as part of a panel of markers to evaluate the risk of MS development and disability progression. The relevance of these markers identified in our study should be verified in larger groups of individuals not only in Slovakia but also in other different populations. The relevant positive or negative prognostic genetic or biochemical markers can improve the diagnostic and therapeutic procedure and can help to minimize neurological damage in predisposed individuals.

Acknowledgements

The work was supported by the projects '"Centre for Translational Medicine' code: 6220220021, 'Identification of Novel Markers in Diagnostic Panel of Neurological Diseases' code: 26220220114, 'Martin Biomedical Center (BioMed Martin)' ITMS code: 26220220187 co-financed from EU sources and European Regional Development Fund and the grant of Ministry of Health, 2012/30-UKMA-7 and APVV No. 15/0107.

Author details

Daniel Čierny[1], Jozef Michalik[2], Ema Kantorová[2], Egon Kurča[2] and Ján Lehotský[3*]

*Address all correspondence to: lehotsky@jfmed.uniba.sk

1 Department of Clinical Biochemistry, Jessenius Faculty of Medicine and University Hospital Martin, Comenius University in Bratislava, Martin, Slovak Republic

2 Department of Neurology, Jessenius Faculty of Medicine and University Hospital Martin, Comenius University in Bratislava, Martin, Slovak Republic

3 Department of Medical Biochemistry and BioMed, Jessenius Faculty of Medicine in Martin, Comenius University in Bratislava, Martin, Slovak Republic

References

[1] Kakalacheva K, Lünemann JD. Environmental triggers of multiple sclerosis. FEBS Lett. 2011; 585(23):3724–9. doi: 10.1016/j.febslet.2011.04.006

[2] International Multiple Sclerosis Genetics Consortium, Hafler DA, Compston A, Sawcer S, Lander ES, Daly MJ, De Jager PL, de Bakker PI, Gabriel SB, Mirel DB, Ivinson AJ, Pericak-Vance MA, Gregory SG, Rioux JD, McCauley JL, Haines JL, Barcellos LF, Cree B, Oksenberg JR, Hauser SL. Risk alleles for multiple sclerosis identified by a genome-wide study. N Engl J Med. 2007;357(9):851-62. PMID: 17660530

[3] Nischwitz S, Müller-Myhsok B, Weber F. Risk conferring genes in multiple sclerosis.FEBS Lett. 2011; 585(23):3789–97. doi: 10.1016/j.febslet.2011.03.037

[4] Stinissen P, Hellings N.Activation of myelin reactive T cells in multiple sclerosis: a possible role for T cell degeneracy? Eur J Immunol. 2008; 38(5):1190–3. doi: 10.1002/eji.200838371

[5] Compston A, Coles A. Multiple sclerosis.The Lancet. 2008; 372(9648):1502–17. doi: 10.1016/S0140-6736(08)61620-7

[6] Levin MC, Douglas JN, Meyers L, Sangmin L, Yoojin S, Gardner LA.Neurodegeneration in multiple sclerosis involves multiple pathogenic mechanisms. DegenerNeurolNeuromuscul Dis. 2014; 2014(4):49–63. doi: http://dx.doi.org/10.2147/DNND.S54391

[7] Kostic MS, Rajkovic JS, PoticFloranovic MS, Dimov ID, Pavlovic DD. Multiple sclerosis and oxidative stress—a clinical perspective.Neurochem J. 2013; 7(1):76–86. doi: 10.1134/S1819712412040083

[8] Roxburgh RH, Seaman SR, Masterman T, Hensiek AE, Sawcer SJ, Vukusic S, Achiti I, Confavreux C, Coustans M, le Page E, Edan G, McDonnell GV, Hawkins S, Trojano M, Liguori M, Cocco E, Marrosu MG, Tesser F, Leone MA, Weber A, Zipp F, Miterski B, Epplen JT, Oturai A, Sørensen PS, Celius EG, Lara NT, Montalban X, Villoslada P, Silva AM, Marta M, Leite I, Dubois B, Rubio J, Butzkueven H, Kilpatrick T, Mycko MP, Selmaj KW, Rio ME, Sá M, Salemi G, Savettieri G, Hillert J, Compston DA. Multiple sclerosis severity score: using disability and disease duration to rate disease severity. Neurology. 2005; 64(7):1144–51. PMID: 15824338

[9] Kurtzke JF. Rating neurologic impairment in multiple sclerosis: an expanded disability status scale (EDSS). Neurology. 1983; 33(11):1444–52. PMID: 6685237

[10] Čierny D, Michalik J, Kurča E, Dobrota D, Lehotský J.FokI vitamin D receptor gene polymorphism in association with multiple sclerosis risk and disability progression in Slovaks. Neurol Res. 2015; 37(4):301–8. doi: 10.1179/1743132814Y.0000000459

[11] Orton SM, Herrera BM, Yee IM, Valdar W, Ramagopalan SV, Sadovnick AD, Ebers GC; Canadian Collaborative Study Group. Sex ratio of multiple sclerosis in Canada: a longitudinal study. Lancet Neurol. 2006; 5(11):932–6. PMID: 17052660

[12] Hayes CE. Vitamin D: a natural inhibitor of multiple sclerosis. ProcNutr Soc. 2000; 59(4): 531–5. PMID: 11115787

[13] Wall JD, Pritchard JK. Assessing the performance of the haplotype block model of linkage disequilibrium.Am J Hum Genet. 2003; 73(3):502–15. PMID: 12916017

[14] De Bakker PI, McVean G, Sabeti PC, Miretti MM, Green T, Marchini J, Ke X, Monsuur AJ, Whittaker P, Delgado M, Morrison J, Richardson A, Walsh EC, Gao X, Galver L, Hart J, Hafler DA, Pericak-Vance M, Todd JA, Daly MJ, Trowsdale J, Wijmenga C, Vyse TJ, Beck S, Murray SS, Carrington M, Gregory S, Deloukas P, Rioux JD. A high-resolution HLA and SNP haplotype map for disease association studies in the extended human MHC. Nat Genet. 2006; 38(10):1166–72. PMID: 16998491

[15] Sombekke MH, Lukas C, Crusius JB, Tejedor D, Killestein J, Arteta D, Martínez A, Uitdehaag BM, Knol DL, Peña AS, Geurts JJ, De Jager PL, Barkhof F, Vrenken H, Polman

CH. HLA-DRB1*1501 and spinal cord magnetic resonance imaging lesions in multiple sclerosis. Arch Neurol. 2009; 66(12):1531–6. doi: 10.1001/archneurol.2009.278

[16] Benešová Y, Vašků A, Stourač P, Hladíková M, Fiala A, Bednařík J. Association of HLA-DRB1*1501 tagging rs3135388 gene polymorphism with multiple sclerosis. J Neuroimmunol. 2013; 255(1–2):92–6. doi: 10.1016/j.jneuroim.2012.10.014

[17] Mehra NK, Kaur G. 2003.Gene map of the human leukocyte antigen (HLA) region.In Expert RevMol Med.2003; 5:1. Available from: http://journals.cambridge.org/fulltext_content/ERM/ERM5_07/S1462399403005957sup001.pdf

[18] Jedlička P. Onemocneníbíléhmotymozkomíšní. In: Jedlička P, Keller O. editors. Speciálníneurologie. 1st ed. Praha: Galén; 2005. p. 203–212. ISBN 80-7262-312-5.

[19] Sundqvist E, Bäärnhielm M, Alfredsson L, Hillert J, Olsson T, Kockum I. Confirmation of association between multiple sclerosis and CYP27B1. Eur J Hum Genet. 2010; 18(12): 1349–52. doi: 10.1038/ejhg.2010.113

[20] Dyment DA, Herrera BM, Cader MZ, Willer CJ, Lincoln MR, Sadovnick AD, Risch N, Ebers GC. Complex interactions among MHC haplotypes in multiple sclerosis: susceptibility and resistance. Hum Mol Genet. 2005; 14(14):2019–26. PMID: 15930013

[21] Oksenberg JR, Barcellos LF, Cree BA, Baranzini SE, Bugawan TL, Khan O, et al. Mapping multiple sclerosis susceptibility to the HLA-DR locus in African Americans. Am J Hum Genet. 2004; 74(1):160–7.

[22] Lincoln MR, Montpetit A, Cader MZ, Saarela J, Dyment DA, Tiislar M, Ferretti V, Tienari PJ, Sadovnick AD, Peltonen L, Ebers GC, Hudson TJ. A predominant role for the HLA class II region in the association of the MHC region with multiple sclerosis. Nat Genet. 2005; 37(10):1108–12.

[23] Sawcer S, Hellenthal G, Pirinen M, Spencer CCA, Patsopoulos NA, Moutsianas L, et al. The International Multiple Sclerosis Genetics Consortium (IMSGC), Wellcome Trust Case Control Consortium 2 (WTCCC2).Genetic risk and a primary role for cell-mediated immune mechanisms in multiple sclerosis.Nature. 2011; 476(7359):214–9. doi: 10.1038/nature10251

[24] Zhang Q, Lin CY, Dong Q, Wang J, Wang W. Relationship between HLA-DRB1 polymorphism and susceptibility or resistance to multiple sclerosis in Caucasians: a meta-analysis of non-family-based studies. Autoimmun Rev. 2011; 10(8):474–81. doi: 10.1016/j.autrev.2011.03.003

[25] Schmidt H, Williamson D, Ashley-Koch A. HLA-DR15 haplotype and multiple sclerosis: a HuGE review. Am J Epidemiol. 2007; 165(10):1097–109. PMID: 17329717

[26] Ramagopalan SV, Morris AP, Dyment DA, Herrera BM, DeLuca GC, Lincoln MR, Orton SM, Chao JM, Sadovnick AD, Ebers GC.The inheritance of resistance alleles in multiple sclerosis.PLoS Genet. 2007; 3(9):e150. doi: 10.1371/journal.pgen.0030150

[27] Masterman T, Ligers A, Olsson T, Andersson M, Olerup O, Hillert J. HLA-DR15 is associated with lower age at onset in multiple sclerosis. Ann Neurol. 2000; 48(2):211–9. PMID: 10939572

[28] Kaimen-Maciel DR, Reiche EM, Borelli SD, Morimoto HK, Melo FC, Lopes J, Dorigon RF, Cavalet C, Yamaguchi EM, Silveira TL, Da Silva WV, Comini-Frota ER, Brum Souza DG, Donadi EA. HLA-DRB1* allele-associated genetic susceptibility and protection against multiple sclerosis in Brazilian patients. Mol Med Rep. 2009; 2(6):993–8. doi: 10.3892/mmr_00000204.

[29] Romero-Pinel L, Pujal JM, Martínez-Yélamos S, Gubieras L, Matas E, Bau L, Torrabadella M, Azqueta C, Arbizu T. HLA-DRB1: genetic susceptibility and disability progression in a Spanish multiple sclerosis population. Eur J Neurol. 2011; 18(2):337–42. doi: 10.1111/j.1468-1331.2010.03148.x

[30] Kouri I, Papakonstantinou S, Bempes V, Vasiliadis HS, Kyritsis AP, Pelidou HS.HLA associations with multiple sclerosis in Greece. J Neurol Sci. 2011; 308(1–2):28–31. doi: 10.1016/j.jns.2011.06.037

[31] Marrosu MG, Murru R, Murru MR, Costa G, Zavattari P, Whalen M, Cocco E, Mancosu C, Schirru L, Solla E, Fadda E, Melis C, Porru I, Rolesu M, Cucca F. Dissection of the HLA association with multiple sclerosis in the founder isolated population of Sardinia. Hum Mol Genet. 2001; 10(25):2907–16. PMID: 11741834

[32] Stankovich J, Butzkueven H, Marriott M, Chapman C, Tubridy N, Tait BD, Varney MD, Taylor BV, Foote SJ; ANZgene Consortium, Kilpatrick TJ, Rubio JP. HLA-DRB1 associations with disease susceptibility and clinical course in Australians with multiple sclerosis. Tissue Antigens. 2009; 74(1):17–21. doi: 10.1111/j.1399-0039.2009.01262.x

[33] Fernández O, Fernández V, Alonso A, Caballero A, Luque G, Bravo M, León A, Mayorga C, Leyva L, de Ramón E. DQB1*0602 allele shows a strong association with multiple sclerosis in patients in Malaga, Spain. J Neurol. 2004; 251(4):440–4. PMID: 15083289

[34] Link J, Kockum I, Lorentzen AR, Lie BA, Celius EG, Westerlind H, Schaffer M, Alfredsson L, Olsson T, Brynedal B, Harbo HF, Hillert J. Importance of human leukocyte antigen (HLA) class I and II alleles on the risk of multiple sclerosis. PLoS One. 2012; 7(5):e36779. doi: 10.1371/journal.pone.0036779

[35] Kaushansky N, Ben-Nun A. DQB1*06:02-associated pathogenic anti-myelin autoimmunity in multiple sclerosis-like disease: potential function of DQB1*06:02 as a disease-predisposing allele. Front Oncol. 2014; 4:280.doi: 10.3389/fonc.2014.00280

[36] Caballero A, Alves-Leon S, Papais-Alvarenga R, Fernandez O, Navarro G. Alonso, A. DQB1*0602 confers genetic susceptibility to multiple sclerosis in Afro-Brazilians. Tissue Antigens. 1999; 54(5):524–26. PMID: 10599893

[37] Kaushansky N, Altmann DM, David CS, Lassmann H, Ben-Nun A. DQB1*0602 rather than DRB1*1501 confers susceptibility to multiple sclerosis-like disease induced by proteolipid protein (PLP). J Neuroinflammation.2012; 9:29.doi: 10.1186/1742-2094-9-29

[38] Isobe N, Gourraud PA, Harbo HF, Caillier SJ, Santaniello A, Khankhanian P, Maiers M, Spellman S, Cereb N, Yang S, Pando MJ, Piccio L, Cross AH, De Jager PL, Cree BA, Hauser SL, Oksenberg JR. Genetic risk variants in African Americans with multiple sclerosis. Neurology. 2013; 81(3):219–27. doi: 10.1212/WNL.0b013e31829bfe2f

[39] Barcellos LF, Sawcer S, Ramsay PP, Baranzini SE, Thomson G, Briggs F, et al. Heterogeneity at the HLA-DRB1 locus and risk for multiple sclerosis. Hum Mol Genet. 2006; 15(18):2813–24. PMID: 16905561

[40] Cocco E, Murru R, Costa G, Kumar A, Pieroni E, Melis C, Barberini L, Sardu C, Lorefice L, Fenu G, Frau J, Coghe G, Carboni N, Marrosu MG. Interaction between HLA-DRB1-DQB1 Haplotypes in Sardinian multiple sclerosis population. PloS One. 2013; 8(4):e59790. doi: 10.1371/journal.pone.0059790

[41] Michalik J, Čierny D, Kantorová E, Kantárová D, Juraj J, Párnická Z, Kurča E, Dobrota D, Lehotský J. The association of HLA-DRB1 and HLA-DQB1 alleles with genetic susceptibility to multiple sclerosis in the Slovak population. Neurol Res. 2015; 37:1060–67 doi: 10.1080/01616412.2015.1115212.

[42] D'Netto MJ, Ward H, Morrison KM, Ramagopalan SV, Dyment DA, DeLuca GC, Handunnetthi L, Sadovnick AD, Ebers GC. Risk alleles for multiple sclerosis in multiplex families.Neurology. 2009; 72(23):1984–8. doi: 10.1212/WNL. 0b013e3181a92c25

[43] Hoffjan S, Akkad DA. The genetics of multiple sclerosis: an update 2010. Mol Cell Probes. 2010; 24(5):237–43. doi: 10.1016/j.mcp.2010.04.006

[44] Akkad DA, Hoffjan S, Petrasch-Parwez E, Beygo J, Gold R, Epplen JT. Variation in the IL7RA and IL2RA genes in German multiple sclerosis patients. J Autoimmun. 2009; 32(2):110–5. doi: 10.1016/j.jaut.2009.01.002

[45] Brynedal B, Bomfim IL, Olsson T, DuvefeltK,Hillert J. Differential expression, and genetic association, of CD58 in Swedish multiple sclerosis patients. ProcNatlAcadSci U S A. 2009; 106(23):E58. doi: 10.1073/pnas.0904338106

[46] De Jager PL, Jia X, Wang J, de Bakker PI, Ottoboni L, Aggarwal NT, Piccio L, Raychaudhuri S, Tran D, Aubin C, Briskin R, Romano S; International MS Genetics Consortium, Baranzini SE, McCauley JL, Pericak-Vance MA, Haines JL, Gibson RA, Naeglin Y, Uitdehaag B, Matthews PM, Kappos L, Polman C, McArdleWL, Strachan DP, Evans D, Cross AH, Daly MJ, Compston A, Sawcer SJ, Weiner HL, Hauser SL, Hafler DA, Oksenberg JR. Meta-analysis of genome scans and replication identify CD6, IRF8 and TNFRSF1A as new multiple sclerosis susceptibility loci. Nat Genet. 2009; 41(7):776–82. doi: 10.1038/ng.401

[47] Dyment DA, Cader MZ, Chao MJ, Lincoln MR, Morrison KM, Disanto G, Morahan JM, De Luca GC, Sadovnick AD, Lepage P, Montpetit A, Ebers GC, Ramagopalan SV. Exome sequencing identifies a novel multiple sclerosis susceptibility variant in the TYK2 gene. Neurology. 2012; 79(5):406–11. doi: 10.1212/WNL.0b013e3182616fc4

[48] Park TJ, Kim HJ, Kim JH, Bae JS, Cheong HS, Park BL, Shin HD. Associations of CD6, TNFRSF1A and IRF8 polymorphisms with risk of inflammatory demyelinating diseases.NeuropatholApplNeurobiol. 2013; 39(5):519–30. doi: 10.1111/j. 1365-2990.2012.01304.x

[49] Fry TJ, Mackall CL. 2002. Interleukin-7: from bench to clinic. Blood. 2002; 99(11):3892–904

[50] Bomprezzi R, Ringnér M, Kim S, Bittner ML, Khan J, Chen Y, Elkahloun A, Yu A, Bielekova B, Meltzer PS, Martin R, McFarland HF, Trent JM. Gene expression profile in multiple sclerosis patients and healthy controls: identifying pathways relevant to disease. Hum Mol Genet. 2003; 12(17):2191–9. PMID: 12915464

[51] Ramanathan M, Weinstock-Guttman B, Nguyen LT, Badgett D, Miller C, Patrick K, Brownscheidle C, Jacobs L. In vivo gene expression revealed by cDNA arrays: the pattern in relapsing–remitting multiple sclerosis patients compared with normal subjects. J Neuroimmunol. 2001; 116(2):213–9.116: 213–219. PMID: 11438176

[52] Lundmark F, Duvefelt K, Iacobaeus E, Kockum I, Wallström E, Khademi M, Oturai A, Ryder LP, Saarela J, Harbo HF, Celius EG, Salter H, Olsson T, Hillert J. Variation in interleukin 7 receptor alpha chain (IL7R) influences risk of multiple sclerosis. Nat Genet. 2007; 39(9):1108-13. PMID: 17660816

[53] Goodwin RG, Friend D, Ziegler SF, Jerzy R, Falk BA, Gimpel S, Cosman D, Dower SK, March CJ, Namen AE, et al. Cloning of the human and murine interleukin-7 receptors: demonstration of a soluble form and homology to a new receptor superfamily. Cell. 1990; 60(6):941–51. PMID: 2317865

[54] Kreft KL, Verbraak E, Wierenga-Wolf AF, van Meurs M, Oostra BA, Laman JD, Hintzen RQ. Decreased systemic IL-7 and soluble IL-7Rα in multiple sclerosis patients. Genes Immun. 2012; 13(7):587–92. doi: 10.1038/gene.2012.34

[55] Zhang Z, Duvefelt K, Svensson F, Masterman T, Jonasdottir G, Salter H, Emahazion T, Hellgren D, Falk G, Olsson T, Hillert J, Anvret M. Two genes encoding immune-regulatory molecules (LAG3 and IL7R) confer susceptibility to multiple sclerosis. Genes Immun. 2005; 6(2):145–52. PMID: 15674389

[56] Teutsch SM, Booth DR, Bennetts BH, Heard RN, Stewart GJ. Identification of 11 novel and common single nucleotide polymorphisms in the interleukin-7 receptor-alpha gene and their associations with multiple sclerosis.Eur J Hum Genet. 2003; 11(7):509–15. PMID: 12825072

[57] Gregory SG, Schmidt S, Seth P, Oksenberg JR, Hart J, Prokop A, Caillier SJ, Ban M, Goris A, Barcellos LF, Lincoln R, McCauley JL, Sawcer SJ, Compston DA, Dubois B, Hauser

SL, Garcia-Blanco MA, Pericak-Vance MA, Haines JL; Multiple Sclerosis Genetics Group. Interleukin 7 receptor alpha chain (IL7R) shows allelic and functional association with multiple sclerosis. Nat Genet. 2007; 39(9):1083–91. PMID: 17660817

[58] O'Doherty C, Kantarci O, Vandenbroeck K. IL7RA polymorphisms and susceptibility to multiple sclerosis. N Engl J Med. 2008; 358(7):753–4. doi: 10.1056/NEJMc0707553

[59] Alcina A, Fedetz M, Ndagire D, Fernández O, Leyva L, Guerrero M, Arnal C, Delgado C, Matesanz F. The T244I variant of the interleukin-7 receptor-alpha gene and multiple sclerosis.Tissue Antigens. 2008; 72(2):158–61. doi: 10.1111/j.1399-0039.2008.01075.x

[60] Weber F, Fontaine B, Cournu-Rebeix I, Kroner A, Knop M, Lutz S, Müller-Sarnowski F, Uhr M, Bettecken T, Kohli M, Ripke S, Ising M, Rieckmann P, Brassat D, Semana G, Babron MC, Mrejen S, Gout C, Lyon-Caen O, Yaouanq J, Edan G, Clanet M, Holsboer F, Clerget-Darpoux F, Müller-Myhsok B. IL2RA and IL7RA genes confer susceptibility for multiple sclerosis in two independent European populations. Genes Immun. 2008; 9(3):259–63. doi: 10.1038/gene.2008.14

[61] Sombekke MH, van der Voort LF, Kragt JJ, Nielsen JM, Guzel H, Visser A, Oudejans CB, Crusius JB, Peña AS, Vrenken H, Polman CH, Killestein J. Relevance of IL7R genotype and mRNA expression in Dutch patients with multiple sclerosis. MultScler. 2011; 17(8):922–30. doi: 10.1177/1352458511402411

[62] Fang L, Isobe N, Yoshimura S, Yonekawa T, Matsushita T, Masaki K, Doi H, Ochi K, Miyamoto K, Kawano Y, Kira J; South Japan Multiple Sclerosis Genetics Consortium. Interleukin-7 receptor alpha gene polymorphism influences multiple sclerosis risk in Asians. Neurology. 2011; 76(24):2125–7. doi: 10.1212/WNL.0b013e31821f466c

[63] Stanković A, Dincić E, Ristić S, Lovrecić L, StarcevićCizmarević N, Djurić T, Sepcić J, Kapović M, Raicević R, Peterlin B, Alavantić D, Zivković M. Interleukin 7 receptor alpha polymorphism rs6897932 and susceptibility to multiple sclerosis in the Western Balkans. MultScler. 2010; 16(5):533–6. doi: 10.1177/1352458509360548

[64] Booth DR, Arthur AT, Teutsch SM, Bye C, Rubio J, Armati PJ, Pollard JD, Heard RN, Stewart GJ; Southern MS Genetics Consortium. Gene expression and genotyping studies implicate the interleukin 7 receptor in the pathogenesis of primary progressive multiple sclerosis. J Mol Med. 2005; 83(10):822–30. PMID: 16075257

[65] Čierny D, Hányšová S, Michalik J, Kantorová E, Kurča E, Škereňová M, Lehotský J. Genetic variants in interleukin 7 receptor α chain (IL-7Ra) are associated with multiple sclerosis risk and disability progression in Central European Slovak population. J Neuroimmunol.2015; 282:80–4.doi: 10.1016/j.jneuroim.2015.03.010

[66] Chaudhuri A. Why we should offer routine vitamin D supplementation in pregnancy and childhood to prevent multiple sclerosis. Med Hypotheses. 2005; 64(3):608–18. PMID: 15617877

[67] Saccone D, Asani F, Bornman L. Regulation of the vitamin D receptor gene by environment, genetics and epigenetics. Gene. 2015; 561(2):171–80. doi: 10.1016/j.gene.2015.02.024

[68] Norman AW.Minireview: vitamin D receptor: new assignments for an already busy receptor. Endocrinology. 2006; 147(12):5542–8. PMID: 16946007

[69] Ascherio A, Munger KL, Simon KC. Vitamin D and multiple sclerosis. Lancet Neurol. 2010; 9(6):599–612. doi: 10.1016/S1474-4422(10)70086-7

[70] Adorini L, Penna G. Control of autoimmune diseases by the vitamin D endocrine system. Nat ClinPractRheumatol. 2008; 4(8):404–12.doi: 10.1038/ncprheum0855

[71] Bikle DD. Vitamin D regulation of immune function.VitamHorm. 2011; 86:1–21.doi: 10.1016/B978-0-12-386960-9.00001-0

[72] Smolders J, Thewissen M, Peelen E, Menheere P, Tervaert JW, Damoiseaux J, Hupperts R. Vitamin D status is positively correlated with regulatory T cell function in patients with multiple sclerosis. PLoS One. 2009; 4(8):e6635. doi: 10.1371/journal.pone.0006635.

[73] Penna G, Adorini L. 1 Alpha,25-dihydroxyvitamin D3 inhibits differentiation, maturation, activation, and survival of dendritic cells leading to impaired alloreactive T cell activation. J Immunol. 2000; 164(5):2405–11. PMID: 10679076

[74] Boonstra A, Barrat FJ, Crain C, Heath VL, Savelkoul HF, O'Garra A. 2001. 1α,25-Dihydroxyvitamin D3 has a direct effect on naive CD4+ T cells to enhance the development of Th2 cells. JImmunol. 2001; 167(9):4974–80. PMID: 11673504

[75] Geldmeyer-Hilt K, Heine G, Hartmann B, Baumgrass R, Radbruch A, Worm M. 1,25-dihydroxyvitamin D3 impairs NF-kB activation in human naïve B cells. BiochemBiophys Res Commun. 2011; 407(4):699–702. doi: 10.1016/j.bbrc.2011.03.078

[76] Chen S, Sims GP, Chen XX, Gu YY, Chen S, Lipsky PE. Modulatory effects of 1,25-dihydroxyvitamin D3 on human B cell differentiation. J Immunol. 2007; 179(3):1634–47. PMID: 17641030

[77] Lemire JM, Archer DC, Beck L, Spiegelberg HL. Immunosuppressive actions of 1,25-dihydroxyvitamin D3: preferential inhibition of Th1 functions. J Nutr. 1995; 125(6 Suppl):1704S–8S. PMID: 7782931

[78] Helming L, Böse J, Ehrchen J, Schiebe S, Frahm T, Geffers R, Probst-Kepper M, Balling R, Lengeling A. 1alpha,25-Dihydroxyvitamin D3 is a potent suppressor of interferon gamma-mediated macrophage activation. Blood. 2005; 106(13):4351–8. PMID: 16118315

[79] Bartels LE, Hvas CL, Agnholt J, Dahlerup JF, Agger R. Human dendritic cell antigen presentation and chemotaxis are inhibited by intrinsic 25-hydroxy vitamin D activation. IntImmunopharmacol. 2010;10(8):922–8. doi: 10.1016/j.intimp.2010.05.003

[80] O'Kelly J, Hisatake J, Hisatake Y, Bishop J, Norman A, Koeffler HP. Normal myelopoiesis but abnormal T lymphocyte responses in vitamin D receptor knockout mice. J Clin Invest. 2002; 109(8):1091–9. PMID: 11956247

[81] Panda DK, Miao D, Tremblay ML, Sirois J, Farookhi R, Hendy GN, Goltzman D. Targeted ablation of the 25-hydroxyvitamin D 1alpha -hydroxylase enzyme: evidence for skeletal, reproductive, and immune dysfunction. ProcNatlAcadSci U S A. 2001; 98(13):7498–503. PMID: 11416220

[82] Cantorna MT, Hayes CE, DeLuca HF. 1,25-Dihydroxyvitamin D3 reversibly blocks the progression of relapsing encephalomyelitis, a model of multiple sclerosis. ProcNatlAcadSci U S A. 1996; 93(15):7861–4. PMCID: PMC38839

[83] Kamen DL, Tangpricha V. Vitamin D and molecular actions on the immune system: modulation of innate and autoimmunity. J Mol Med (Berl). 2010; 88(5):441–450. doi: 10.1007/s00109-010-0590-9

[84] Mattner F, Smiroldo S, Galbiati F, Muller M, Di Lucia P, Poliani PL, Martino G, Panina-Bordignon P, Adorini L. Inhibition of Th1 development and treatment of chronic-relapsing experimental allergic encephalomyelitis by a non-hypercalcemic analogue of 1,25-dihydroxyvitamin D(3). Eur J Immunol. 2000; 30(2):498–508. PMID: 10671205

[85] Haynes RC Jr. Vitamin D. In Gilman AG, Rall TW, Nies AR, Taylor P. editors. Goodman and Gilman's the pharmacological basis of therapeutics. 8th ed. New York: McGraw-Hill; 1992. p. 1515

[86] Pierrot-Deseilligny C, Souberbielle JC. Widespread vitamin D insufficiency: a new challenge for primary prevention, with particular reference to multiple sclerosis. Presse Med. 2011; 40(4 Pt 1):349–56. doi: 10.1016/j.lpm.2011.01.003

[87] Burton JM, Kimball S, Vieth R, Bar-Or A, Dosch HM, Cheung R, Gagne D, D'Souza C, Ursell M, O'Connor P. A phase I/II dose-escalation trial of vitamin D3 and calcium in multiple sclerosis. Neurology. 2010; 74(23):1852–9. doi:10.1212/WNL.0b013e3181e1cec2

[88] Kimball SM, Ursell MR, O'Connor P, Vieth R. Safety of vitamin D3 in adults with multiple sclerosis. Am J ClinNutr. 2007; 86(3):645–51. PMID: 17823429

[89] Munger KL, Zhang SM, O'Reilly E, Hernán MA, Olek MJ, Willett WC, Ascherio A.Vitamin D intake and incidence of multiple sclerosis. Neurology. 2004; 62(1):60–5. PMID: 14718698

[90] Munger KL, Levin LI, Hollis BW, Howard NS, Ascherio A. Serum 25-hydroxyvitamin D levels and risk of multiple sclerosis. JAMA. 2006; 296(23):32–8. PMID: 17179460

[91] Soilu-Hänninen M, Airas L, Mononen I, Heikkilä A, Viljanen M, Hänninen A. 25-Hydroxyvitamin D levels in serum at the onset of multiple sclerosis. MultScler. 2005; 11(3):266–71.

[92] Ozgocmen S, Bulut S, Ilhan N, Gulkesen A, Ardicoglu O, Ozkan Y. Vitamin D deficiency and reduced bone mineral density in multiple sclerosis: effect of ambulatory status and functional capacity. J Bone MinerMetabol. 2005; 23(4):309–13. PMID: 15981027

[93] Smolders J, Menheere P, Kessels A, Damoiseaux J, Hupperts R. Association of vitamin D metabolite levels with relapse rate and disability in multiple sclerosis.MultScler. 2008; 14(9):1220–4. doi: 10.1177/1352458508094399

[94] Runia TF, Hop WC, de Rijke YB, Buljevac D, Hintzen RQ. Lower serum vitamin D levels are associated with a higher relapse risk in multiple sclerosis. Neurology. 2012; 79(3): 261–6. doi: 10.1212/WNL.0b013e31825fdec7

[95] Cadden MH, Koven NS, Ross MK. Neuroprotective effects of vitamin D in multiple sclerosis.NeurosciMed. 2011; 2(3):198–207. doi: 10.4236/nm.2011.23027

[96] Simon KC, Munger KL, Kraft P, Hunter DJ, De Jager PL, Ascherio A. Genetic predictors of 25-hydroxyvitamin D levels and risk of multiple sclerosis. J Neurol. 2011; 258(9): 1676–82. doi: 10.1007/s00415-011-6001-5

[97] Smolders J, Damoiseaux J, Menheere P, Tervaert JW, Hupperts R. Fok-I vitamin D receptor gene polymorphism (rs10735810) and vitamin D metabolism in multiple sclerosis. J Neuroimmunol. 2009; 207(1–2):117–21. doi: 10.1016/j.jneuroim.2008.12.011

[98] Simon KC, Munger KL, Xing Yang, Ascherio A. Polymorphisms in vitamin D metabolism related genes and risk of multiple sclerosis. MultScler. 2010; 16(2):133–8. doi: 10.1177/1352458509355069

[99] Orton SM, Morris AP, Herrera BM, Ramagopalan SV, Lincoln MR, Chao MJ, Vieth R, Sadovnick AD, Ebers GC. Evidence for genetic regulation of vitamin D status in twins with multiple sclerosis.Am J ClinNutr. 2008; 88(2):441–7. PMID: 18689381

[100] Holick MF, Chen TC. Vitamin D deficiency: a worldwide problem with health consequences. Am J ClinNutr. 2008; 87(4):1080S–6S. PMID: 18400738

[101] Ramagopalan SV, Dyment DA, Cader MZ, Morrison KM, Disanto G, Morahan JM, Berlanga-Taylor AJ, Handel A, De Luca GC, Sadovnick AD, Lepage P, Montpetit A, Ebers GC. Rare variants in the CYP27B1 gene are associated with multiple sclerosis. Ann Neurol. 2011; 70(6):881–6. doi: 10.1002/ana.22678

[102] Meehan TF, DeLuca HF. The vitamin D receptor is necessary for 1alpha,25-dihydroxyvitamin D(3) to suppress experimental autoimmune encephalomyelitis in mice. Arch BiochemBiophys. 2002; 408(2):200–4. PMID: 12464272

[103] Miyamoto K, Kesterson RA, Yamamoto H, Taketani Y, Nishiwaki E, Tatsumi S, Inoue Y, Morita K, Takeda E, Pike JW. Structural organization of the human vitamin D receptor chromosomal gene and its promoter.MolEndocrinol. 1997; 11(8):1165–79. PMID: 9212063

[104] Wang TT, Tavera-Mendoza LE, Laperriere D, Libby E, MacLeod NB, Nagai Y, Bourdeau V, Konstorum A, Lallemant B, Zhang R, Mader S, White JH. Large-scale in silico

and microarray-based identification of direct 1,25-dihydroxyvitamin D3 target genes. MolEndocrinol. 2005; 19(11):2685–95. PMID: 16002434

[105] Uitterlinden AG, Fang Y, Van Meurs JB, Pols HA, Van Leeuwen JP. Genetics and biology of vitamin D receptor polymorphisms. Gene. 2004; 338(2):143–56. PMID: 15315818

[106] Jurutka PW, Remus LS, Whitfield GK, Thompson PD, Hsieh JC, Zitzer H, Tavakkoli P, Galligan MA, Dang HT, Haussler CA, Haussler MR. The polymorphic N terminus in human vitamin D receptor isoforms influences transcriptional activity by modulating interaction with transcription factor IIB. MolEndocrinol. 2000; 14(3):401–20. PMID: 10707958

[107] Tajouri L, Ovcaric M, Curtain R, Johnson MP, Griffiths LR, Csurhes P, Pender MP, Lea RA. Variation in the vitamin D receptor gene is associated with multiple sclerosis in an Australian population. J Neurogenet. 2005; 19(1):25–38. PMID: 16076630

[108] Morrison NA, Qi JC, Tokita A, Kelly PJ, Crofts L, Nguyen TV, Sambrook PN, Eisman JA. Prediction of bone density from vitamin D receptor alleles.Nature. 1994; 367(6460): 284–7. PMID: 8161378

[109] Fukazawa T, Yabe I, Kikuchi S, Sasaki H, Hamada T, Miyasaka K, Tashiro K. Association of vitamin D receptor gene polymorphism with multiple sclerosis in Japanese. J Neurol Sci. 1999; 166(1):47–52. PMID: 10465499

[110] Niino M, Fukazawa T, Yabe I, Kikuchi S, Sasaki H, Tashiro K. Vitamin D receptor gene polymorphism in multiple sclerosis and the association with HLA class II alleles. J Neurol Sci. 2000; 177(1):65–71. PMID: 10967184

[111] Partridge JM, Weatherby SJ, Woolmore JA, Highland DJ, Fryer AA, Mann CL, Boggild MD, Ollier WE, Strange RC, Hawkins CP. Susceptibility and outcome in MS: associations with polymorphisms in pigmentation-related genes. Neurology. 2004; 62(12): 2323–5. PMID: 15210908

[112] Cox MB, Ban M, Bowden NA, Baker A, Scott RJ, Lechner-Scott J. Potential association of vitamin D receptor polymorphism Taq1 with multiple sclerosis. MultScler. 2012; 18(1):16–22. doi: 10.1177/1352458511415562

[113] Steckley JL, Dyment DA, Sadovnick AD, Risch N, Hayes C, Ebers GC. Genetic analysis of vitamin D related genes in Canadian multiple sclerosis patients. Canadian Collaborative Study Group.Neurology. 2000; 54(3):729–32. PMID: 10680811

[114] Smolders J, Damoiseaux J, Menheere P, Tervaert JW, Hupperts R. Association study on two vitamin D receptor gene polymorphisms and vitamin D metabolites in multiple sclerosis. Ann N Y Acad Sci. 2009; 1173:515–20. doi: 10.1111/j.1749-6632.2009.04656.x

[115] Sioka C, Papakonstantinou S, Markoula S, Gkartziou F, Georgiou A, Georgiou I, Pelidou SH, Kyritsis AP, Fotopoulos A.Vitamin D receptor gene polymorphisms in

multiple sclerosis patients in northwest Greece. J Negat Results Biomed.2011; 10:3.doi: 10.1186/1477-5751-10-3

[116] Irizar H, Muñoz-Culla M, Zuriarrain O, Goyenechea E, Castillo-Triviño T, Prada A, Saenz-Cuesta M, De Juan D, Lopez de Munain A, Olascoaga J, Otaegui D. HLA-DRB1*15:01 and multiple sclerosis: a female association? MultScler. 2012; 18(5):569–77. doi: 10.1177/1352458511426813

[117] García-Martín E, Agúndez J. A. G., Martínez C, Benito-León J, Millán-Pascual J, Calleja P, Díaz-Sánchez M, Pisa D, Turpín-Fenoll L, Alonso-Navarro H, Ayuso-Peralta L, Torrecillas D, Plaza-Nieto JF, Jiménez-Jiménez FJ. Vitamin D3 Receptor (VDR) Gene rs2228570 (Fok1) and rs731236 (Taq1) variants are not associated with the risk for multiple sclerosis: results of a new study and a meta-analysis. PLoS One. 2013; 8(6): e65487. doi: 10.1371/journal.pone.0065487

[118] Dickinson JL, Perera DI, van der Mei AF, Ponsonby AL, Polanowski AM, Thomson RJ, Taylor BV, McKay JD, Stankovich J, Dwyer T. Past environmental sun exposure and risk of multiple sclerosis: a role for the Cdx-2 vitamin D receptor variant in this interaction. MultScler. 2009; 5(5):563–70. doi: 10.1177/1352458509102459

[119] Niksresht AR, Dadkhah B, KamaliSarverstani E. The association of vitamin D receptor gene BsmIpolymorphism with multiple sclerosis in Iranian patients.J Kerman Univ MedSci Health Serv. 2009; 16(2):116–23. doi: http://jkmu.kmu.ac.ir/en/index.php/kmus/article/view/245

[120] Agliardi C, Guerini FR, Saresella M, Caputo D, Leone MA, Zanzottera M, Bolognesi E, Marventano I, Barizzone N, Fasano ME, Al-Daghri N, Clerici M. Vitamin D receptor (VDR) gene SNPs influence VDR expression and modulate protection from multiple sclerosis in HLA-DRB1*15-positive individuals. Brain Behav Immun. 2011; 25(7):1460–7. doi: 10.1016/j.bbi.2011.05.015

6

Cognitive Deficits and Neuropsychological Assessment in Multiple Sclerosis

Alena Javůrková, Denisa Zimová,
Katarína Tomašovičová and Jaroslava Raudenská

Abstract

The aim of this chapter was to introduce the contents of neuropsychological assessment in multiple sclerosis, which should include the functional evaluation of cognitive domains, the psychopathology of personality, levels of depression, and the assessment of psychosocial aspects and quality of life with multiple sclerosis. Further, the most commonly used neuropsychological diagnostics are described. The chapter hopes to draw attention to the importance of neuropsychological assessment which should be a part of neurological diagnostics and therapy, including rehabilitation and psychotherapy.

Keywords: neuropsychology, multiple sclerosis, cognitive deficit, neuropsychiatry, neurorehabilitation

1. Introduction

Multiple sclerosis (lat. sclerosis multiplex) is a chronic disease of the central nervous system caused by the damage of the myelin sheath. The symptoms of the disease depend on the location of the damage in the nervous system and can vary: optic neuritis, paresthesia, motor symptoms (spasticity), impairment of cranial nerves, oculomotor disorders, cerebellar disorders, vertigo, urinary disorders, defecation, sexual dysfunctions, fatigue, depression, cognitive disorders, and paroxysmal symptoms. Multiple sclerosis is the most common cause of chronic neurological disabilities in young adults. The onset of the disease is usually between the ages of 20 and 40. Its prevalence is higher among women. The highest susceptibility to the disease is among Caucasians; the geographic gradient of the incidence increases together with the distance from the equator. Genetic predisposition plays a role.

1.1. Types of the disease

Four types of the disease are recognized according to their clinical course. In the early years of the disease, the most common type is relapsing-remitting MS (RRMS), occurring in 80–85% of patients and characterized by attacks and remissions. If a previous attack left no neurological deficit, remissions may be completely asymptomatic at the beginning of the disease. Half of these patients develop into the stage of secondary progression (SPMS) during the first 10 years of the disease's progression. This stage is characterized by a gradual increase in neurological deficits that are already irreversible, with both the presence and absence of relapses that are not as dramatic as in the remitting stage. The relapsing-progressive (RPMS) form of the disease is characterized by an increased neurological deficit also evident between the relapses; it is thus prognostically the most unfavorable form of the disease. The primary progressive (PPMS) form affects about 10–15% of patients and is characterized by a gradual increase in neurological deficit. This form occurs more frequently among males and with a later onset of the disease [1].

In the relapsing-remitting forms, approximately 20–30% of patients continue working following their first attack. It is uncommon for patients in the early stages of this form of MS to be physically disabled or to have noticeable alternations in terms of dementia. It is primarily the progressive form of MS, developing at a later age that tends to pose more difficulty in the cognitive domains, compared to the remitting one. Patients with the spinal form of the disease have trouble mostly with motor skills and mobility. This form often occurs in the primary progressive form. Cognitive deficits include impaired attention. The typical cognitive domains impaired in the cerebral forms of MS are described below. Psychosocial and maladaptive problems are described in the case report.

1.1.1. Case report 1

A woman of 47 years reported the first symptoms of MS (optic neuritis and paresthesia) at the age of 17; later, the attacks recurred about once a year; the problems worsened after two child deliveries. Therefore, she did not breastfeed her children, for which she blames herself for until today. She underwent an abortion 2 years after the second birth due to the above-mentioned difficulties, then was psychiatrically treated, and still has feelings of guilt. The diagnosis of MS was definitely confirmed about 4 years ago. The patient has since been considerably anxious, unreconciled with the diagnosis, dominated by hostility and distrust of the medical staff (the disease was not diagnosed correctly). MRI scans of the brain and spinal cord showed multiple demyelinating lesions or plaques in the white matter. Nobody in the family had MS. She was entitled to disability pension and has been taking antidepressants for 4 years, based on the psychiatrist's indication of anxiety and depressive problems. Formerly, she worked as a teacher. She feels very tired after only about a 3–4 km walk. She is married, has two adult sons, and lives with her family. When she learned about MS, she was overtaken by fear of dying and felt mentally ill, and thus stopped working. She did not observe any difficulties with cognition. Gradually, a panic anxiety developed; when she wakes up, she feels scared, but this panic is also present while traveling; family members take her everywhere by car. The patient is recommended to systematic cognitive-behavioral psychotherapy.

2. Cognitive functions and MS

The most characteristic feature of cognitive dysfunction in MS is the slowing down of processing speed [2]. Another often affected domain is long-term episodic memory and attention (alternating and maintained). Less frequent but significant cognitive disorders include disorders of executive functions (especially abstract and conceptual reasoning and problem-solving) [3].

2.1. Outline of basic neuropsychological techniques

Due to the high incidence of cognitive disorders in patients with MS, the adequate evaluation and diagnosis of such deficits is of great importance. Their existence is often under diagnosed during an ordinary neurological examination. Various tests are used to identify these.

One of the most significant neuropsychological studies of MS patients was carried out by Rao [4]. The Brief Repeatable Battery (BRB) for neuropsychological impairment in MS [5] was created based on a set of highly sensitive tests, with a few modifications. The BRB tests were chosen with regard to time restrictions, and so the administration of the entire battery lasts only about 40–45 min. It contains the following subtests: The Paced Auditory Serial Addition Test (PASAT); The Symbol Digit Modalities Test (SDMT) measuring attention, visual accuracy, and executive functions; The Selective Reminding Test (SRT) measuring verbal memory and delayed recall periods; The Spatial Recall Test (SPART) measuring visuospatial memory and delayed recall; and The Word List Generation (WLG) measuring verbal fluency. The battery has 15 versions and is thus, despite its longer duration, the most commonly used battery for the longitudinal monitoring of patients with MS. Clinical research supports the high sensitivity of the battery. Its abbreviated version with 3 subtests has been under verification recently.

For cognitive screenings, Beatty [6] developed the Screening Examination for Cognitive Impairment (SEFCI) neuropsychological battery, which proved to confirm cognitive deficits typical of MS in a comparative study (duration 22 min) with other time-consuming neuropsychological batteries. It does not have variants and is thus not suitable for longitudinal observations. The study compared the battery with the Neuropsychological Screening Battery for Multiple Sclerosis (NPSBMS) for which the administration period lasted 31 min. Both batteries identified significantly more patients with cognitive impairment in MS than the Mini-Mental State Exam (MMSE) [7]. The Multiple Sclerosis Functional Composite (MSFC) is a score used in clinical studies, measuring the function of the lower limb—timed walk, upper limb function (nine-hole peg test), and cognitive function (PASAT) [8, 9].

In 2001, the battery Minimal Assessment of Cognitive Function in MS (MACFIMS) [10] was created with respect to neglected domains (higher cognitive functions and spatial processing), and its reliability and validity has been verified in several studies. The MACFIMS battery includes the following tests: Controlled Oral Word Association Test (COWAT); Judgement of Line Orientation Test (JLO); California Verbal Learning Test, Second edition (CVLT-II); Brief Visuospatial Memory Test-Revised (BVMT-R); Paced Auditory Serial Addition Test (PASAT); Symbol Digit Modalities Test (SDMT); and the Sorting Test from the Delis-Kaplan Executive Function System (D-KEFS). However, the MACFIMS battery is limited by time constraints and for its need to be carried out by an experienced neuropsychologist. For this reason, a shorter battery of cognitive tests has recently been designed. This consists of three subtests from the MACFIMS battery and may be administered by neuropsychological workers without training —International Brief Cognitive Assessment for Multiple Sclerosis—BICAMS [11]. It is suitable for use in routine clinical practices in centers with no neuropsychologist to administrate the MACFIMS. The BICAMS screening battery consists of three tests that are included in the MACFIMS battery: SDMT, CVLT-II (the first five experiments), BVMT-R (the first three trials).

2.2. Cognitive domains and their examination

Cognitive deficits observed within MS can have almost any composition [12]; a typical profile shows impairment of processing speed, memory, and often of executive skills as well [2].

2.2.1. *Intellectual skills*

Over the past two decades, numerous studies using neuropsychological assessment showed that approximately half the patients exhibit some degree of cognitive impairment. We also know that cognitive disorders may occur at any time during the illness and are not bound to the presence of physical disorders [13]. Generally, a substantial variability of cognitive impairments in MS in terms of their gravity and types has been described. Although approximately 10% of MS patients have severe problems that display extensive impairment even when measuring overall intelligence, the vast majority (90%) of patients is affected only mildly to moderately [14]. It should be emphasized that patients with MS as a group display a relatively small decline on intelligence measures, and overall dementia is rare in MS [13]. Cognitive deficits in MS are usually more focal than generalized. Verbal IQ, therefore, often remains intact during the first signs of MS [4].

2.2.2. *Visuomotor skills, visuospatial skills, and attention*

Visual disorders including diplopia, reduced color discrimination, blurred vision, and transient blindness, and motor symptoms such as limb weakness, spasticity, incoordination, or a combination of all the problems, as well as sensory disorders including numbness or paresthesia, contribute to the alteration of visuomotor skills in neuropsychological examinations. Deficits of visual attention in MS patients significantly influence their level of visuomotor skills. When evaluating visual attention, it is thus necessary to take into account the visual disorders. For example, test results in automatic attention (reaction time) and focused attention may be in norm in terms of errors, but the patient completes them in a longer period of time. In contrast, controlled attention and divided attention are often deficient [15].

2.2.3. *Memory and learning*

Long-term memory is related to the learning and retrieval of new information. Patients with MS often have difficulties with memory—the prevalence is reported between 40 and 65%. The most common verbal memory tests are tasks in which the patient learns a wordlist [16]. Visuospatial memory, too, is affected in patients with MS [13]. Patients with MS have significant abnormalities of the hippocampal functional connectivity, even before spatial memory impairment is apparent [17]. Patients with MS in the initial stages of the disease display a relatively intact short-term memory and learning ability, measured by tests of memory skills. More patients experience problems in recalling new material, while recognition is rarely altered.

2.2.4. *Verbal ability and executive functions*

Executive functions are related to planning and goal-directed behavior. Drew and colleagues [18] reported a series of executive dysfunctions—including disinhibition, poor fluency, and an inability to shift sets. Overall, 17% of their sample of MS patients displayed this kind of deficit. Language functions typically remain intact in MS; however, some minor deficits in understanding were demonstrated. Weakened sentence comprehension has been associated with slower information processing. Deficits in semantic memory and visual processing were also observed [19].

Overall verbal skills in patients with MS are usually preserved for a long time, depending on premorbid mental performance, flexibility, and vocabulary; a low level of verbal fluency is observed. Dysarthria or problems with articulation are more prevalent in speech. The best and longest preserved of all verbal skills is naming. Recalling information from long-term memory, vocabulary, and conceptual reasoning are often normal. If these abilities are altered, it is usually the result of a generalized deterioration, or of the patient having low levels of premorbid education and of cognitive reserve. Some studies have found lower levels of conceptual reasoning in patients with chronic progressive MS. A more detailed examination of verbal and oral skills is possible with a complex speech assessment.

Cognitive impairment in MS, however, does not correlate with the degree of physical disability (Expanded Disability Status Scale EDSS Kurtzke [20]); some studies showed a correlation with disease duration, yet other studies did not prove this. The impairment of cognitive functions correlates positively with some MRI abnormalities—mostly concerning atrophy, ventricular dilatation, and the total volume of impaired white matter on W T2 lesion load. The sites of predilection are areas of the corpus callosum, and extensive demyelination further affects circuits linking the prefrontal and subcortical areas. Large confluent periventricular lesions are also typical. As a whole, the huge variability in cognitive impairment may depend on many factors, such as the patient's age, sex, age at disease onset, level of education, and cognitive reserve [3]. Dysexecutive and prefrontal behavioral syndromes in a patient with a cerebral, relapsing–remitting form are illustrated in the following case report.

2.3. Case report 2

A woman of 54 years was treated for MS and migraine for 15 years. A cognition and personality assessment was recommended by a neurologist for her memory problems. MRI of the brain showed unique plaque lesions in the white matter, predominantly in the right frontal lobe; the spinal cord was not affected. There has been improvement when comparing MRI scans, the lesions were less apparent. The patient was entitled to a full disability pension 10 years ago. She was a skilled saleswoman. She has been married for 35 years; her sons are adults. There is no report of MS in the family. She commutes to a psychiatric clinic where antidepressants are prescribed. She is oriented in contact, talkative, often gets lost, and exhibits signs of the prefrontal syndrome. Memory problems have occurred for a longer period, approximately 10 or even more years. She misplaces thing and then cannot find them, someone talks about something and she does not know about it, and she does not remember old information. She also experiences sudden interruptions of activities when she goes off to do another one, although she had not planned it; it is impulsive. She experiences confusions in her mind; she wanted something and suddenly does not know what she was thinking about. It troubles her. She "masks" these difficulties in front of her family and friends. Headaches occur daily. Neuropsychologically, it is mainly attention that is impaired, and the generalized deterioration of intellect is also striking, considering her education. It is possible to explain the problems behaviorally, mainly through the prefrontal behavioral and dysexecutive syndromes, which might be related to the largest findings of plaques in the frontal lobes. Cognitive behavioral therapy and training of cognitive functions was advised.

3. The course of cognitive deficit

Studies on large MS patient samples have shown that the range of cognitive impairment prevalence in MS is between 40 and 70% and appears in all stages and types of the disease (which also includes the clinically isolated syndrome—CIS) [21]. It seems that observations carried out for long enough are able to show cognitive impairment in progressive stages [22]. Several studies have confirmed the relationship between the dysexecutive syndrome and frontal lesions, and others have focused on deficits in interhemispheric transfer (i.e., disconnection syndrome) in the atrophy of the corpus callosum.

The course of a cognitive deficit without progression but with behavioral disorders is illustrated in the following case report.

3.1. Case report 3

A 43-year-old man with the relapsing-remitting form, treated for MS for 18 years, was initially assessed due to problems with memory, concentration, exhaustion, and no sexual appetite. An MRI scan of the brain showed small plaque lesions subcortically, compared with no progression found on MRI scans 4 years ago. The patient had been treated with interferons for 3 years. He is left-handed, a skilled auto-mechanic, has his own workshop at home, and works

17 h a day. He has been married for 22 years, has two children and "does not get on well" with his wife, and he admits to extramarital relations. They are currently in a divorce proceeding. The main problem is with his erection. Neuropsychologically, no striking impairment of cognitive domains was found, and only anxiety and a conflictive family environment were found. Marriage counseling, a sexologist, and conflict solving were recommended. The patient refused the proposed recommendations and increasingly adopted strange and promiscuous behaviors; he forced his wife and their children to move out of the house. He was incapable of rational thinking; he explained the promiscuity as a verification of his sexual functions. A 1-year follow-up neuropsychological assessment showed no impairment of cognitive domains and intellect, but a psychiatric examination was recommended due to paranoid thinking and aggressiveness.

On the contrary, a rapid development of cognitive deficits into dementia can be seen in the following case report.

3.2. Case report 4

A 42-year-old woman diagnosed with chronic progressive MS for 10 years was treated by interferons for 6 years. At the time of her visit, eye problems are dominant for the first time; she uses a white cane. She also experiences hearing difficulties, but does not complain about memory at all. A former governess, now entitled to full disability pension, divorced, with two children, both studying, not in contact with her ex-husband. Her mother and brother help her mostly, but the patient feels dependent and helpless. According to an MRI scan of the brain, periventricular plaque lesions are apparent in the white matter of both hemispheres. There has been a slight progression of plaque and atrophy when compared to an MRI from 4 years ago. The initial psychological examination suggested a multi-domain impairment, a decrease of more than 2 SDs (verbal mnestic and visual skills, construction, executive functioning), with severe anosognosia. The performance may have been influenced by her impaired visual and auditory perception. Two years later, she comes fundamentally oriented, and the right eye is blind. The outcome of the examination is a multi-domain cognitive disorder; cognitive abilities are significantly impaired across the whole profile.

4. Cognitive abilities and imaging methods

Magnetic resonance imaging (MRI) is used as one of the basic methods for diagnostics, visualization, and monitoring of the inflammatory lesion dynamics in the brain and spinal cord. The first MRI studies in patients with MS were published in 1981. It was found that inflammatory lesions occur 5–10 times more than MS clinical attacks. Commonly used images for the diagnosis of MS are those in which lesions of hyperintense signal of size from 1 mm to several cm are apparent, located in the white matter of both hemispheres, mostly in the cerebral ventricles, as well as in the brain stem, medulla, cerebellum, and upper cervical spinal cord. If the radiologist wants to depict the active lesions, he/she applies gadolinium. The range of lesions visible in this way does not correlate with clinical disability as it is not known whether the lesion is currently in the stage of reparation or destruction.

The only areas described as hypodensities ("black holes") are areas where a loss of axons, thus the definitive loss of tissue, has occurred. The typical brain damage in the white matter in MS patients is clearly associated with a loss of axons [23]. Loss of axons is also a natural sign of brain aging, and its verification is only possible postmortem.

Recent neuropsychological studies especially use functional magnetic resonance imaging (fMRI) to assess the plasticity of functional cognitive deficits in patients with MS. The method consists of recording the activation of brain areas during the presentation of various simple neuropsychological tests. Compensatory mechanisms of cognitive functions already in the early stages of chronic MS are described. The results of fMRI scans in a group of MS patients with mild cognitive impairment and a healthy control group were compared. The functional activation areas of the brain were completely distinct during the presentation of the verbal naming test in each group (in MS patients in the frontal part of the right cortex and in the left Brodmann's area, and in the right cingulate gyrus in the healthy group). The functional reorganizations of motor functions are also described in fMRI assessments of MS patients, when compared to healthy subjects. MS patients with mild cognitive deficits assessed by neuropsychological tests were presented with auditory memory tests during an fMRI and were found to display heightened activity in different areas. Patients with greater neuropsychological deficits were found to exhibit lower activation of brain areas during the fMRI assessment, which probably supports the theory of adaptive mechanisms resulting from neural disorganization or inhibition associated with MS [24]. It is therefore also possible to explain the unproven relationship between the extent of morphological findings of gliosis and plaques in the white matter, and the severity and location of neuropsychological deficits in terms of this plasticity of neuropsychological functions. The range of specific cognitive deficits, such as memory disorders, reduced processing speed, and attention disorders, can be better explained by the cortical gray matter lesions (lesions and atrophy) than subcortical white matter lesions [25]. It has been shown that neocortical atrophy is associated with impaired verbal memory, visual episodic and working memory, verbal fluency, attention/concentration, and processing speed [26]. It is also possible that the neocortical atrophy is further responsible for slight personality changes, such as euphoria, that are seen in MS patients [27]. The left frontal atrophy occurs in patients with impaired verbal/auditory memory, while the right frontal atrophy is associated with impaired visual episodic and working memories. The medial temporal cortex atrophy is associated with a decrease in processing speed and impaired episodic and verbal memories. The most important within the subcortical gray mater are atrophy, structural changes, and an altered metabolism of the thalamus, which are associated with the impairment of many cognitive domains [28]. Generally, it can be concluded that the cognitive impairment observed in MS patients is caused by inflammatory lesions and a widespread loss of gray matter. Although it is not possible to define the neuropsychological profile of MS patients as strictly "cortical" or "subcortical", it seems that it is the disruption of the cortical gray matter which determines the degree and nature of cognitive dysfunction. Instead of the term subcortical dementia, often associated with a severe multi-domain cognitive impairment, the term multiple disconnection syndrome is also used for cognitive deficits in MS [29].

5. Neuropsychiatric aspects of MS

Cognitive and affective disorders in MS have largely been ignored for many years, yet they occur in 5% of the patients early in the disease, while in its advanced stages, this can be up to 70% of cases. MS is associated with a variety of behavioral changes. These may be associated with emotional disorders and cognitive distortions and may often overlap. The prevalence of depression is at least 50%; it is often manifested in parallel with the MS attack, and suicidal tendencies may occur. The causes of depression are probably neuropathological changes associated with the limbic system, neuroendocrinological, and psychoneuroimmunological changes, responses to life change, or a side effect of MS therapy (especially corticosteroids). The prevalence of bipolar disorders in MS is approximately 15%, and the prevalence of anxiety disorders in MS is about 36%. The occurrence of bipolar disorder and psychosis in MS is twice as common as in the general population, and the so-called pseudobulbar affectation (involuntary emotional expression disorder) affects one in ten patients. It is likely that the interruption of frontolimbic and temporolimbic connections plays a role in the pathogenesis of euphoria. Euphoric patients tend to have higher EDSS and a significantly more impaired cognition, including anosognosia. The incidence of euphoria is lower (approximately 2%) than is described in the older literature, thanks to an earlier diagnosis and treatment of MS. Symptoms of depression do not correlate with neurological findings or with disease severity, as measured by the sum of symptoms of physical disability and cognitive dysfunction [30]. However, depression positively correlates with subjective experience of stress, memory deficits, and with age in elderly patients over 65 years of age, in patients with the chronic progressive form and in patients with a predominance of spinal distortion. The neuropsychological assessment should therefore, in addition to cognitive domains, also include assessments of emotional alterations, especially depression and anxiety scales (e.g., methods HAD–Hospital Anxiety and Depression Scale, BDI-II) and their development over time [31].

Other changes in patients with MS, particularly changes in values and attitudes, progress together with the psychosocial adjustment and are mostly associated with the subjective perception of a physical handicap, but do not correlate with the duration of MS or other demographic indicators. Specific quality of life with MS questionnaires is used to measure the quality of life in these patients, such as the MSQOL-54 [32], which measures 12 subscales: physical function, role limitations—physical, role limitations—emotional, pain, emotional well-being, energy, health perceptions, social function, cognitive function, health distress, overall quality of life, and sexual function.

The Multi-domain battery Multiple Sclerosis Quality of Life Inventory (MSQLI) contains 10 scales, both generic and specific to MS [33]; some scales also have a shortened version: Health Status Questionnaire (SF-36), Modified Fatigue Impact Scale (MFIS), MOS Pain Effects Scale (PES), Sexual Satisfaction Scale (SSS), Bladder Control Scale (BLCS), Bowel Control Scale

(BWCS), Impact of Visual Impairment Scale (IVIS), Perceived Deficits Questionnaire (PDQ), Mental Health Inventory (MHI), and MOS Modified Social Support Survey (MSSS). The scales can also be presented individually.

6. Multi-disciplinary MS treatment

6.1. Cognitive disorders therapy in MS

Pharmacotherapy for cognitive impairment in MS is currently the subject of intense research. First and foremost, a preventive effect of early initiation and immunomodulatory therapy, in association with the possible development of cognitive disorders, is assumed. The primary point is to prevent axonal loss and the development of atrophy. Very few randomized trials have been carried out so far. Acetylcholinesterase inhibitors have currently been examined, through only with questionable or entirely negative results. No effective pharmacological treatment for cognitive disorders in MS has yet been found [34]. The pharmacological manipulation of depression is also significant, however, and should always be combined with psychotherapy in MS patients. Moreover, depression can be enhanced by a variety of biopsychosocial factors, such as reduced work performance or increased neurological symptoms.

6.2. Neuropsychological rehabilitation and the cognitive deficit psychotherapy

Kalb and Reitman [35] report the so-called cognitive rehabilitation as the basic therapy for cognitive deficits. They present two approaches: The first is to restore functions, such as through direct training and exercising of skills that are altered in neuropsychological tests (this approach, however, has a limited benefit in improving daily activities in MS patients) and the second approach is more compensatory, and closer to current neuropsychology, with its desire to improve a function through substitution, that is, the individual use of residual cognitive abilities in order to improve the quality of life through behavioral and cognitive therapy. The first approach is based on a more experimental approach, while the second is more clinical. It concerns creating an individual plan, "customized" for each patient.

This plan is based on neuropsychological assessment and interviews with the patient and their family. The evidence for the efficacy of cognitive rehabilitation in MS is, unfortunately, quite limited and contradictory. Memory rehabilitation studies suggest that individualized computer programs focused on patient-specific difficulties could be most effective. The most beneficial in the rehabilitation of executive functions is perhaps a direct instruction by a therapist, that is, paper and pencil method. The main problem of cognitive training in MS remains to be particularly its unavailability for patients and their often low motivation. It is therefore very important to maintain employability of patients for as long as possible and motivate them toward mental activity.

For these purposes, teams of multi-disciplinary experts work with people with MS, where a neurologist, psychologist, psychiatrist, speech therapist, occupational therapist, physiotherapist, and a psychotherapist cooperate in complex, holistic, all-day programs, based on cognitive as well as emotional, behavioral, and physiological changes. Even though it is impossible to increase one's premorbid IQ and brain volume, we can work on cognitively stimulating leisure activities. It is also very important to motivate the patient to lead an active life that includes adherence to the prescribed pharmacotherapy, but also an active attitude toward physiotherapy, psychotherapy, and cognitive training. It is the combination of physiotherapy and cognitive training that has the correct effect on the neurogenesis and formation of new synapses.

The specific model of psychosocial support for patients with MS at different levels, which has the characteristics of a cognitive-behavioral supportive therapy and family therapy, includes [35]: (1) psychoeducation, that is, education leading to the understanding of the disease, explanation of adaptive coping strategies; (2) diagnostics/treatment of emotional or cognitive problems; (3) family intervention, that is, how to organize family support for members with MS for adaptive coping with the illness; (4) work support for MS patients, that is, to work productively in a field for as long as they are able and interested, and vice versa, to stop working if necessary; (5) individual psychosocial assistance to individuals with MS. In addition to professional psychotherapy, a support group of people with the same disease, but also of family, friends, possibly a cultural-social or religious community, is appropriate.

6.3. Disability, employability, and MS

The organization of care for MS patients is similar around the world. A patient with a benign course of the disease is usually checked by a neurologist twice a year; more complicated patients are consulted in centers for MS that are a part of most university neurological clinics. In the case of a more severe disability, it is advisable to contact social services or long-term care. Neuropsychological approaches, however, show that employability can also be predicted by a short battery of tests that focuses on relevant domains, such as the aforementioned battery BICAMS [36]. The issue of employment restrictions, disability, work, and life disability due to MS is illustrated in the following case report.

6.3.1. Case report 5

A doctor, surgeon specialist, formerly a chief physician, 50 years old, with remitting MS. MRI scans revealed the cerebrospinal form with multiple plaques in the white matter of the brain and spinal cord; the demyelinating plaque findings are unchanged for 3 years. The patient was recommended to a cognition assessment for his memory problems, was dismissed from the surgical specialty, and thus works as a GP, which does not satisfy him. He is divorced and has problems with his second wife, who is a nurse, approximately 25 years younger. The wife is hostile, blames him for the change of social status. Neuropsychologically, only his psychomotor speed and motor dexterity are slightly reduced, which exhibits moderate depression in emotional experience, not suicidal. Couples therapy was recommended to address the changes in his professional situation and partner quality of life, together with a psychiatric consultation.

7. Conclusion

This article summarizes a neuropsychologist's perspective on cognitive skills in MS. When evaluating the cognitive level of patients, the comprehensive or screening assessment should examine specific domains that may not correlate with the length of the illness, neurological objective findings, the amount of plaque on MRI scans, and the MS form or type. Cognitive disorders are a significant predictor of quality of life during all stages of MS; they reduce physical independence and the ability to perform both activities of daily life and of employment, they influence one's coping and compliance to the treatment and their rehabilitation potential. The employability of people with MS can thus be easily predicted by the severity of cognitive disorders and their premorbid cognitive reserves, rather than by physical disability. The neuropsychological assessment of cognitive functions in MS should be a part of care for patients with MS and a part of a multi-disciplinary approach to neurorehabilitation.

Acknowledgements

The authors would like to express their sincere gratitude toward Lucie Steinerova from the University of Edinburgh for helping out with the language revision.

This article is supported by Ministry of Health, Czech Republic—conceptual development of research organization, Motol University Hospital, Prague, Czech Republic, 00064203.

Author details

Alena Javůrková[1,2*], Denisa Zimová[3], Katarína Tomašovičová[4] and Jaroslava Raudenská[2,5]

*Address all correspondence to: alena.javurkova@post.cz

1 Department of Clinical Psychology, University Hospital FNKV, Prague, Czech Republic

2 Department of Nursing, 2nd Medical Faculty, Charles University, University Hospital Motol, Prague, Czech Republic

3 Department of Neurology, 3rd Medical Faculty, Charles University, University Hospital FNKV, Prague, Czech Republic

4 Department of Psychology, Faculty of Arts, Charles University, Prague, Czech Republic

5 Department of Clinical Psychology, University Hospital Motol, Prague, Czech Republic

References

[1] Weinshenker BG, Bass B, Rice GP, Noseworthy J, Carriere W, Baskerville J, Ebers GC: The natural history of multiple sclerosis: a geographically based study I. Clinical course and disability. Brain. 1989;112(Pt1):133–146. doi: 10.1093/brain/112.1.133

[2] DeLuca J, Chelune GJ, Tulsky DS, Lengenfelder J, Chiaravalloti ND: Is speed of processing or working memory the primary information processing deficit in multiple sclerosis? J Clin Exp Neuropsychol. 2004;26(4):550–562. doi: 10.1080/13803390490496641

[3] Benedict RH, Zivadinov R: Risk factors for and management of cognitive dysfunction in multiple sclerosis. Nat Rev Neurol. 2011;7(6):332–342. doi: 10.1038/nrneurol.2011.61

[4] Rao SM, Leo GJ, Bernardin L, Unverzagt F: Cognitive dysfunction in multiple sclerosis. I. Frequency, patterns, and prediction. Neurology. 1991;41(5):685–691.doi: 10.1212/WNL.41.5.685

[5] Rao SM: A Manual for the Brief, Repeatable Battery of Neuropsychological Tests in Multiple Sclerosis. New York: National Multiple Sclerosis Society; 1991

[6] Beatty WW, Paul RH, Wilbanks SL, Hames KA, Blanco CR, Goodkin DE: Identifying multiple sclerosis patients with mild or global cognitive impairment using the Screening Examination for Cognitive Impairment (SEFCI). Neurology. 1995;45(4):718–723. doi: 10.1212/WNL.45.4.718

[7] Aupperle RL, Beatty WW, Shelton Fde N, Gontkovsky ST: Three screening batteries to detect cognitive impairment in multiple sclerosis. Mult Scler. 2002;8:382–389. doi: 10.1191/1352458502ms832oa

[8] Rudick R, Antel J, Confavreux C, Cutter G, Ellison G, Fischer J, Lublin F, Miller A, Petkau J, Rao S, Reingold S, Syndulko K, Thompson A, Wallenberg J, Weinshenker B, Willoughby E: Recommendations from the national multiple sclerosis society clinical outcomes assessment task force. Ann Neurol. 1997;42: 379–382. doi: 10.1002/ana.410420318

[9] Rudick RA, Cutter G, Baier M, Fisher E, Dougherty D, Weinstock-Guttman B, Mass MK, Miller D, Simonian NA: Use of the multiple sclerosis functional composite to predict disability in relapsing MS. Neurology. 2001; 56(10):1324–1330. doi: 10.1212/WNL.56.10.1324

[10] Benedict RH, Fischer JS, Archibald CJ, Arnett PA, Beatty WW, Bobholz J, Chelune GJ, Fisk JD, Langdon DW, Caruso L, Foley F, LaRocca NG, Vowels L, Weinstein A, DeLuca J, Rao SM, Munschauer F: Minimal neuropsychological assessment of MS patients: a consensus approach. Clin Neuropsychol. 2002;16(3):381–397. doi: 1385-4046/02/1603-381

[11] Langdon DW, Amato MP, Boringa J, Brochet B, Foley F, Fredrikson S, Hämäläinen P, Hartung HP, Krupp L, Penner IK, Reder AT, Benedict RH: Recommendations for a Brief

International Cognitive Assessment for Multiple Sclerosis (BICAMS). Mult Scler. 2012;18(6):891–898. doi: 10.1177/1352458511431076

[12] Prakash RS, Snook EM, Lewis JM, Motl RW, Kramer AF: Cognitive impairments in relapsing-remitting multiple sclerosis: a meta-analysis. Mult Scler. 2008;14(9):1250–1261. doi: 10.1177/1352458508095004

[13] Langdon DW: Cognition in multiple sclerosis. Curr Opin Neurol. 2011;24(3):244–249. doi: 10.1097/WCO.0b013e328346a43b

[14] Patti F: Cognitive impairment in multiple sclerosis. Mult Scler. 2009;15(1):2–8. doi: 10.1177/1352458508096684

[15] Beatty WW: Assessment of cognitive and psychological functions in patients with multiple sclerosis: considerations for databasing. Mult Scler. 1999;5(4):239–243. doi: 10.1177/135245859900500408

[16] Stegen S, Stepanov I, Cookfair D, Schwartz E, Hojnacki D, Weinstock-Guttman B, Benedict RH: Validity of the California Verbal Learning Test-II in multiple sclerosis. Clin Neuropsychol. 2010;24(2):189–202. doi: 10.1080/13854040903266910

[17] Roosendaal SD, Hulst HE, Vrenken H, Feenstra HE, Castelijns JA, Pouwels PJ, Barkhof F, Geurts JJ: Structural and functional hippocampal changes in multiple sclerosis patients with intact memory function. Radiology. 2010;255(2):595–604. doi: 10.1148/radiol.10091433

[18] Drew M, Tippett LJ, Starkey NJ, Isler RB: Executive dysfunction and cognitive impairment in a large community-based sample with multiple sclerosis from New Zealand: a descriptive study. Arch Clin Neuropsychol. 2008;23(1):1–19. doi: 10.1016/j.acn.2007.09.005

[19] Laatu S, Revonsuo A, Hämäläinen P, Ojanen V, Ruutiainen J: Visual object recognition in multiple sclerosis. J Neurol Sci. 2001;185(2):77–88. doi: 10.1016/S0022-510X(01)00461-0

[20] Kurtzke JF. Rating neurologic impairment in multiple sclerosis: an expanded disability status scale (EDSS). Neurology. 1983;33(11):1444–1452. doi: 10.1212/WNL.33.11.1444

[21] Potagas C, Giogkaraki E, Koutsis G, Mandellos D, Tsirempolou E, Sfagos C, Vassilopoulos D: Cognitive impairment in different MS subtypes and clinically isolated syndromes. J Neurol Sci. 2008;267(1–2):100–106. doi: 10.1016/j.jns.2007.10.002

[22] Denney DR, Sworowski LA, Lynch SG: Cognitive impairment in three subtypes of multiple sclerosis. Arch Clin Neuropsychol. 2005;20(8):967–981. doi: 10.1016/j.acn.2005.04.012

[23] Evangelou N, Konz D, Esiri MM, Smith S, Palace J, Matthews PM: Regional axonal loss in the corpus callosum correlates with cerebral white matter lesion volume and

distribution in multiple sclerosis. Brain. 2000;123 (Pt 9):1845–1849. doi: 10.1093/brain/123.9.1845

[24] Mainero C, Caramia F, Pozzilli C, Pisani A, Pestalozza I, Borriello G, Bozzao L, Pantano P: fMRI evidence of brain reorganization during attention and memory tasks in multiple sclerosis. Neuroimage. 2004; 21(3): 858–867. doi: 10.1016/j.neuroimage.2003.10.004

[25] Calabrese M, Rinaldi F, Grossi P, Gallo P: Cortical pathology and cognitive impairment in multiple sclerosis. Expert Rev Neurother. 2011;11(3):425–432. doi: 10.1586/ern.10.155

[26] Batista S, Zivadinov R, Hoogs M, Bergsland N, Heininen-Brown M, Dwyer MG, Weinstock-Guttman B, Benedict RH: Basal ganglia, thalamus and neocortical atrophy predicting slowed cognitive processing in multiple sclerosis. J Neurol. 2012; 259(1):139–146. doi: 10.1007/s00415-011-6147-1

[27] Benedict RH, Hussein S, Englert J, Dwyer MG, Abdelrahman N, Cox JL, Munschauer FE, Weinstock-Guttman B, Zivadinov R: Cortical atrophy and personality in multiple sclerosis. Neuropsychology. 2008;22(4):432–441. doi: 10.1037/0894-4105.22.4.432

[28] Benedict RH, Ramasamy D, Munschauer F, Weinstock-Guttman B, Zivadinov R: Memory impairment in multiple sclerosis: correlation with deep grey matter and mesial temporal atrophy. J Neurol Neurosurg Psychiatry. 2009;80(2):201–206. doi: 10.1136/jnnp.2008.148403

[29] Calabrese P, Penner IK: Cognitive dysfunctions in multiple sclerosis–a "multiple disconnection syndrome"? J Neurol. 2007;254 Suppl 2:II18–II21. doi: 10.1007/s00415-008-0901-z

[30] Feinstein A: Neuropsychiatric syndromes associated with multiple sclerosis. J Neurol. 2007;254 Suppl 2:II73–II76. doi: 10.1007/s00415-008-0901-z

[31] Javůrková A, Amlerová J, Raudenská J: Long-term observation of cognitive, emotional and behavioral changes in patient with multiple sclerosis—a case report (In Czech). Cesk Slov Neurol N. 2014;77(4):501–504

[32] Vickrey BG, Hays RD, Harooni R, Myers LW, Ellison GW: A health-related quality of life measure for multiple sclerosis. Qual Life Res. 1995;4(3):187–206.

[33] Fischer JS, LaRocca NG, Miller DM, Ritvo PG, Andrews H, Paty D: Recent developments in the assessment of quality of life in multiple sclerosis (MS). Mult Scler. 1999;5(4):251–259. doi: 10.1177/135245859900500410

[34] Patti F, Leone C, D'Amico E: Treatment options of cognitive impairment in multiple sclerosis. Neurol Sci. 2010;31(Suppl 2):S265–S269. doi: 10.1007/s10072-010-0438-7

[35] Kalb , R, Reitman, N: Multiple Sclerosis: A model of Psychosocial Support [Internet]. 2012. http://www.nationalmssociety.org/NationalMSSociety/media/MSNationalFiles/Brochures/Book-A-Model-of-Psychosocial-Support.pdf

[36] Benedict RH, Cookfair D, Gavett R, Gunther M, Munschauer F, Garg N, Weinstock-Guttman B: Validity of the minimal assessment of cognitive function in multiple sclerosis (MACFIMS). J Int Neuropsychol Soc. 2006;12(4):549–558

7

Multiple Sclerosis and its Relationship with Oxidative Stress, Glutathione Redox System, ATPase System and Membrane Fluidity

Genaro G. Ortiz, Fermín P. Pacheco-Moisés, Erandis D. Torres-Sánchez, Tanya E. Sorto-Gómez, Mario Mireles-Ramírez, Alfredo León-Gil, Héctor González-Usigli, Luis J. Flores-Alvarado, Erika D. González-Renovato, Angelica L. Sánchez-López, Margarita Cid-Hernández and Irma E. Velázquez-Brizuela

Abstract

Multiple sclerosis (MS) is an autoimmune disease of the central nervous system (CNS) with a focus on inflammation, demyelination, and damage to axons leading to neurological deficits. MS pathology is associated with excessive reactive oxygen species (ROS) and generation of reactive nitrogen species (RNS), causing oxidative/nitrosative stress. Deregulation of glutathione homeostasis and alterations in glutathione-dependent enzymes are implicated in MS. Reactive oxygen species enhance both monocyte adhesion and migration across brain endothelial cells. In addition, ROS can activate the expression of the nuclear transcription factor-kappa, which upregulates the expression of many genes involved in MS, such as tumor necrosis factor-α and nitric oxide synthase, among others, leading to mitochondrial dysfunction and energy deficits that result in mitochondrial and cellular calcium overload. Loss of mitochondrial membrane potential can increase the release of cytochrome c, one pathway that leads to neuronal apoptosis. Clinical studies suggest that omega-3 long-chain polyunsaturated fatty acids (PUFAs) including eicosapentaenoic acid (EPA) and docosahexaenoic acid (DHA) have anti-inflammatory, antioxidant, and neuroprotective effects in MS and animal models of MS. Here, we review the relationship of oxidative stress, the glutathione redox system, the ATPase system, and membrane fluidity with the development of MS. In addition, we describe the main findings of a clinical trial conducted with relapsing-remitting MS patients who received a diet supplemented with 4 g/day of fish oil or olive oil. The effects of PUFAs supplementation on the parameters indicated above are analyzed in this work.

Keywords: multiple sclerosis, oxidative stress, mitochondria, membrane fluidity, ATPase

1. Introduction

Multiple sclerosis (MS) is a chronic inflammatory demyelinating disease of the central nervous system (CNS) with partially known etiology. It is the most common cause of neurological disability in young adults. Nutrition is commonly accepted as one of the possible environmental factors involved in the pathogenesis of MS. Omega-3 polyunsaturated fatty acids (PUFAs) such as eicosapentaenoic acid (EPA) and docosahexaenoic acid (DHA) are fatty acids that possess several carbon–carbon double bonds. A diet supplemented with PUFAs has clinical and biochemical effects in patients with autoimmune diseases such as MS. Eicosapentaenoic acid and DHA are found in high proportions in fish oil, and these molecules may have anti-inflammatory, antithrombotic, antioxidant, immunomodulatory functions, and neuroprotective effects on the synaptogenesis and biogenesis of the neuronal membrane. Oxidative stress (OS) that is characterized by excessive production of reactive oxygen species and a reduction in antioxidant defense mechanisms have been implicated in the pathogenesis of MS. In consequence, a reduction in this phenomenon could be beneficial for MS patients [1]. In this work, we describe the relationship of several oxidative stress markers (glutathione redox system, mitochondrial ATPase activity, and membrane fluidity) with the development of MS. Furthermore, we describe the main findings of a clinical trial conducted with relapsing–remitting MS patients who received a diet supplemented with 4 g/day of fish oil or olive oil.

Pathologically, MS is characterized by perivenous infiltration of lymphocytes and macrophages in the brain parenchyma. There are four clinical manifestations of MS: relapsing–remitting, primary progressive, secondary progressive, and progressive-relapsing. The MS lesions are typically scattered, and the clinical picture can vary from a benign self-limiting disorder to severe and highly disabling disease. MS is a multifactorial disease involving genetic, immunological, and environmental factors that trigger the autoimmune process leading to the pathological changes of the disease. In this regard, it has been proposed that a viral infection in which self-antigens that generate molecular mimicry with myelin proteins cause a loss of tolerance against it, which results in the destruction of myelin mediated by activated T lymphocytes in white matter of the brain and sometimes extending into the gray matter, resulting in defects in the conduction of nerve impulses that leads to symptoms, depending on the affected site of the brain or spinal cord [1] (**Figure 1**).

According to the areas of myelin destruction, sensory or motor symptoms are affected (balance or vision disorders). The symptoms can change between an "outbreak" or relapse (emergence of new neurological symptoms or worsening of previous ones) and remission. Demyelinating lesions or "plaques" of different sizes and locations are spread throughout the CNS, and the onset of symptoms and response to treatment is unique to each patient [2].

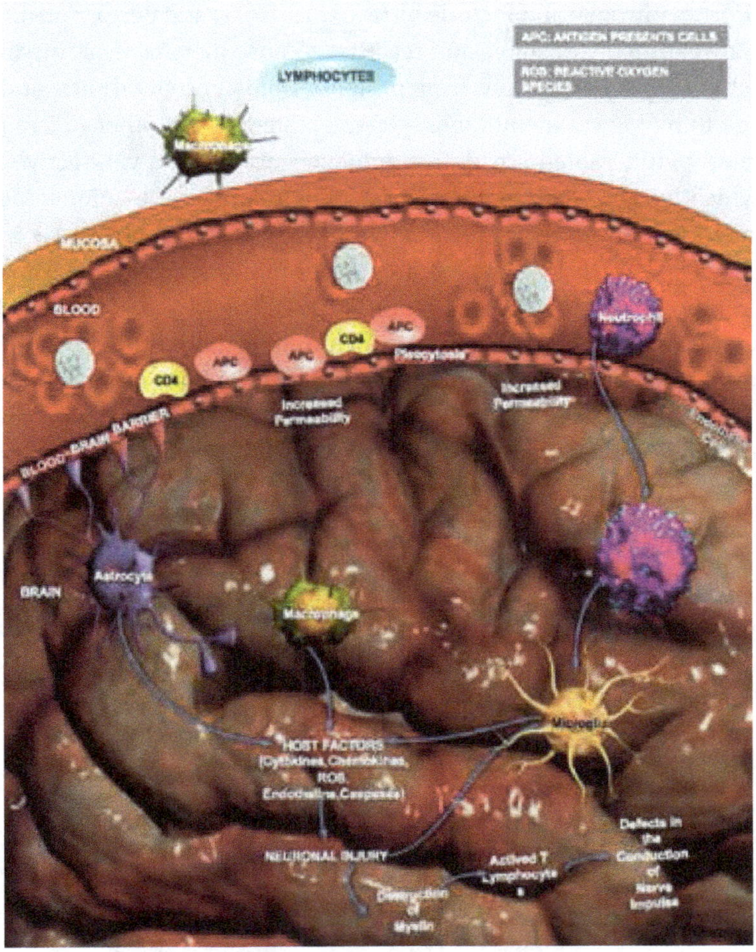

Figure 1. Immune-mediated destruction of myelin components in multiple sclerosis. Pathway Builder Online Tool was used to draw the figure [27].

2. Oxidative stress and multiple sclerosis

OS is a cellular state where the homeostasis of redox reactions is altered when the production of reactive oxygen (ROS) and reactive nitrogen species (RNS) exceed their elimination. These reactive species are generated, among other causes, by oxidative metabolism. Neurons of the CNS are very active in oxidative metabolism, as they are constantly exposed to low-to-moderate levels of ROS, and these species are removed by antioxidants (melatonin, vitamin D, vitamin E, glutathione) and antioxidant enzymes (superoxide dismutase, catalase, glutathione peroxidase, etc.). In chronic inflammatory diseases, such as MS, antioxidant defenses are overcome, which leads to oxidative stress [3].

Collectively, the ROS are reactive species derived from oxygen that include the superoxide anion (O^-), hydrogen peroxide (H_2O_2), and the hydroxyl radical (•OH). The RNS are reactive species derived from nitrogen and include nitric oxide (NO•) and peroxynitrite ($ONOO^-$). The ROS and RNS are extremely unstable and reactive because they have an unpaired electron in their outer orbital. They take electrons from proteins, lipids, carbohydrates, and nucleic acids, causing damage to biological membranes, genetic material, and other macromolecules. The CNS is particularly vulnerable to oxidative damage since it has a very active mitochondrial metabolism, which leads to high levels of intracellular superoxide anions. Moreover, oligodendrocytes have low levels of antioxidant enzymes and a high concentration of iron. Unsaturated fatty acids are the most vulnerable to free radicals, and because myelin has a high lipid-to-protein ratio, it is a preferred target of ROS [4]. The ROS are generated by a number of cellular oxidative and metabolic processes including activity of the enzymes of the mitochondrial respiratory chain, xanthine oxidase, NADPH oxidase, monoamine oxidases, and metabolism of arachidonic acid (AA) mediated by the activity of lipoxygenases (LOX), and ROS are produced primarily by leakage of electrons in the mitochondrial respiratory chain [3].

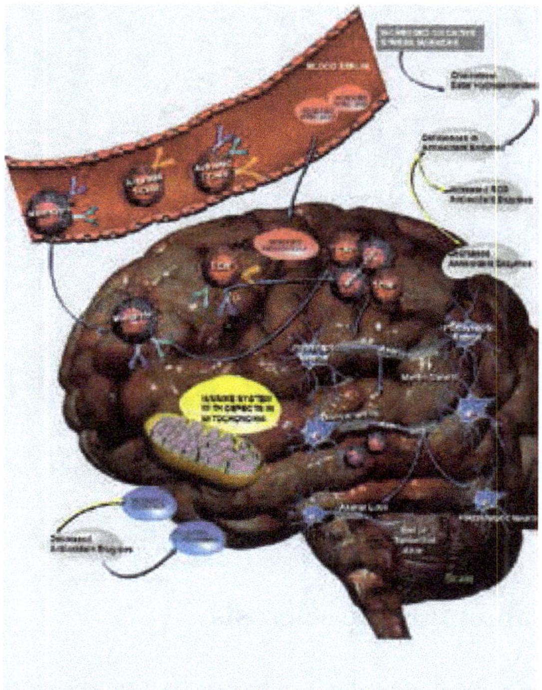

Figure 2. Oxidative stress levels are directly related to the progression of MS. Pathway Builder Online Tool was used to draw the figure [27].

Numerous studies in MS patients have shown an increase in the production of OS markers (such as cholesteryl ester hydroperoxides) and lower levels of uric acid (a $ONOO^-$ scavenger). These changes are accompanied by significant deficiencies in antioxidant enzymes compared to healthy subjects. The increase in ROS coupled with decreased antioxidant capacity is not enough to entirely explain the pathogenesis of MS [4, 5]. Other reports suggest that the loss of myelin nerve sheath is possible because the immune system participates in combination with defects in the mitochondria, and these defects cause the generation of ROS and RNS. Macrophages and monocytes release mediators of OS that degrade the unsaturated fatty acids. The ROS have also been implicated as a mediator of demyelination of axonal damage in MS and experimental autoimmune encephalomyelitis (EAE) [6]. It is important to mention that in assessing platelets in MS patients, increased activity of free radicals with decreased levels of important antioxidants such as glutathione and alpha-tocopherol has been reported [7] (**Figure 2**).

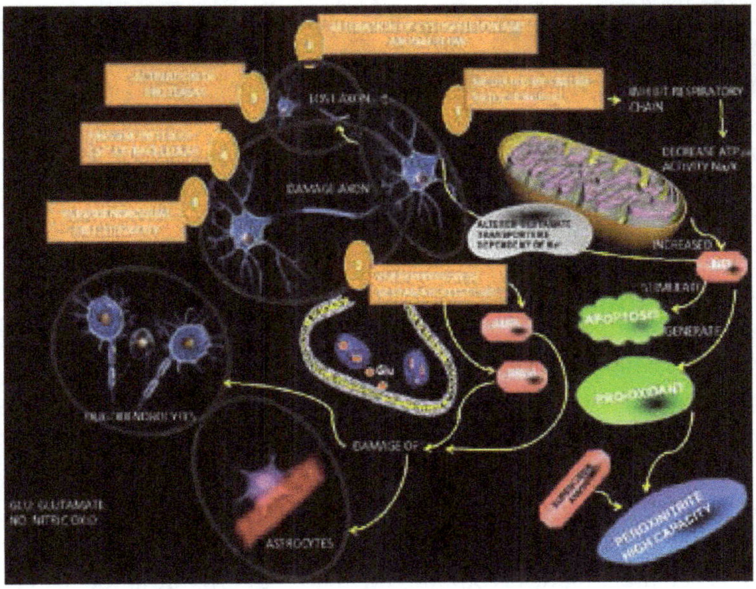

Figure 3. Damage to axons. Pathway Builder Online Tool was used to draw the figure [27].

The molecular mechanisms proposed to explain how ROS could specifically mediate brain damage are the following: (1) The lower levels of antioxidants can promote increased activity of lipoxygenase in CNS stimulating leukotriene production, thereby increasing the immunoinflammatory processes in the cerebral cortex; (2) the damage to myelin can be caused by activation of T cells that may be activated for the presence of free radicals produced by the synthesis route of AA. Then appear the markers of OS associated with reduced activity of superoxide dismutase and the increase in glutamine, followed by increases of •OH and the production of peroxides which ultimately has a negative impact on myelin. After that, the evident changes in mitochondrial activity and finally changes in membrane fluidity (particularly, mitochondrial membranes) appear [8].

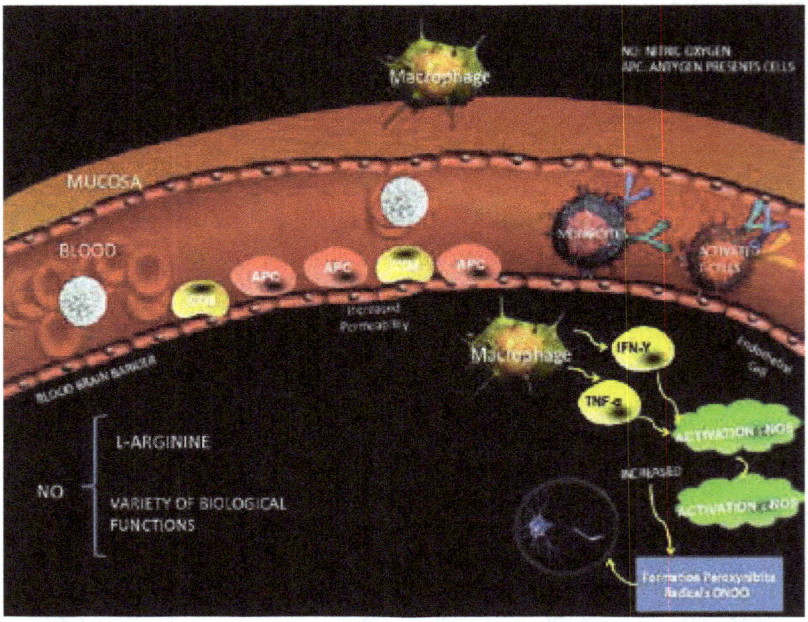

Figure 4. Effect of nitric oxide in inflammation. Pathway Builder Online Tool was used to draw the figure [27].

Paraclinical studies have shown an increased metabolism of the RNS in serum, lymphocytes, and cerebrospinal fluid of MS patients, which correlate to pathology studies. $ONOO^-$ is also closely associated with acute inflammatory lesions [9]. Damage to axons is mediated by the following: (1) failure in mitochondrial energy metabolism due to inhibition of the respiratory chain by nitric oxide, which in turn causes a decrease in Na^+/K^+ ATPase activity and alters Na^+-dependent glutamate transporters, (2) over-expression of glutamate receptors, (3) oligodendroglial excitotoxicity, (4) massive influx of extracellular Ca^{++}, (5) activation of proteases, and (6) impaired axonal transport. These mechanisms produce glutamate excitotoxicity and increased generation of nitric oxide leading to nitrosative stress. Nitric oxide is a highly toxic element that by itself blocks nerve conduction, especially in demyelinated axons, and stimulates apoptosis. When nitric oxide is combined with the superoxide anion, it generates a potent free radical, the pro-oxidant peroxynitrite. Glutamate in turn causes neurodegeneration through the AMPA and NMDA receptors in oligodendrocytes and astrocytes (**Figure 3**). It is possible to explain the role of mediators using an experimental model of autoimmune encephalitis: Protection against the experimental disease occurs after administration of a glutamate antagonist [10].

Under physiologic conditions, nitric oxide is produced from L-arginine by constitutive nitric oxide synthase (cNOS) and participates in a variety of important biological functions such as immunoregulation of inflammatory reactions, the downregulation of tumor necrosis factor (TNF)-α production, MHC II expression in macrophages, induction of apoptosis in CD4 cells, physiological regulation of the mitochondrial respiratory chain, inhibition of antigen presentation, and leukocyte adhesion and migration. However, during inflammatory reactions, exposure of macrophages to interferon (IFN)-γ and TNF-α results in the activation of the inducible isoenzyme of NOS (iNOS), which increases up to 10 times the levels of nitric oxide. Nitric oxide facilitates the formation of peroxynitrite radicals. Only cells capable of generating a high flow of NO• have the potential for causing nitrosative stress. The role of nitric oxide in MS is therefore complex, and in fact, peroxynitrite is definitely more toxic than nitric oxide [9] (**Figure 4**).

3. Reactive oxygen species, cytokines, and axonal damage in multiple sclerosis

Mechanisms of axonal damage are the consequence of the presence of TNF-α, matrix metalloproteinases (MMPs), ROS, antibodies, increased glutamate, and aspartate, and these molecules cause excitotoxicity in MS patients. Glutamate is increased in MS patients (active lesions) especially in white matter of normal appearance. Mature oligodendrocytes and astrocytes are highly sensitive to glutamate due to the expression of AMPA and NMDA receptors [9]. The myelin sheath can be damaged by cytokines, autoantibodies, ROS, proteolytic enzymes, and phagocytosis. Increased ROS by activated microglia (specialized macrophages of the CNS) during the immune response gives a state of increased lipid peroxidation, and the oligodendrocyte cell is the cell most susceptible to damage by ROS. Myelin degradation may be the result of lipid peroxidation mediated by peroxides, but the role of these specific toxic factors in the pathogenesis of MS remains partially elusive [9].

4. Glutathione system and multiple sclerosis

In a recent study, the oxidation of DNA in the nucleus of oligodendrocytes and oxidation of lipids in the myelin of oligodendrocytes and axons were observed. This oxidation was associated with the active process of demyelination and neurodegeneration. Active lesions in relapsing-remitting MS (RRMS) and progressive course patients were associated with inflammation, lipid peroxidation, and DNA oxidation [11]. Similarly, Ortiz et al. [12] observed an increase in serum lipid peroxides and nitrite/nitrate levels and the activity of glutathione peroxidase in patients with RRMS compared to healthy individuals.

Reduced ubiquinone and vitamin E levels, and reduced activity of the enzyme glutathione peroxidase in lymphocytes and granulocytes were reported (with a decrease in 51 and 78%, respectively), as well as a decrease in glutathione reductase activity in granulocytes (27%) and lymphocytes (8%) [13]. In contrast, in 2012, Tasset et al. [14] found an increase in activity of the glutathione reductase in patients with RRMS when compared to control subjects (1.3 ± 0.9 vs 0.3 ± 0.19, $P < 0.01$), and an increased ratio of reduced glutathione to oxidized glutathione (GSH/GSSG) in these patients (28.2 ± 39.6 vs 4.0 ± 2.9, $P < 0.01$). Similarly, an increase was found in the levels of oxidized glutathione and also increased concentrations of isoprostanes and malondialdehyde (MDA) in patients with MS [15, 16].

4.1. Glutathione deficiency and multiple sclerosis

There are several reports in the literature that relate the decrease or alteration of glutathione (GSH) metabolism with several neurodegenerative diseases. Biochemical analysis of postmortem brains has provided evidence for the generation of oxidative stress during the course of the disease since the total GSH content is reduced by 40–50% compared to controls. Also in several brain regions, we have found increased levels of lipid peroxidation [17]. The ratio GSH/GSSG (usually 10:1) is considered consistent with the concept of oxidative stress as an important part in the pathogenesis of MS. Moreover, low concentrations of GSH appear to be an important indicator of oxidative stress during the progression of MS. Although the decrease in GSH alone is not responsible for the degeneration of glial cells and neurons, reduced GSH could increase the susceptibility to other stressful factors and contribute to neuronal damage at glia and neuron cells. Glutathione has been reported to protect mitochondrial complex I activity against nitrosative stress, as S-nitrosoglutathione is formed. When this complex increases its content of nitrotyrosine and nitrosothiol groups in response to nitrosative stress, its activity is inhibited and therefore ATP production is diminished, which causes neuronal degeneration [10]. The role of glial cells in generating ROS in MS and the selective vulnerability of neurons is due to activated glial cells surrounding these neurons, as these glial cells are also directly involved in GSH levels. The engagement of the glutathione system in astroglial cells contributes to the reduction in its antioxidant defenses and so poor glial defense could contribute to existing neuronal damage (**Figure 5**) [10]. Furthermore, the specific activities of some enzymes that metabolize GSH are high, as in the case of glutathione peroxidase, glutathione reductase, and glutathione S-transferase. Other products of OS are also elevated, as in the case of 4-hydroxynonenal (4-HNE, a product of lipid peroxidation of polyunsaturated omega-6 fatty acids) [17].

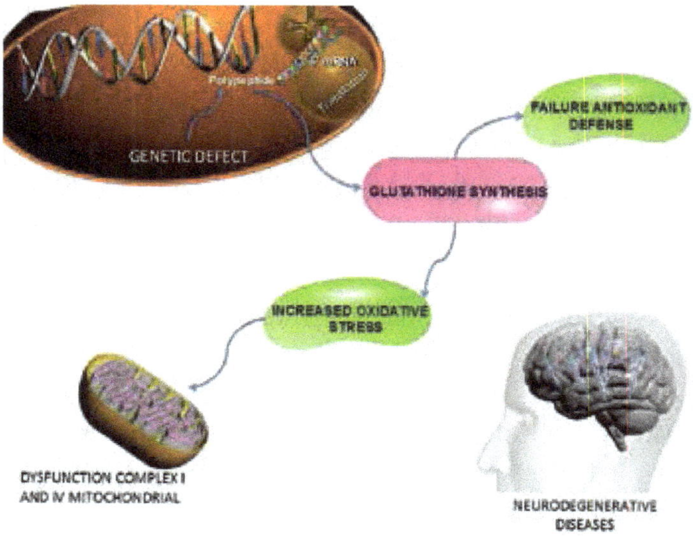

Figure 5. Genetic defect in glutathione synthesis and neurodegenerative diseases. Pathway Builder Online Tool was used to draw the figure [27].

A new proposal is that a genetic defect of glutathione synthesis may be the initial event in the failure of the antioxidant defenses. In neurodegenerative diseases, a decreased GSH level is accompanied by dysfunction of the mitochondrial complex I and complex IV and promotes oxidative stress [18]. We found a significant decrease in GSH levels in the cerebrospinal fluid of patients with this disease, and, in addition, proton magnetic resonance studies have shown a 50% decrease in GSH levels in the frontal cortex of patients with MS (**Figure 5**).

5. Mitochondria

Mitochondria are granular and filamentous organelles found in the cytoplasm of all eukaryotic cells and are the main site of adenosine triphosphate (ATP) synthesis by the processes of oxidative phosphorylation. These organelles vary in size and shape depending on the source and metabolic status, but are often ellipsoids of about 5 microns in diameter and 1 micron long. A typical eukaryotic cell contains more than 2,000 mitochondria, which takes up about one-fifth of the cell volume, an amount that is needed to meet the energy demands of the cell. Its main function is the mitochondrial respiration process in which the reducing power produced in the oxidation reactions enters the electron transport chain and energy is captured in the form of adenosine triphosphate (ATP). Mammalian tissues containing more mitochondria are the heart and brain [19]. The mitochondrion is formed by two membranes: the outer membrane and the inner membrane, which is highly folded, and the inner matrix is gel (approximately 50% water) [20].

The outer mitochondrial membrane contains porin, a pore-forming protein that allows diffusion of up to 10 kD molecules). The inner membrane contains approximately 75% protein and 25% lipids by weight, and it is much richer in outer membrane proteins. The inner membrane is permeable only to carbon dioxide (CO_2), oxygen (O_2), and water (H_2O). The passage of metabolites such as ATP, adenosine diphosphate (ADP), pyruvate, calcium ions (Ca^{2+}), and phosphate (PO_4) is regulated by controlling the transport proteins. This controlled permeability allows the generation of ionic gradients and results in the compartmentalization of metabolic functions between the cytoplasm and mitochondria. The inner membrane components of the respiratory chain are responsible for the synthesis of ATP (ATP synthase F_oF_1) [22], where the enzyme complex is housed. The inner membrane is arranged in ridges, giving it a large surface area: A single mitochondrion may have more than 10,000 sets of electron transfer systems (respiratory chain) and ATP synthase molecules distributed throughout the membrane's internal surface [21]. The inner membrane is, from the functional point of view, the most important because it contains the components of the respiratory chain and proteins necessary for the synthesis of ATP [21]. The mitochondrial matrix is the space delimited by the inner membrane and contains the pyruvate dehydrogenase complex and the enzymes of the tricarboxylic acid cycle (TCA), the fatty acid oxidation, and the oxidation of amino acids [21] (**Figure 6**).

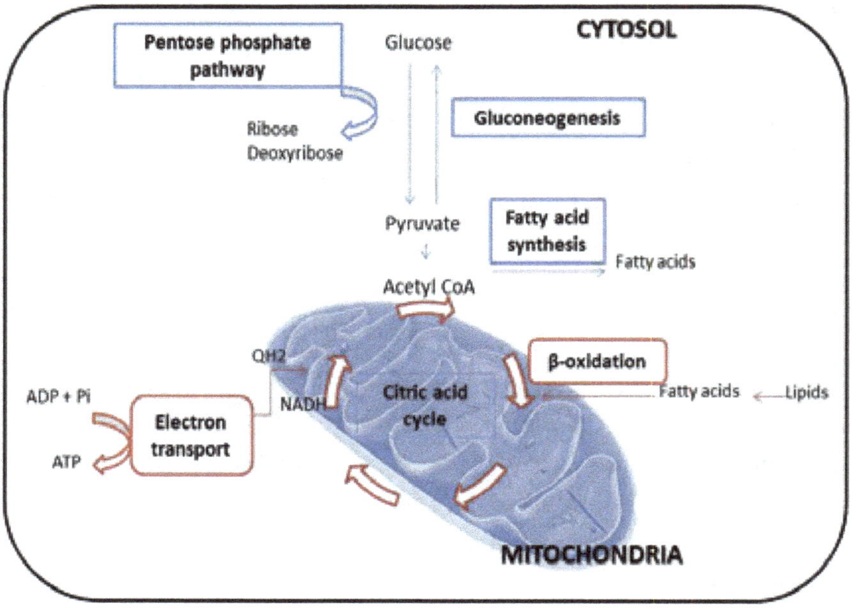

Figure 6. Main mitochondrial metabolic pathways. An important component of metabolic regulation is specialization. Mitochondria have a role in biosynthesis, catabolism, and energy metabolism, including citric acid cycle, oxidative phosphorylation, and fatty acid breakdown pathways.

The chemical energy required for cellular activities such as biosynthesis, transportation of ions and molecules, and mechanical work comes from ATP. Mitochondria generate more than 90% of the energy needed for the proper functioning of tissues that are highly dependent on aerobic metabolism, such as the brain and heart. This subcellular organelle provides the energy necessary for the production of ATP [22]. Depending on cell type and metabolic state, mitochondria consume approximately 90–95% of the oxygen consumed by the cell. The energy of this process, in which electrons are transferred from the substrates of the TCA to oxygen, is coupled to vectorial transport of H^+ from the mitochondrial matrix space [22].

The electron carriers, reduced nicotinamide dinucleotide adenine (NADH) and reduced flavin dinucleotide adenine ($FADH_2$), originating mainly in the TCA cycle, confer the energy that electrons carry. This energy is released gradually along the respiratory chain in the mitochondrial inner membrane. In this membrane, an exchange of electrons between the enzymatic complexes is given by NADH or $FADH_2$ [20].

The complexes are as follows: I (NADH-ubiquinone reductase), II (succinate-ubiquinone reductase), III (ubiquinol-cytochrome c reductase), IV (cytochrome oxidase), and V (ATP synthase complex F_0F_1) [20]. Electron transport is carried out by complexes I, III, and IV that produce a flow of electrons accompanied by a movement of protons from the mitochondrial matrix to the intermembrane space (space between the inner and outer mitochondrial membrane). This produces a difference in proton concentration and a difference in charge across the membrane [20]. The proton-motive force generated thereby drives protons through the F_0F_1-ATP synthase, allowing condensation of a phosphate group to ADP, with the formation of ATP [23]. Meanwhile, the complex F_0F_1-ATP synthase is an enzyme located in the inner membrane of the mitochondria, responsible for ATP synthesis from ADP and a phosphate group (Pi), and the energy is supplied by a flow of protons (H^+). The difference between the terms ATPase and ATP synthase is that the enzyme has a dual function: It breaks down ATP to ADP and Pi (activated ATPase), and it also allows for catalyzing Pi binding of ADP using the proton gradient for ATP synthesis (ATP synthase activity). As complex V has both functions, we can name it indiscriminately when speaking in general terms of the enzyme [23]. This enzyme is constituted by two components: a soluble portion (F_1), located in aqueous medium, and another portion (F_o), which is lipid soluble. The F_o part is inserted into the lipid bilayer and is sensitive to the antibiotic oligomycin (**Figure** 7).

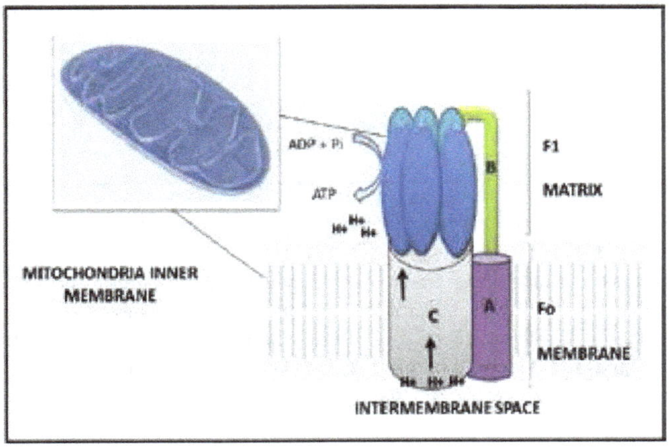

Figure 7. ATP synthase complex structure. The ATP synthase complex plays a central role in energy transduction in living cells that uses energy released by the movement of protons down a transmembrane electrochemical gradient to drive the synthesis of ATP. This enzyme is located in the inner membrane of mitochondria and is constituted by two parts: a soluble portion (F1) in aqueous medium and another portion (Fo) lipid soluble. The Fo part is inserted into the lipid bilayer.

On the other hand, pathophysiological features exhibited the association between mitochondrial dysfunction, decreased activity of complex I and complex IV of the electron transport chain, and the glutathione system in MS [23].

6. Mitochondria and multiple sclerosis

In acute phases of the disease, axonal degeneration correlates with the severity of inflammation. This type of injury has been used in an experimental model of autoimmune encephalomyelitis (EAE), where acute mitochondrial damage within axons is detected and later suffers from focal damage as a preliminary pathological step of axonal damage [15].

Complex IV of the mitochondrial electron transport chain has a binding site for O_2 (The final acceptor in the respiratory chain) and catalyzes the reduction in O_2 to H_2O. Interestingly, nitric oxide inhibits mitochondrial respiration by reacting with either the reduced or the oxidized binuclear site of cytochrome c oxidase, leading to ATP depletion. In cases of excessive nitric oxide production, complete inhibition of cytochrome c oxidase has been shown to contribute to pathology.

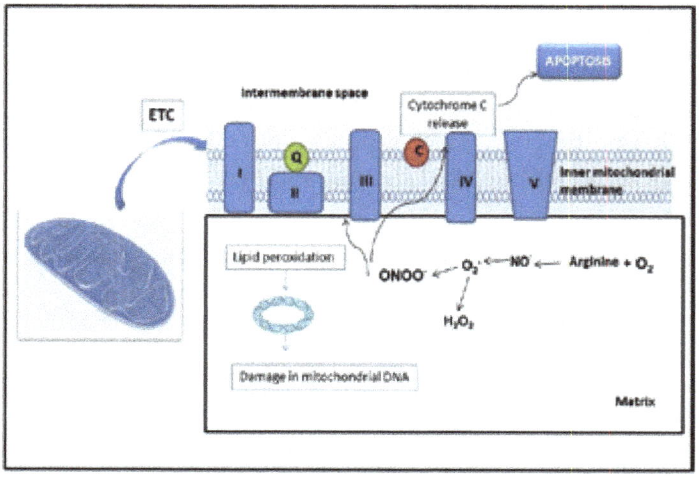

Figure 8. Association of mitochondrial electron transport chain with oxidative stress. The mitochondrial electron transport chain (ETC), which is composed of four multiprotein complexes named complex I–IV, has been recognized as one of the major cellular generators of free radicals. Leakage of electrons directly from the intermediate electron carriers generates reactive oxygen species that leads to membrane lipid peroxidation, mitochondrial DNA damage, and the release of cytochrome C to the cytosol triggering apoptosis.

At the same time, interrupting the electron transport chain by binding of NO to complex IV increases electron release, thus facilitating the formation of reactive oxygen species, firstly superoxide anion and subsequently H_2O_2 and OH.·Peroxynitrite has a direct effect on mitochondria leading to lipid peroxidation of membrane lipids and thus damaging the complexes of the respiratory chain and mitochondrial DNA. Opening of permeability transition pores and release of cytochrome C from mitochondria initiate apoptosis (**Figure 8**).

At the stage of acute inflammation, a set of mechanisms that alter mitochondrial function is produced. The energy deficit causes structural and functional damage to macromolecules by increased ROS that ultimately leads to severe axonal damage. In these events, the mitochondria has an important role; therefore, if we know what the mechanisms involved in glial and neuronal alterations are, we must be able to identify the elements that can be used as effector elements and design drugs to control and reduced harm during the stage of relapse [14].

Many demyelinated axons survive during a relapse, and these can become chronically demyelinated axons, in which case axonal mitochondria develop compensatory mechanisms to cope with the lack of myelin. There are reports in which inactive lesions from chronic demyelinated axons of patients with MS are observed. In such reports, they have found an increase in the activity of mitochondrial complex IV and increased synphilin anchoring protein [19]. However, axons progressively degenerate in chronic lesions of MS patients. In the absence of myelin, redistribution of Na^+ occurs to maintain the transmission of nerve impulses that increases energy demand, and this produces a situation of "virtual hypoxia." At the end, the demand exceeds the capacity of axonal mitochondria to produce enough ATP, which causes an increase in the concentration of Ca^{2+} in the axon. Ca^{2+} pumping and extended levels of intramitochondrial calcium leads to opening pores, rupture of the outer mitochondrial membrane, and release of cytochrome C, finally leading to apoptosis (**Figure 8**).

One of the questions we have not answered is: Why are mitochondria helpless and overwhelmed by the energy demand and how does this happen? Are the axons unable to maintain stable mitochondrial activity in demyelination?. This reflects the inability of the cell to carry and generate mitochondria. Dutta et al. [23] have shown decreased gene expression of 26 nuclear-encoded subunits of the oxidative phosphorylation chain in non-demyelinated motor cortex from MS patients, which coincided with a significant reduction in activity of NADH dehydrogenase and ubiquinol-cytochrome c reductase . In the progressive phase of MS, it is postulated that chronically demyelinated axons are unable to maintain mitochondrial function, and thus, a deficit of ATP synthesis coupled with oxidative stress results in irreversible axonal damage.

7. Effect of fish oil (Omega3) and olive oil on membrane fluidity, ATPase activity in relapsing-remitting multiple sclerosis.

The mechanism of action for omega-3 PUFAs is suggested to be attributed to immunomodulation and antioxidant action [24]. For instance, omega-3 PUFAs decrease the production of inflammatory mediators (eicosanoids, cytokines, and ROS) and the expression of adhesion molecules. They both act directly by replacing AA as an eicosanoid substrate and inhibiting AA metabolism and indirectly by altering the expression of inflammatory genes through effects on transcription factor activation. Omega-3 PUFAs also give rise to anti-inflammatory mediators (resolvins and protectins) [25]. Effects of resolvins and protectins include reducing neutrophil trafficking, cytokine, and ROS regulation and lowering the magnitude of the inflammatory response [26].

Previously, we developed a twelve-month randomized double-blind controlled clinical trial in 50 patients with relapsing-remitting MS. Patients received an oral dose of 4 g/day of fish oil (containing a total of 800 mg of EPA and 1600 mg of DHA) or olive oil. Fasting blood samples were collected at baseline and after 6 and 12 months of the trial, in order to evaluate the effect of consumption of omega-3 PUFAs on some markers of oxidative stress at the peripheral level. The initial findings of this work were the decrease in serum levels of TNFα, IL-1β, IL-6, and nitric oxide metabolites compared with the placebo group [27].

On the other hand, after 12 months of intervention, supplementation with omega-3 PUFAs significantly enhanced the quantities of serum omega-3 highly unsaturated fatty acids compared with baseline values. Additionally, the levels of medium-chain monounsaturated fatty acids were significantly decreased. The olive oil supplementation induced minor decreases in EPA and DHA levels after 12 months of intervention. There were significant increases in both EPA and DHA in the group given fish oil supplementation compared to the control group receiving olive oil. These increases were associated with a concomitant decrease in AA. Consequently, the omega-3 fatty acid index in the fish oil group increased significantly, and the ratios of n-6/n-3 and AA/EPA were decreased [28].

No differences in glutathione reductase activity and content of reduced glutathione, oxidized glutathione, and oxidized/reduced glutathione ratio were seen after 12 months of supplementation with omega-3 PUFAs. However, a trend in favor of omega-3 PUFAs supplementation was observed in GSSG levels and glutathione reductase activity at 12 months of intervention between the study groups [28].

A steady decrease in mitochondrial ATPase activity in platelets was observed in the groups given omega-3 fatty acid and the control group receiving olive oil. Membrane fluidity of platelets was significantly reduced in MS patients. Interestingly, a significant increase in platelet membrane fluidity was observed in the groups receiving omega-3 fatty acid and the control group receiving olive oil. As well, the fluidity of erythrocyte membranes was unchanged for both treatments (Unpublished results).

Epidemiological and experimental studies suggest an increased incidence of MS in populations with a high intake of saturated fats mainly from animal sources. Therefore, by consuming a diet high in fatty acids, without an appropriate number of unsaturates, a shift is produced in the integrity and functionality of the membrane [29]. An optimal balance in the consumption of fatty acids includes 35% polyunsaturated fatty acids and 65% saturated fatty acids, and the appropriate proportion of PUFA to maintain membrane balance is 50% omega-3 with 50% omega-6. The above ratio was a factor that inactivated the CD4 autoreactive cells in the CNS, a phenomenon that prevents the production of proinflammatory cytokines and free radicals [30].

Membrane fluidity depends on the temperature, the ratio of saturated/PUFA fatty acids, the presence of "lipid rafts," and the proportion of cholesterol present at the membrane [31]. Previous studies in patients with rheumatoid arthritis had increased cell membrane rigidity compared to membranes from those receiving immunomodulatory treatment. Our results showed diminished platelet membrane fluidity in MS patients and that proper membrane fluidity is restored with treatment of omega3 PUFAs. The increase in platelet membrane fluidity is directly related to the incorporation of PUFA's. Furthermore, the increase in membrane fluidity is accompanied with a significant decrease in mitochondrial ATPase activity. This ensures that the activity of ATP synthesis in mitochondria remains elevated.

8. Conclusions

The inflammatory process seen in MS is due to an excess production of pro-inflammatory cytokines, which leads to increased secretion of ROS. Oxidative stress plays a preponderant, key role in the pathogenesis of MS. Reactive oxygen species generated by macrophages have been implicated as mediators of demyelination and axonal damage in EAE and MS. The main findings of a clinical trial conducted with relapsing-remitting MS patients who received a diet supplemented with 4 g/day of fish oil or olive oil are the following:

1. Fish oil supplementation resulted in a high increase in proportions of EPA and DHA, leading to a decrease in AA concentrations as well as the AA/EPA ratio. These changes in fatty acids are indicative of a reduction in the production of inflammatory eicosanoids from AA and an increase in anti-inflammatory mediators such as resolvins and protectins.
2. No differences in glutathione reductase activity, content of reduced and oxidized glutathione, and GSH/GSSG ratio were seen after 12 months of supplementation. However, fish oil supplementation resulted in a smaller increase in GR compared with the control group. In addition, there was a significant change in glutathione reductase activity within subjects in the fish oil group after 6 months of treatment, while no significant differences within subjects were observed in the control group, suggesting a possible effect of fish oil on antioxidant defense mechanisms of the cell. Although glutathione reductase activity was not significantly different between the groups, fish oil supplementation resulted in a smaller increase in GR compared with the control group, suggesting a possible antioxidant effect of fish oil supplementation.
3. Membrane fluidity of platelets was significantly reduced in MS patients. That membrane property steadily increased in the groups given omega-3 fatty acid and the control group receiving olive oil. The increases in membrane fluidity of platelets were associated with a decrease in mitochondrial ATPase. As well, the fluidity of erythrocyte membranes was unchanged for both treatments (unpublished results).

Author details

Genaro G. Ortiz[1*], Fermín P. Pacheco-Moisés[2], Erandis D. Torres-Sánchez[1], Tanya E. Sorto-Gómez[1], Mario Mireles-Ramírez[3], Alfredo León-Gil[3], Héctor González-Usigli[3], Luis J. Flores-Alvarado[4], Erika D. González-Renovato[1], Angelica L. Sánchez-López[1], Margarita Cid-Hernández[2] and Irma E. Velázquez-Brizuela[5]

*Address all correspondence to: genarogabriel@yahoo.com

1 Laboratory of Mitochondria-Oxidative Stress and Pathology, Neurosciences Division, Occidental Biomedical Research Center, The Mexican Social Security Institute, Guadalajara, Jalisco, México

2 Department of Chemistry, Centre of Exact Sciences and Engineering, University of Guadalajara, Guadalajara, Jalisco, México

3 Department of Neurology, Sub-specialty Medical Unit, National Occidental Medical Center, The Mexican Social Security Institute, Guadalajara, Jalisco, México

4 Department of Biochemistry, Health Sciences Center, University of Guadalajara, Guadalajara, Jalisco, México

5 Health Sciences Center, University of Guadalajara, Guadalajara, Jalisco, México

References

[1] Mejía BL, Agudelo RC, Gómez HJC, Cabrera HD. Genética de la EM: An epidemiological and molecular perspective. Archivos de medicina 2009;5(1:5).

[2] Lassmann H. The pathology of MS and its evolution. Phil Trans R. Soc. Lond B 1999;354:1635–40.

[3] Coronado HM, Vega y León S, Gutiérrez TR, García FB, Díaz G. omega-3 and omega-6 fatty acids Nutrición, Bioquímica y Salud 2009;REB 25(3):72–79.

[4] Reinhart GA. (1996), Review of w-3 Fatty acids and dietary influences on tissue concentration en recent advances en canine and feline nutritional research. Edit Carey D. P., Ohio 235–242.

[5] Villegas P, Vidal S, Bray GM, Aguayo T. (2005), Axonal regeneration and synapse formation in the superior colliculus by retinal ganglion cells in the adult rat. Journal of Neuroscience 2005;7:2894–2909.

[6] Valenzuela A, Nieto S. Ácido docosahexanoico (DHA) en el desarrollo fetal y en la nutrición materno infantil. Revista Médica de Chile 2001;129:1203–1211.

[7] Bazan G, Bodker M, Serhan N, Marcheselli V, Lukiw W. A role for docosahexaenoic acid-derived neuroprotectin D1 in neural cells survival and Alzheimer disease. Journal Clinic Investigation 2005;115:2774–2780.

[8] White P. (1995) Essential fatty acids in medicine veterinary, Bayer AG. S Business group animal health supplement, Germany.

[9] Li S, Vana AC, Ribeiro R, Zhang Y. Distinct role of nitric oxide and peroxynitrite in mediating oligodendrocyte toxicity in culture and in experimental autoimmune encephalomyelitis. Neuroscience 2011;184:107–119.

[10] Ferreira B, Mendes F, Osório N, et al. Glutathione in multiple sclerosis. Br J Biomed Sci 2013;70(2):75–79.

[11] Fischer MT, Sharma R, Lim JL et al. NADPH oxidase expression in active multiple sclerosis lesions in relation to oxidative tissue damage and mitochondrial injury. Brain: A Journal of Neurology 2012;135:886–899.

[12] Ortiz GG, Macias-Islas MA, Pacheco-Moises FP, et al. Oxidative stress is increased in serum from Mexican patients with relapsing-remitting multiple sclerosis. Dis Markers 2009;26:35–39.

[13] Jensen GE, Clausen J. Glutathione peroxidase and reductase, glucose-6-phosphate dehydrogenase and catalase activities in multiple sclerosis. Journal of the Neurological Sciences, 1984;63:45–53.

[14] Tasset I, Agüera E, Sánchez-López F, et al. Peripheral oxidative stress in relapsing–remitting multiple sclerosis. Clinical Biochemistry 2012;45:440–444.

[15] Greco A, Minghetti L, Sette G, et al. Cerebrospinal fluid isoprostane shows oxidative stress in patients with multiple sclerosis. Neurology 1999 Nov 10;53(8):1876–1879.

[16] Karg E, Klivényi P, Németh I, et al. Nonenzymatic antioxidants of blood in multiple sclerosis. J Neurol. 1999;246(7):533–539.

[17] Hauser S, Oksenberg J. The neurobiology of multiple sclerosis: genes, inflammation, and neurodegeneration. Neuron 2006;52:61–76.

[18] Correale J, Tenembaum S. Myelin basic protein and myelin oligodendrocyte glycoprotein T-cell repertoire in childhood and juvenile multiple sclerosis. Multiple sclerosis 2006;12:1–9.

[19] Westermann B. (2002), Merging mitochondria matters: Cellular role and molecular machinery of mitochondrial fusion. European Molecular Biology Organization, 2002;3(6):527–531.

[20] Frey Terrence G, Mannella Carmen A. The internal structure of mitochondria, Review. TIBS 2000;Jul;25(7) 319–24

[21] Lehninger (2000) Principles of Biochemistry 3rd, Ed. Worth Publishers, pp. 389, 391, Capitulo 5, Capitulo 8, Capitulo 1, Capitulo 14, Capitulo 19.

[22] Lee CL, Hanay J, Hrachovy R. (2001) Spatial learning deficits without hippocampal loss in a model of early-onset epilepsy. Neuroscience 2001;107:71–84.

[23] Dutta R, McDonough J, Yin X, Peterson J, Chang A, et al. Mitochondrial dysfunction as a cause of axonal degeneration in multiple sclerosis patients. Ann Neurol 2006;59:478–489.

[24] Mehta LR, Dworkin RH, Schwid SR. Polyunsaturated fatty acids and their potential therapeutic role in multiple sclerosis. Nat Clin Pract Neurol 2009;5:82–92.

[25] Calder PC. n-3 Polyunsaturated fatty acids, inflammation, and inflammatory diseases. Am J Clin Nutr 2006;83(6 suppl):1505S–19S.

[26] Serhan CN, Ariel A. Resolvins and protectins in the termination program of acute inflammation. Trends Immunol 2007;28:176–183.

[27] Ramirez-Ramirez V, Macias-Islas MA, Ortiz GG, Pacheco-Moises F, Torres-Sanchez ED, et al. Efficacy of fish oil on serum of TNF-α, IL-1 β, and IL-6 oxidative stress markers in multiple sclerosis treated with interferon beta-1b. Oxid Med Cell Longev. 2013;2013:709493.

[28] Effect of Fish Oil on glutathion redox system in multiple sclerosis. Am J Neurodegenertive Dis 2016; 5(2): 145–151.

[29] Shinitzky M. Membrane fluidity and cellular functions. Physiology of membrane fluidity. Boca Raton: CRC Press 1984;1–151.

[30] Kantarci OH, Weinshenker BG. Natural history of multiple sclerosis. Neurol Clin 2005;23(1):17–38.

[31] Comparán A, Interés de los brotes en la EM, Fisiopatología y tratamiento. Rev Neurol 2003;36:1058–64.

8

Therapeutic and Prophylactic Potential of Vitamin D for Multiple Sclerosis

Sofia F.G. Zorzella-Pezavento, Larissa L.W. Ishikawa, Thais F.C. Fraga-Silva, Luiza A.N. Mimura and Alexandrina Sartori

Abstract

A plethora of investigations demonstrated that vitamin D (VitD) has a broad immunomodulatory potential. It induces tolerogenic dendritic cells *in vitro* leading to the development of regulatory T cells that have a key role in immunomodulation of autoimmune diseases including multiple sclerosis (MS). Studies showed that many MS patients present lower serum levels of VitD than healthy subjects. In addition, VitD supplementation has been associated with a reduced relative risk of developing MS. Considering the alterations in VitD levels in patients and also the immunomodulatory properties of VitD, it would be interesting to evaluate VitD potential as a tolerogenic adjuvant in experimental models of MS. In this context, our research team has been investigating strategies employing VitD to establish an *in vivo* tolerance state toward central nervous system antigens in experimental autoimmune encephalomyelitis (EAE). We observed that the association between a myelin peptide and VitD determined both therapeutic and prophylactic effects on EAE development.

Keywords: vitamin D, multiple sclerosis, experimental autoimmune encephalomyelitis, immunomodulation, myelin peptides

1. Introduction

The immune system is well known by its ability to defend the host against infections. In this sense, it is academically subdivided into innate and adaptive immune responses. Innate immunity is the first defense line and includes the microbicidal activity of macrophages and polymorphonuclear cells. Host defense against microorganisms is dependent upon recognition of pathogen-associated molecular patterns, mainly by toll-like receptors (TLRs) present in these cells. Otherwise, adaptive immunity requires specific antigen recognition by B and T lymphocytes. Differently from B cells that can directly recognize the antigens, T cells require previous antigen processing and interaction of epitopes with major histocompatibility complex proteins that are then expressed at the surface of antigen-presenting cells (APCs) as, for example, dendritic cells (DCs). Due to their strong potential for proliferation and activation, B and T cell activity needs to be regulated. A special T-cell subpopulation called regulatory T (Treg) cell plays a major role in controlling inflammatory immune responses. To maintain its homeostasis, the immune system has to manage a balance between inflammatory and anti-inflammatory responses. The imbalance of these immune responses leads to the development of many diseases such as autoimmune pathologies. In this context, other T-cell subpopulations such as T helper type 1 (Th1) and type 17 (Th17) cells, which are inflammatory, and type 2 cells (Th2), which are predominantly anti-inflammatory, are also involved. Besides its ability to eliminate pathogens and restore the host homeostasis, the immune system has also a mechanism to hamper the development of an immune response against the body's own tissues. This mechanism, called self-tolerance, can be disrupted by the combination of a variety of genetic, environmental, and immunological factors that lead to autoimmunity. The relevance of vitamin D (VitD) in multiple sclerosis (MS), which is an autoimmune disease involving the central nervous system (CNS), is discussed in this chapter.

2. VitD metabolism

The history of VitD is strongly linked to rickets and its treatment with cod liver oil. In 1922, McCollum [1] coined the term vitamin D to refer to the antirachitic factor found in cod liver oil [2]. For this reason and for a long time, the most widely accepted physiological role of VitD was related to calcium and phosphorus metabolism and bone mineralization [3]. However, since the 1980s, many researches implicated VitD on the cardiovascular, endocrine, and central nervous system (CNS), as well as on the immune system physiology. The active form of VitD (1α,25-dihydroxyvitamin D_3) determines pleiotropic effects in human body through binding to vitamin D receptor (VDR), which is a member of the steroid hormone receptor superfamily found in a variety of human cells. The biological effects of VitD can be elicited by non-genomic and genomic mechanisms depending on the cell location of VDR. The non-genomic (rapid) mechanisms consist in VitD direct effect on the cells through membrane VDR binding. These effects include, for example, the activation of protein kinase C in different organs [4]. The genomic mechanism is determined by intracellular VDR that heterodimerizes with retinoic X receptor after binding to active VitD. This heterodimer is then translocated to the nucleus leading to activation or inhibition of a vast diversity of genes [5].

Some of the most important aspects of VitD epidemiology have been established by the scientist Michael Holick and his collaborators. As many people do not have an adequate sunlight exposure due to skin cancer risk, sedentary lifestyle, darker skin, or during the winter in countries far from the equator, there is an increasing number of persons with VitD deficiency around the world [6]. In the past few years, VitD deficiency has been associated with the etiology of many chronic diseases, like Crohn's disease, infections of the upper respiratory tract, cancer, myocardial infarction, Alzheimer's disease, autoimmune diseases, and others [7]. According to current knowledge, VitD serum levels should be between 30 and 100 ng/mL in healthy humans. VitD insufficiency is related to levels between 21 and 29 ng/mL, whereas a pronounced VitD deficiency is considered in individuals whose VitD levels are below 20 ng/mL. On the other hand, serum levels over 150 ng/mL can determine intoxication VitD intoxication [8]. Excessive oral intake of VitD may cause a hypervitaminosis condition with toxic effects such as hypercalcemia and hypercalciuria. Theories concerning the mechanisms of VitD toxicity involve elevated plasma concentration of VitD itself or its metabolites that culminates in overexpression of a variety of genes [9]. Although solubility of vitamins (fat or water) has no direct effect on toxicity, the ability of fat-soluble vitamins such as VitD to accumulate in the adipose tissue determines their higher toxic potential than water-soluble vitamins. For example, subcutaneous fat necrosis releases tissue-accumulated VitD that leads to hypervitaminosis and its toxic effects [10].

The highest amounts of VitD are synthesized by the skin exposed to sunlight. Ultraviolet radiation converts 7-dehydrocholesterol in pre-vitamin D3. Then pre-vitamin D3 suffers a spontaneous thermal isomerization into vitamin D3, named cholecalciferol [11]. Due to this essential role of sunlight, this vitamin has been called "sunshine vitamin" [12]. Smaller amounts of VitD can be obtained from intake of certain foods such as mushrooms, fish, milk, and eggs [13]. To become a metabolically active hormone, cholecalciferol needs to be hydroxylated twice. The first hydroxylation takes place in the liver and converts cholecalciferol into 25-dyhidroxyvitamin D (calcidiol) via the enzyme 25-hydroxilase [14]. Plasma calcidiol levels are usually used as a parameter of VitD status because it increases in proportion to VitD intake [15]. After that, calcidiol binds to a carrier molecule, known as the vitamin D-binding protein, to be systemically transported to tissues that express 1α-hydroxylase (CYP27B1) [16]. The second hydroxylation, which generates the bioactive metabolite 1,25-dihydroxyvitamin D3 (calcitriol), occurs at the renal proximal tubular cells that are rich in CYP27B1 [17]. This reaction involves the sequential reduction of flavoprotein, renal ferredoxin, and cytochrome P-450 [18]. A critical physiological role in skeletal homeostasis is mediated by calcitriol. Concisely, hypocalcemia stimulates parathyroid glands to release parathyroid hormone, which activates renal CYP27B1 enzyme function, resulting in calcitriol production. Besides, parathyroid hormone stimulates osteoclast maturation to release calcium and phosphate from the bones. Calcitriol also reduces renal calcium excretion and increases calcium absorption from foods in the intestine. When normal calcium levels are obtained, calcitriol exerts a feedback regulation in the parathyroid gland, downregulating CYP27B1 activity to avoid VitD intoxication [14]. Besides the kidneys, 1α-hydroxylase has been reported in many tissues including bone, placenta, prostate, and parathyroid gland. In addition, several cancer cells and immune cells, such as macrophages, T lymphocytes, and DCs, are also able to produce this enzyme [19,20].

3. Immunomodulatory properties of VitD

First evidences of VitD role in the immune system regulation date from the 80s. Haq [21] demonstrated that active VitD, but not its non-active form, blocked the production of IL (interleukin)-2 and consequently inhibited T-cell proliferation. Based on this downmodulatory effect, the potential of VitD to increase organ survival in experimental allograft transplantation was also evaluated. First studies in this field were based on the *in vitro* immunosuppressive effects of VitD and its analogs. One of the most evident toxic effects of high VitD doses, which are usually required to avoid transplant rejection, is hypercalcemia. To avoid this and other toxic effects such as bone resorption, many efforts were done to develop synthetic structural analogs of active VitD that still preserved its immunomodulatory properties [22]. When tested *in vivo*, a 20-epi-vitamin D3 analog did not prolong renal allograft survival in Lewis rats and also led to the development of hypercalcemia [23]. These authors emphasized the importance of more experimental studies to evaluate the potential of VitD and its analogs to prevent graft rejection. Later, Hullett et al. [24] successfully demonstrated that Lewis rats orally receiving active VitD presented prolonged survival heart allografts without hypercalcemia. Over the years, a much broader role of VitD in the immune system was disclosed and the mechanisms underlying its immunomodulatory effects were progressively elucidated. Currently, calcitriol is largely known to modulate both innate and adaptive immunity through its binding to VDR, which is present in a multitude of immune cells. Although VitD can bind to both genomic and non-genomic targets, the most important immunomodulatory properties are elicited by genomic mechanisms [25].

It is well known that VitD stimulates the innate immune system by enhancing the antimicrobial ability of monocytes and macrophages. This effect is mainly associated with TLRs activation and increased release of cathelicidin and IL-1β by these cells [26]. Clinical evidences suggested a strong correlation between a poor VitD status and an increased susceptibility to infections. VitD has also been linked to more severe infectious diseases [27–29]. Moreover, Nouari et al. [30] recently demonstrated that active VitD can enhance the microbicidal activity of human monocyte-derived macrophages against *Pseudomonas aeruginosa*.

Conversely, VitD has an inhibitory effect on the adaptive immune system. It directly targets APCs, which are a very important link between the innate and adaptive immunity. In this sense, conventional APCs as DCs are profoundly affected by VitD. The mechanisms underlying the effects of VitD on DC function were recently reviewed by Barragan et al. [31]. *In vitro* treatment with active VitD or its analogs inhibits both differentiation and maturation of human and murine DCs leading to changes in its phenotype and function [32]. The immature or semi-mature state induced by VitD is generally characterized by a decreased expression of co-stimulatory molecules such as CD40, CD80, and CD86. This state determines a tolerogenic DC phenotype associated with reduced IL-12 and increased IL-10 production. The addition of VDR agonists or active VitD during differentiation of DCs *in vitro* determines a reduction in subsequent T-cell proliferation and also in interferon-gamma (IFN-γ) production [33]. Tolerogenic DCs are also able to induce the development of Treg cells that are mainly characterized by the expression of CD4 and CD25 molecules and production of anti-inflammatory cytokines such as IL-10 and transforming growth factor-β (TGF-β) [34]. As mentioned before, Treg cells play a major role in controlling inflammatory immune responses. The main mechanisms underlying their suppressive activity include the induction of inhibitory molecules such as cytotoxic T-lymphocyte antigen 4, the production of inhibitory cytokines that leads to impaired T-cell expansion and the release of granzymes and perforin that trigger T-cell death [35]. Chambers et al. [36] demonstrated that addition of active VitD on human CD4+ T lymphocytes significantly increased the expression of forkhead box protein P3 (Foxp3) that characterizes Treg cells.

The direct effect of VitD on T cells was the first evidence of the immunomodulatory activity of this hormone. Active VitD suppresses Th1 inflammatory immune response through inhibition of IL-2 and IFN-γ production, which are the main cytokines produced by this Th cell subset. This subject was revised by Lemire et al. [37]. These authors described that VitD preferentially inhibited Th1 functions having little effects over Th2 cells. At that time, they already suggested that this vitamin could have a potential therapeutic application in Th1-mediated diseases as is the case of some autoimmune pathologies.

Many inflammatory responses are also related to the development of Th17 cells and its signature cytokine named IL-17. It is largely known that this T-cell subpopulation is involved in the pathogenesis of a variety of inflammatory and autoimmune disorders [38]. In this context, Th17 cell pathogenicity is frequently related to a Th17-Th1 functional plasticity that is regulated by the cytokine milieu [39]. The immunomodulatory effects of VitD on Th17 cells are not clear and depend upon the disease. Most of what is known concerning VitD effect on these cells is based on experimental studies. For example, oral treatment with active VitD prevented and partly reversed experimental autoimmune uveitis in mice. This effect was related to both decreased IL-17 production and impaired development of Th17 cells [40]. Moreover, Chang et al. [41] demonstrated that active VitD treatment protected mice from experimental autoimmune encephalomyelitis (EAE) by inhibiting the differentiation and further migration of Th17 cells to the central nervous system (CNS). Even though the effect of VitD on animal models is evident, human data are controversial and there is not a consensus in the literature yet.

Data on the effects of VitD on the development of Th2 cells are also conflicting. This T-cell subset is able to suppress Th1 inflammatory immune response through the production of anti-inflammatory cytokines such as IL-4 and IL-5. A direct effect of active VitD on Th2 cells was demonstrated by Boonstra et al. [42]. Even in the absence of APCs, these authors observed an increased frequency of IL-4-, IL-5-, and IL-10-producing murine CD4+ T cells after *in vitro* stimulation with VitD. In addition, there was a decrease in the frequency of IFN-γ-producing cells. However, Staeva-Vieira and Freedman [43] demonstrated that active VitD inhibited the *in vitro* production of both, IFN-γ and IL-4 by murine CD4+ T cells.

Other T-cell subsets such as CD8+ T cells and natural-killer T cells (NKT) are also targets of VitD. Chen et al. [44] demonstrated that active VitD signaling through VDR is essential to control pathogenic CD8+ T cells in inflammatory bowel diseases. The importance of VDR was also highlighted by Yu et al. [45] who demonstrated a critical role of VDR expression in the development of induced NKT cells from mice fed with synthetic diets containing active VitD.

There are few studies concerning the impact of VitD on B cells. *In vitro* assays indicated that the active form of VitD inhibited the production of immunoglobulin E and increased IL-10 production by B cells [46,47]. Similarly to the effect over DCs, active VitD also downregulated the expression of co-stimulatory molecules at the surface of human B cells. Drozdenko et al. [48] demonstrated that the antigen-presenting function of B cells was compromised by *in vitro* addition of active VitD to B and T cell co-cultures. The authors detected a reduced expression of the co-stimulatory molecule CD86 in B cells along with diminished T-cell expansion and lower cytokine production by these cells. A general scheme indicating some of the most relevant effects of VitD on innate and adaptive immunity is displayed in **Figure 1**.

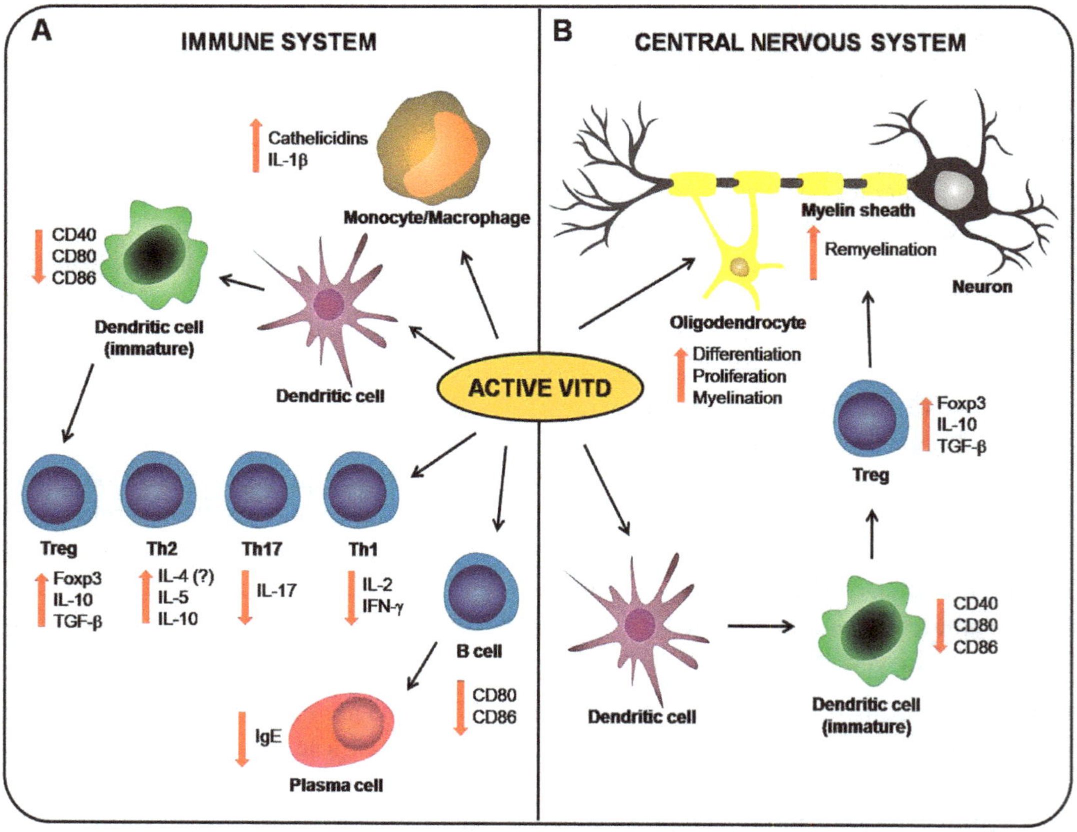

Figure 1. VitD action on the immune and the central nervous systems. (A) Effect of active VitD on the innate and the adaptive immunity cells and (B) direct and indirect effects of active VitD on the central nervous system.

The immunomodulatory potential of VitD has been widely explored in the field of autoimmune diseases. Epidemiological studies demonstrated that low VitD is correlated with a higher incidence of autoimmune diseases. Besides, genetic factors as VDR polymorphisms are also linked to autoimmune disorder susceptibility. The association between VitD and systemic and organ-specific autoimmune diseases, including multiple sclerosis (MS), was carefully reviewed by Agmon-Levin et al. [49].

4. Epidemiological evidence that VitD is relevant in MS

MS is an autoimmune disease characterized by the activation of self-reactive T cells specific for CNS antigens. This immune response triggers an initial inflammation in brain and spinal cord that is then followed by demyelination, axonal damage, and scar formation [50]. The pathogenic immune response observed in MS is mainly mediated by Th1 and Th17 [51]. About 85% of MS patients present with a biphasic disease characterized by alternating episodes of neurological disability and recovery, which is entitled as relapsing remitting MS (RRMS). Within 20–25 years, 60–70% of these patients progress to a secondary-progressive disease that is characterized by progressive neurological deterioration. Approximately 10% of the patients display a disease course classified as primary progressive MS, which is characterized by a continuous decline in neurological performance without any recovery episode [52]. Magnetic resonance imaging (MRI) is playing a prominent role in the diagnosis and also in the analysis of MS therapy efficacy [53]. As mentioned before, autoimmune diseases result from the interactions of environmental and genetic risk factors. Environmental risk factors considered essential for MS development include infections and non-infectious factors that comprise differences in diet and other behaviors, such as cigarette smoking and sunlight exposure [54,55]. The development of MS has been strongly associated with viral and bacterial infections [54,56]. More recently, a possible relationship between MS and Candida species was proposed [57–59]. Our research team recently demonstrated that previous infection with *Candida albicans*, a commensal and opportunistic human pathogen, aggravates the clinical signs of EAE [60].

Epidemiological data on MS incidence and prevalence drew attention to a possible link between the geographical distribution of the disease and exposure to the sun, UV radiation/intensity, and VitD levels. This sunshine hypothesis also known as latitude-gradient effect was initially proposed by Limburg [61] that suggested a correlation between higher MS occurrence and increasing distance from the equator. According to the World Health Organization [62], the highest prevalence of MS occurs in Europe (80 per 100,000 people) and the lowest prevalence in Africa (0.3 per 100,000). More recently it was reported that, until 2013, the number of MS was higher in northern hemisphere and lower in southern hemisphere, with the exception of Australia and New Zealand [63]. A latitudinal variation was also identified in the continents. For example, geospatial analysis carried out in North American regions showed an inverse correlation between MS and UV radiation, that is, higher MS rates have been associated with lower UV radiation due to a south-north latitudinal gradient [64]. Interestingly, a series of lifestyle changes that include sun evasion associated with skin protection and extra time indoors, or increased charter tourism to warmer countries during the winter, seems to abolish latitude effects on UV radiation exposure [65]. According to these authors, this association between sun exposure and MS can be determined by distinct effects: by the VitD generated by sun exposure, by direct sun effects, or by a combination of both. These possibilities are reinforced by data from experimental animals and also from dietary studies in human populations. Dermal application of VitD ointments and UV radiation in VDR knockout mice were both able to induce Treg cells [66]. Further study indicated that these UV-induced Treg cells were able to migrate to the CNS of mice with EAE where they downregulated the inflammatory activity [67].

A lower prevalence of MS in some northern countries, which in a general way are expected to have a higher number of patients with the disease, could be explained by VitD-related dietary factors. For example, VitD sufficiency could be achieved through a traditional diet that includes fatty fish and cod liver oil. This possibility has been suggested to explain the reduced risk of MS in Norway that is located at the north of the Arctic Circle [68]. The relevant role of dietary VitD intake in MS was examined in two large cohorts of women: the Nurses' Health Study (NHS; 92,253 women followed between 1980 and 2000) and the Nurses' Health Study II (NHS II; 95,310 women followed between 1991 and 2001). The authors concluded that intake of VitD from supplements had a protective effect on the risk of developing MS [69]. A recent study with 953 MS patients indicated an inverse association between MS risk and the dose of cod liver oil during adolescence, suggesting that this stage of life is an important susceptible period for adult-onset MS, reinforcing the importance of dietary VitD as a risk factor for MS [70]. Altogether these data supported the possibility that MS patients could have lower levels of VitD. Regarding this, the largest study to date compared VitD levels present in Iranian MS patients (n = 700) to the ones found in healthy individuals (n = 1000) and demonstrated that VitD levels were significantly lower in patients with MS [71]. Strong evidences also support the likelihood that low VitD levels can be related to disability and progression of this disease. In a study with 267 patients, lower serum VitD levels were also associated with higher rates of both relapse and disability [72]. Other authors showed an association between a low VitD status at the start of RRMS and the early conversion to secondary progressive MS [73]. The possible effect of VitD levels in the therapeutic efficacy of interferon beta 1b(IFN-β-1b), fingolimod (FTY), and glatiramer acetate (GA) was also investigated. Among patients treated with IFN-β-1b, higher VitD levels were associated with a reduced risk of relapse [74], whereas lower VitD levels early in the disease course correlated with a strong risk factor for long-term MS activity and progression [75]. In a similar way, in FTY-treated patients, higher VitD levels were associated with an approximately 50% reduction in new inflammatory events and in relapses [76]. By contrast, there was no significant benefit of higher VitD levels with respect to inflammatory events, relapses, or disability progression in GA-treated patients [76]. The strong correlation between low VitD levels and higher MS susceptibility reinforces the hypothesis that VitD deficiency leads to MS and/or disease progression and stimulates new researches focused on supplementation of these patients with VitD.

5. Supplementation of MS patients with VitD

The recent identification of VitD as a risk factor for MS susceptibility, and more recently as a potential modifier of disease course, inspired several clinical trials in relapsing MS [77]. It has been proposed that VitD supplementation is a low-cost and a low-risk intervention that may potentiate the efficacy of certain treatments against MS, without the risk of provoking serious adverse events as occurs with other combination therapies [76]. In effect, many patients are being already supplemented with VitD. However, it is not known whether supplementation has a significant impact on MS progression. A clinical trial (NCTO1339676) employing oral supplementation with active VitD (20,000 IU/week, cholecalciferol, Dekristol) administered once a week during 12 months together with IFN-β-1b resulted in reduction of MRI lesions in the brain of MS patients [78]. In another clinical trial (NCT 00785473), this same dose (20,000 IU/week, cholecalciferol, Dekristol) was administered during 24 months in RRMS patients under treatment with IFN-β-1b, GA, or natalizumab. Even though the patients presented a significant increase in serum VitD levels, the markers of systemic inflammation were not modified. The authors suggested that the anti-inflammatory effects of VitD supplementation are limited to RRMS patients with VitD insufficiency or to earlier stages of the disease [79]. A higher dose of VitD3 (50,000 IU/week) administered by oral route during a short period (2 months) reduced disability in RRMS patients and surprisingly upregulated IL-6 and IL-17 gene expression in the peripheral blood mononuclear cells of these patients [80]. Similarly, the same VitD dose (50,000 IU) administered by oral route every five days for 3 months in 94 RRMS patients under treatment with IFN-β-1b reduced disability of these patients but also increased IL-17 serum levels in comparison to a placebo group [81]. Investigations in this area suggested that changes in IL-17 levels could be related to the adopted VitD doses. For example, Golan et al. [82] demonstrated that IL-17 serum levels were significantly increased in a lower dose group (800 IU/per day), whereas patients that were taking higher doses (4370 IU/per day) presented heterogeneous IL-17 responses: 40% of them had decreased serum IL-17 levels, whereas 45% had increased IL-17 levels after three months of supplementation. These authors suggested that IL-17 data must be interpreted with caution as serum IL-17 is not an established biomarker of MS disease activity. Furthermore, IL-17 serum levels before treatment with IFN-β could not be correlated to disease activity parameters [83]; IL-17 also showed a trend toward higher levels in MS patients with inactive disease compared to those with active disease [84]. More recently, 40 patients with RRMS were randomized to receive 10,400 IU or 800 IU of cholecalciferol daily for 6 months. Mean increase of VitD levels from baseline to the ones detected at final visit was larger in the high-dose group than in the low-dose one and adverse events were minor and did not differ between the two groups. Interestingly, in the high-dose group, but not in the low-dose one, there was a reduction in the proportion of IL-17+CD4+ T cells. The authors concluded that daily cholecalciferol supplementation with 10,400 IU is safe and well tolerated in patients with MS and determines *in vivo* pleiotropic immunomodulatory effects [85]. Considering that IL-17 is an important cytokine involved in MS pathogenesis, further studies are needed to clarify the role of VitD on these unexpected elevated IL-17 levels. Therefore, until nowadays it is not possible to consider IL-17 as a biological marker for VitD levels in human body.

The researches done so far strongly suggest that VitD supplementation could be useful in MS treatment. However, the exact doses to be prescribed to patients presenting different clinical symptoms are still waiting to be determined [86]. Regarding the side effects of VitD that include hypercalcemia [87] and the imbalance in serum concentration of parathyroid hormone [88], monitoring serum VitD would also be extremely important. In spite of the findings that VitD directly regulates the nervous system development and function [89], there is no scientific evidence to support its use as a monotherapy for MS in clinical practice [90]. Recent human trials concerning VitD supplementation in MS patients suggest that higher VitD doses are more efficient to control the symptoms and disease inflammatory markers. Nonetheless, to fix the ideal dose, it is essential to measure VitD serum levels before supplementation and to follow up the patients by constantly monitoring side effects. It is important, however, to highlight that the ideal dose could vary from one patient to another. The possible use of VitD analogs devoid of side effects must be also evaluated. World Health Organization (WHO) and Multiple Sclerosis International Federation (MSIF) published in 2008 the first Atlas of MS [62], correlating the epidemiology, diagnosis, and therapy. To the best of our knowledge, WHO did not define a specific VitD dose to treat MS.

6. Therapeutic effect of VitD in EAE

Experimental autoimmune encephalomyelitis (EAE) is an animal model universally employed to investigate mechanisms of inflammation in the CNS in the context of MS. EAE is mainly induced in rodents either by active immunization with CNS antigens associated with adjuvant or by passive transfer of CNS-specific T cells. Most of the therapeutic procedures adopted nowadays were initially tested in murine EAE [91]. In 1991, it was demonstrated that VitD administration every other day for 15 days, starting 3 days before EAE induction, significantly prevented disease development and prolonged the survival of SJL/J mice [92]. This was the first report concerning the therapeutic potential of VitD on EAE. To avoid undesirable hypercalcemia *in vivo*, the immunomodulatory activity of VitD analogs were confirmed and they were equally efficient to suppress EAE development [93,94]. Since then, EAE has been widely employed to understand the mechanisms involved in VitD efficacy against MS. In this regard, one of the first studies was done with the Lewis rat model. The authors observed that VitD administered after the beginning of clinical signs determined significant clinical improvement. This therapeutic effect was associated with a striking decrease in the number of CD4+ cells, macrophages, and activated microglia in the CNS [95]. VDR is also essential for the beneficial effects of VitD on EAE since VitD treatment was not able to prevent disease manifestations in VDR-knockout mice [96]. The efficacy of VitD over EAE has also been attributed to effects on cells from the innate immunity. It decreases macrophage accumulation [97], inhibits chemokine synthesis and inducible NOS, and also suppresses CD11b+ monocyte recruitment into the CNS [98]. NKT cells also contribute to the protective effect of VitD on murine EAE. All mice lacking NKT cells [CD1d(−/−)] presented EAE symptomatology upon VitD administration, whereas the same treatment completely avoided EAE development in wild-type mice [99]. More recent data revealed that VitD administration induces tolerogenic DCs in the lymph nodes, which leads to suppression of encephalitogenic T cells, resulting in less inflammatory response in the CNS [100].

Critical effects of VitD on CD4+ T cells have been reported, whereas it is not evident if this vitamin affects CD8+ T cells, which express the highest concentrations of VDR. The effect of VitD on CD8+ T cells in EAE was evaluated in one report. The authors demonstrated that VitD inhibits EAE development even in mice lacking functional CD8+ cells, suggesting that they were not essential for VitD-suppressive effect in murine EAE [101]. The conception that the CD4+ T-cell subset was the main VitD target during EAE therapy was then established. VitD treatment triggered a reduction in the total number of lymphocytes, while the amount of IL-4 and TGF-β-1 transcripts increased in the CNS of EAE mice [102]. Still regarding anti-inflammatory cytokines, VitD therapy was reported to be much less effective in preventing EAE symptoms in IL-4-deficient mice [103] and also failed to inhibit EAE in mice with a disrupted IL-10 or IL-10R gene [104]. A more recently described profile of CD4+ T cells termed Th17 plays a critical role in numerous inflammatory conditions and autoimmune diseases. In this context, researchers showed that VitD can inhibit the differentiation and migration of Th17 cells to the CNS, ameliorating EAE symptoms [41,105].

After the first demonstration that VitD leads to induction of CD4+CD25+Foxp3+ cells with suppressive activity *in vitro* [106] and that these regulatory cells are directly involved in the natural resolution of EAE [107], many studies validated the correlation between VitD treatment and the increment of a Foxp3+ regulatory profile in EAE [99,103,104] (**Figure 1B**). The potential for reversing inflammatory and demyelinating processes in the CNS has been attributed to an augmented generation of Foxp3+ Treg cells in the periphery and their further migration to the CNS [100,108]. New therapeutic approaches have also been tested to improve VitD efficacy in EAE. A synergistic effect was found by association of VitD with estrogen, which determined more CD4+Helios+Foxp3+ Treg cells and fewer CD4+ T cells among CNS mononuclear cells, preventing EAE development [109]. In addition to the large contribution of VitD immunomodulatory activity in EAE, this treatment can also directly act on neural cells promoting CNS remyelination and other neuroprotective effects (**Figure 1B**). *In vitro* assays indicated that this vitamin significantly enhanced proliferation of neural stem cells and their differentiation into neurons and oligodendrocytes [110]. In addition, VitD treatment modulated autophagic activity and neuroapoptosis in EAE mice. As autophagy is an evolutionarily conserved cellular catabolic process that recycles damaged organelles and its inhibition causes neurodegeneration in mature neurons, this process plays an essential role in maintaining neuronal homeostasis [111]. In summary, VitD controls EAE symptoms through reduction of inflammatory immune response and elicitation of a regulatory profile. As EAE reproduces specific features of the histopathology and neurobiology of MS [112], highlighting these mechanisms in rodent models is essential to translate VitD supplementation to MS patients.

Emphasis has been given to specific therapies, that is, to procedures that target CNS antigen and that would be, therefore, more efficient and devoid of side effects. In this context, MOG administration by different routes as intravenous [113], oral [114] or nasal [115], was able to suppress EAE symptoms. Various formulations containing myelin antigens were tested to control EAE. MOG conjugated with nanoparticles [116], mannan, [117] or inserted into a plasmid DNA [118] reduced EAE symptoms through induction of Foxp3+ Treg cells and dowmodulation of Th17 and Th1 cells. Our research group has been working in this context. Considering that an antigen from the CNS can provide the required specificity and that VitD is endowed with a strong downmodulatory potential, we anticipated that VitD could work as a tolerogenic adjuvant. Differently from the conventional immunogenic adjuvants that reinforce the immune response, the denominated tolerogenic adjuvants have the ability to downmodulate or modify the specific immune response when associated with specific antigens. Confirming this hypothesis, we recently demonstrated that a combined therapy with MOG + VitD blocked EAE development. This elevated efficacy was correlated with reduced production of IL-6 and IL-17 by spleen and CNS cell cultures stimulated with MOG, reduced splenic DC maturation, and also a striking decline in CNS inflammation [119] (**Figure 2**).

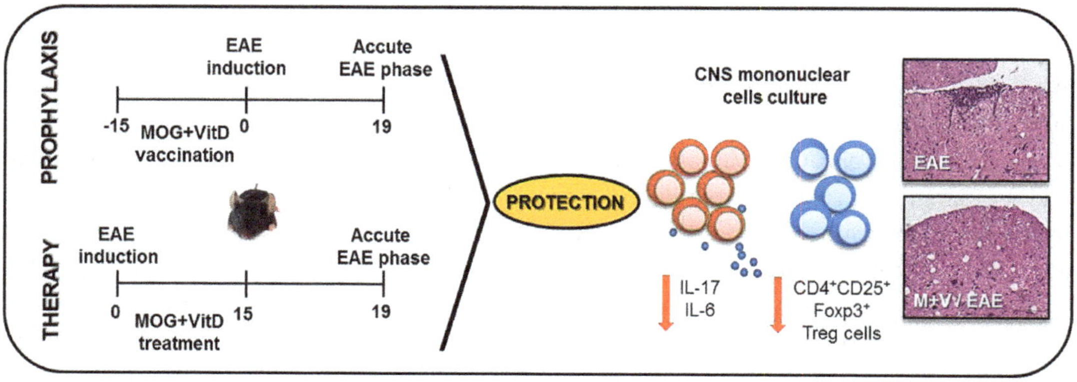

Figure 2. MOG + active vitamin D3 association strategy for EAE prophylaxis and treatment. C57BL/6 mice were vaccinated or treated with this association and the effect on EAE was evaluated in the acute EAE phase. Both strategies decreased production of inflammatory cytokines by CNS mononuclear cells, frequency of CD4+CD25+Foxp3+ Treg cells, and inflammation in the CNS.

7. Prophylactic effect of VitD on EAE

Prophylactic strategies in EAE, and also in other autoimmune pathologies, are based in the concept of "inverse vaccination." This procedure refers to the use of an immunization protocol that, differently from classical vaccination, aims to achieve an antigen-specific tolerogenic state [120]. Even though the term "inverse vaccination" could also be used as a therapeutical strategy, in this text we applied it only in the context of prophylactic vaccination. The majority of the prophylactic strategies in EAE have been done by administration of a diversity of MOG formulations delivered by distinct routes. A few examples of these procedures and the main histological and immunological findings are illustrated in **Table 1**.

The prophylactic potential of VitD (or analogs) alone or associated with other pharmaceuticals has been tested in EAE. The adopted experimental protocols are not standardized and therefore, different amounts of VitD are administered by distinct routes. Time periods chosen for VitD administration in relation to EAE induction are also variable and some procedures consist in prolonged administration periods, even reaching the disease clinical phase. However, a general consensus is that VitD is able to improve clinical disease manifestation and also to trigger evident effects on the CNS and the immune system. Some of the effects observed in mice with EAE that were previously injected with VitD are exemplified in **Table 2**.

Peptide formulation	Animal model	Effects	References
Plasmid DNA vaccines encoding MOG35–55	C57BL6/J mice	↓Microglia/macrophage activation, astrogliosis, and axonal damage ↑CD4+CD25+Foxp3+ Treg	Fissolo et al. [118]
MOG35–55 conjugated to mannan, intradermally	C57BL/6 and SJL/J mice	↓Demyelination ↓Inflammatory infiltrates	Tseveleki et al. [117]
Tolerogenic DC pulsed with MOG40–55	C57BL/6 mice	↑IL-10 production by MOG-stimulated splenocytes ↑CD3+CD4+CD25+FoxP3+ cells	Mansilla et al. [121]
MOG35–55-PLGA + IL-10-PLGA, subcutaneously	C57Bl/6 mice	↓IL-17 and IFN-α production by splenocytes↓Demyelination score	Cappellano et al. [122]

Table 1. MOG prophylactic procedures in EAE.

Route	Animal model	Effects	References
Diet	CD8+ $^{-/-}$ mice	Protection independent of TCD8+ cells	Meehan and DeLuca [101]
Intraperitoneally	C57BL/6 mice	↓MyD88, IRF-4, IRF-7 and NF-kB expression ↓Several TLRs	Li et al. [123]
Oral, gavage	C57BL/6 mice	Intact blood–CNS barrier ↓Inflammatory infiltrates in the CNS	Grishkan et al. [124]
Intraperitoneally	C57BL/6 mice	↓Demyelination ↑Beclin-1 expression in neurons	Zhen et al. [111]

Table 2. Vitamin D3 prophylactic procedures in EAE.

The combination of VitD with other substances as calcitonin [125], IFN-β [126], bisphosphonate [127], rapamycin [128], and cyclosporine [129] has determined cooperative effects over EAE control. We recently tested the association of VitD with MOG as a prophylactic approach to control EAE development. Again, in this procedure, we explored the concept of VitD as a tolerogenic adjuvant. This concept and its potential application to trigger self-tolerance in autoimmune diseases were conceived by Kang et al. [130]. These authors validated this hypothesis by demonstrating that FK506 (tacrolimus) associated with MOG was prophylactic in encephalomyelitis [131]. In this context, we hypothesized that active VitD could also behave as a tolerogenic adjuvant if associated with a CNS-specific antigen. Vaccination with MOG associated with VitD, before EAE induction in C57BL/6 female mice, determined a significant clinical improvement characterized by absence of clinical score and no body weight loss. An impressive reduction in CNS inflammation, DC maturation and also cytokine production by CNS and spleen cell cultures was detected in these vaccinated animals [132]. As described in Section 6 of this chapter, this combination of MOG with VitD was also very efficient as a therapeutic procedure in the EAE model. This prophylactic and therapeutic potential of the MOG/VitD association in EAE is illustrated in **Figure 2**. The possible use of VitD as a tolerogenic adjuvant in association with other self-antigens, as a strategy to control autoimmune pathologies, warrants future investigation. In our opinion, the fact that VitD is already accepted for human supplementation will facilitate its adoption for MS treatments based on its association with neuronal self-antigens.

Acknowledgments

The authors are thankful for the financial support from São Paulo State Foundation (FAPESP) —Grant #2013/26257-8, Conselho Nacional de Desenvolvimento Científico e Tecnológico (CNPq)—Grant #302710/2013-2 and also Pró-Reitoria de Pesquisa—Universidade Estadual Paulista (PROPe—UNESP). Special thanks are given to Danilo Sanches Moreno for his substantial contribution to the art of drawing and figures.

Author details

Sofia F.G. Zorzella-Pezavento, Larissa L.W. Ishikawa, Thais F.C. Fraga-Silva, Luiza A.N. Mimura and Alexandrina Sartori*

*Address all correspondence to: sartori@ibb.unesp.br

Department of Microbiology and Immunology, Institute of Biosciences of Botucatu, Sao Paulo State University (UNESP), Botucatu, São Paulo, Brazil

References

[1] McCollum EV, Simmonds N, Becker JE, Shipley PG. Studies on experimental rickets, XXI: an experimental demonstration of the existence of a vitamin which promotes calcium deposition. The Journal of Biological Chemistry. 1922;53:293–312.

[2] Rajakumar K, Greenspan SL, Thomas SB, Holick MF. SOLAR ultraviolet radiation and vitamin D: a historical perspective. American Journal of Public Health. 2007;97:1746–1754.

[3] Holick, MF. Vitamin D and bone health. The Journal of Nutrition. 1996;126:1159S–1164S.

[4] Norman AW, Okamura WH, Bishop JE, Henry HL. Update on biological actions of 1alpha,25(OH)2-vitamin D3 (rapid effects) and 24R,25(OH)2-vitamin D3. Molecular and Cellular Endocrinology. 2002;197:1–13. DOI: 10.1016/S0303-7207(02)00273-3

[5] Kongsbak M, Levring TB, Geisler C, von Essen MR. The vitamin D receptor and T cell function. Frontiers in Immunology. 2013;4:148. DOI: 10.3389/fimmu.2013.00148

[6] Holick, MF. Vitamin D deficiency. The New England Journal of Medicine. 2007;357:266–281.

[7] Holick MF. Vitamin D deficiency in 2010: Health benefits of vitamin D and sunlight: a D-bate. Nature Reviews. Endocrinology. 2011;7:73–75. DOI: 10.1038/nrendo.2010.234

[8] Holick MF, Binkley NC, Bischoff-Ferrari HA, Gordon CM, Hanley DA, Heaney RP, Murad MH, Weaver CM, Endocrine Society. Evaluation, treatment, and prevention of vitamin D deficiency: an Endocrine Society clinical practice guideline. The Journal of Clinical Endocrinology and Metabolism. 2011;96:1911–1930. DOI: 10.1210/jc.2011-0385

[9] Jones G. Pharmacokinetics of vitamin D toxicity. The American Journal of Clinical Nutrition. 2008;88:582S–586S.

[10] Ozkan B, Hatun S, Bereket A. Vitamin D intoxication. The Turkish Journal of Pediatrics. 2012;54:93–98.

[11] Holick MF. Vitamin D: a millennium perspective. Journal of Cellular Biochemistry. 2003;88:296–307

[12] Nair R, Maseeh A. Vitamin D: the "sunshine" vitamin. Journal of Pharmacology & Pharmacotherapeutics. 2012;3:118–126. DOI: 10.4103/0976-500X.95506

[13] Lamberg-Allardt C. Vitamin D in foods and as supplements. Progress in Biophysics and Molecular Biology. 2006;92:33–38.

[14] Dusso, Brown, Slatopolsky E. Vitamin D. American Journal of Physiology. Renal Physiology. 2005;289:F8–F28.

[15] Holick MF. The cutaneous photosynthesis of previtamin D3: a unique photoendocrine system. The Journal of Investigative Dermatology. 1981;77:51–58.

[16] Zhang J, Habiel DM, Ramadass M, Kew RR. Identification of two distinct cell binding sequences in the vitamin D binding protein. Biochimica et Biophysica Acta. 2010;1803:623–629. DOI: 10.1016/j.bbamcr.2010.02.010

[17] Suzuki Y, Landowski CP, Hediger MA. Mechanisms and regulation of epithelial Ca^{2+} absorption in health and disease. Annual Review of Physiology. 2008;70:257–271. DOI: 10.1146/annurev.physiol.69.031905.161003

[18] DeLuca HF, Schnoes HK. Metabolism and mechanism of action of vitamin D. Annual Review of Biochemistry. 1976;45:631–666. DOI: 10.1146/annurev.bi.45.070176.003215

[19] Hewison M, Zehnder D, Chakraverty R, Adams JS. Vitamin D and barrier function: a novel role for extra-renal 1a-hydroxylase. Molecular and Cellular Endocrinology. 2004;215:31–38.

[20] Baeke F, Takiishi T, Korf H, Gysemans C, Mathieu C. Vitamin D: modulator of the immune system. Current Opinion in Pharmacology. 2010;10:482–596. DOI: 10.1016/j.coph.2010.04.001

[21] Haq AU. 1,25-Dihydroxyvitamin D3 (calcitriol) suppresses IL-2 induced murine thymocyte proliferation. Thymus. 1986;8:295–306.

[22] Mathieu C, Adorini L. The coming of age of 1,25-dihydroxyvitamin D(3) analogs as immunomodulatory agents. Trends in Molecular Medicine. 2002;8:174–179. DOI: 10.1016/S1471-4914(02)02294-3

[23] Lewin E, Olgaard K. The in vivo effect of a new, *in vitro*, extremely potent vitamin D3 analog KH1060 on the suppression of renal allograft rejection in the rat. Calcified Tissue International. 1994;54:150–154.

[24] Hullett DA, Cantorna MT, Redaelli C, Humpal-Winter J, Hayes CE, Sollinger HW, Deluca HF. Prolongation of allograft survival by 1,25-dihydroxyvitamin D3. Transplantation. 1998;66:824–828.

[25] O'Brien MA, Jackson MW. Vitamin D and the immune system: beyond rickets. Veterinary Journal. 2012;194:27–33. DOI: 10.1016/j.tvjl.2012.05.022

[26] van Etten E, Mathieu C. Immunoregulation by 1,25-dihydroxyvitamin D3: basic concepts. The Journal of Steroid Biochemistry and Molecular Biology. 2005;97:93–101. DOI:10.1016/j.jsbmb.2005.06.002

[27] Griffin AT, Arnold FW. Review of metabolic, immunologic, and virologic consequences of suboptimal vitamin D levels in HIV infection. AIDS Patient Care and STDs. 2012;26:516–525. DOI: 10.1089/apc.2012.0145

[28] Pareek M, Innes J, Sridhar S, Grass L, Connell D, Woltmann G, Wiselka M, Martineau AR, Kon OM, Dedicoat M, Lalvani A. Vitamin D deficiency and TB disease phenotype. Thorax. 2015;70:1171–1180. DOI: 10.1136/thoraxjnl-2014-206617

[29] Furuya-Kanamori L, Wangdi K, Yakob L, McKenzie SJ, Doi SA, Clark J, Paterson DL, Riley TV, Clements AC. 25-hydroxyvitamin D concentrations and clostridium difficile infection: a meta-analysis. JPEN Journal of Parenteral and Enteral Nutrition. 2015. DOI: 10.1177/0148607115623457 [Epub ahead of print]

[30] Nouari W, Ysmail-Dahlouk L, Aribi M. Vitamin D3 enhances bactericidal activity of macrophage against *Pseudomonas aeruginosa*. International Immunopharmacology. 2016;30:94–101. DOI: 10.1016/j.intimp.2015.11.033

[31] Barragan M, Good M, Kolls JK. Regulation of dendritic cell function by vitamin D. Nutrients. 2015;7:8127–8151. DOI: 10.3390/nu7095383

[32] Berer A, Stöckl J, Majdic O, Wagner T, Kollars M, Lechner K, Geissler K, Oehler L. 1,25-Dihydroxyvitamin D(3) inhibits dendritic cell differentiation and maturation in vitro. Experimental Hematology. 2000;28:575–583. DOI:10.1016/S0301-472X(00)00143-0

[33] Adler HS, Steinbrink K. Tolerogenic dendritic cells in health and disease: friend and foe! European Journal of Dermatology. 2007;17:476–491. DOI: 10.1684/ejd.2007.0262

[34] Sakaguchi S, Sakaguchi N, Shimizu J, Yamazaki S, Sakihama T, Itoh M, Kuniyasu Y, Nomura T, Toda M, Takahashi T. Immunologic tolerance maintained by CD25+ CD4+ regulatory T cells: their common role in controlling autoimmunity, tumor immunity, and transplantation tolerance. Immunological Reviews. 2001;182:18–32. DOI: 10.1034/j.1600-065X.2001.1820102.x

[35] Vignali DA, Collison LW, Workman CJ. How regulatory T cells work. Nature Reviews Immunology. 2008;8:523–532. DOI: 10.1038/nri2343

[36] Chambers ES, Suwannasaen D, Mann EH, Urry Z, Richards DF, Lertmemongkolchai G, Hawrylowicz CM. 1α,25-dihydroxyvitamin D3 in combination with transforming growth factor-β increases the frequency of Foxp3$^+$ regulatory T cells through preferential expansion and usage of interleukin-2. Immunology. 2014;143:52–60. DOI: 10.1111/imm.12289

[37] Lemire JM, Archer DC, Beck L, Spiegelberg HL. Immunosuppressive actions of 1,25-dihydroxyvitamin D3: preferential inhibition of Th1 functions. The Journal of Nutrition. 1995;125:1704S–1708S.

[38] Singh RP, Hasan S, Sharma S, Nagra S, Yamaguchi DT, Wong DT, Hahn BH, Hossain A. Th17 cells in inflammation and autoimmunity. Autoimmunity Reviews. 2014;13:1174–1181. DOI: 10.1016/j.autrev.2014.08.019

[39] Kleinewietfeld M, Hafler DA. Regulatory T cells in autoimmune neuroinflammation. Immunology Reviews. 2014;259:231–244. DOI: 10.1111/imr.12169

[40] Tang J, Zhou R, Luger D, Zhu W, Silver PB, Grajewski RS, Su SB, Chan CC, Adorini L, Caspi RR. Calcitriol suppresses antiretinal autoimmunity through inhibitory effects on the Th17 effector response. Journal of Immunology. 2009;182:4624–4632. DOI: 10.4049/jimmunol.0801543

[41] Chang JH, Cha HR, Lee DS, Seo KY, Kweon MN. 1,25-Dihydroxyvitamin D3 inhibits the differentiation and migration of T(H)17 cells to protect against experimental autoimmune encephalomyelitis. PLoS One. 2010;5:e12925. DOI: 10.1371/journal.pone.0012925

[42] Boonstra A, Barrat FJ, Crain C, Heath VL, Savelkoul HF, O'Garra A. 1alpha,25-Dihydroxyvitamin d3 has a direct effect on naive CD4(+) T cells to enhance the development of Th2 cells. Journal of Immunology. 2001;167:4974–4980. DOI: 10.4049/jimmunol.167.9.4974

[43] Staeva-Vieira TP, Freedman LP. 1,25-dihydroxyvitamin D3 inhibits IFN-gamma and IL-4 levels during in vitro polarization of primary murine CD4+ T cells. Journal of Immunology. 2002;168:1181–1189.

[44] Chen J, Bruce D, Cantorna MT. Vitamin D receptor expression controls proliferation of naïve CD8+ T cells and development of CD8 mediated gastrointestinal inflammation. BMC Immunology. 2014;15:6. DOI: 10.1186/1471-2172-15-6

[45] Yu S, Zhao J, Cantorna MT. Invariant NKT cell defects in vitamin D receptor knockout mice prevents experimental lung inflammation. Journal of Immunology. 2011;187(9): 4907–4912. doi: 10.4049/jimmunol.1101519

[46] Heine G, Anton K, Henz BM, Worm M. 1alpha,25-dihydroxyvitamin D3 inhibits anti-CD40 plus IL-4-mediated IgE production in vitro. European Journal of Immunology. 2002;32:3395–3404. DOI: 10.1002/1521-4141(200212)32:12<3395::AID-IMMU3395>3.0.CO;2-#

[47] Heine G, Niesner U, Chang HD, Steinmeyer A, Zügel U, Zuberbier T, Radbruch A, Worm M. 1,25-dihydroxyvitamin D(3) promotes IL-10 production in human B cells. European Journal of Immunology. 2008;38:2210–2218. DOI: 10.1002/eji.200838216

[48] Drozdenko G, Scheel T, Heine G, Baumgrass R, Worm M. Impaired T cell activation and cytokine production by calcitriol-primed human B cells. Clinical and Experimental Immunology. 2014;178:364–372. DOI: 10.1111/cei.12406

[49] Agmon-Levin N, Theodor E, Segal RM, Shoenfeld Y. Vitamin D in systemic and organ-specific autoimmune diseases. Clinical Reviews in Allergy and Immunology. 2013;45:256–266. DOI: 10.1007/s12016-012-8342-y

[50] Loleit V, Biberacher V, Hemmer B. Current and future therapies targeting the immune system in multiple sclerosis. Current Pharmaceutical Biotechnology. 2014;15:276–296. DOI: 10.2174/1389201015666140617104332

[51] Domingues HS, Mues M, Lassmann H, Wekerle H, Krishnamoorthy G. Functional and pathogenic differences of Th1 and Th17 cells in experimental autoimmune encephalomyelitis. PLoS One. 2010;5:e15531. DOI: 10.1371/journal.pone.0015531

[52] Dutta R, Trapp BD. Relapsing and progressive forms of multiple sclerosis: insights from pathology. Current Opinion in Neurology. 2014;27:271–278. DOI: 10.1097/WCO.0000000000000094

[53] Brown JW, Chard DT. The role of MRI in the evaluation of secondary progressive multiple sclerosis. Expert Review of Neurotherapeutics. 2016;16:157–171. DOI: 10.1586/14737175.2016.1134323

[54] Ascherio A, Munger KL. Environmental risk factors for multiple sclerosis. Part I: the role of infection. Annals of Neurology. 2007a;61:288–299. DOI: 10.1002/ana.21117

[55] Ascherio A, Munger KL. Environmental risk factors for multiple sclerosis. Part II: noninfectious factors. Annals of Neurology. 2007b;61:504–513. DOI: 10.1002/ana.21141

[56] Gilden DH. Infectious causes of multiple sclerosis. The Lancet Neurology. 2005;4:195–202. DOI: 10.1016/S1474-4422(05)01017-3

[57] Benito-León J, Pisa D, Alonso R, Calleja P, Díaz-Sánchez M, Carrasco L. Association between multiple sclerosis and Candida species: evidence from a case-control study. European Journal of Clinical Microbiology & Infectious Diseases. 2010;29:1139–1145. DOI: 10.1007/s10096-010-0979-y

[58] Pisa D, Alonso R, Carrasco L. Fungal infection in a patient with multiple sclerosis. European Journal of Clinical Microbiology & Infectious Diseases. 2011;30:1173–1180. DOI: 10.1007/s10096-011-1206-1

[59] Pisa D, Alonso R, Jiménez-Jiménez FJ, Carrasco L. Fungal infection in cerebrospinal fluid from some patients with multiple sclerosis. European Journal of Clinical Microbiology & Infectious Diseases. 2013;32:795–801. DOI: 10.1007/s10096-012-1810-8

[60] Fraga-Silva TF, Mimura LA, Marchetti CM, Chiuso-Minicucci F, França TG, Zorzella-Pezavento SF, et al. Experimental autoimmune encephalomyelitis development is aggravated by *Candida albicans* infection. Journal of Immunology Research. 2015;2015:635052. DOI: 10.1155/2015/635052

[61] Limburg CC. The geographic distribution of multiple sclerosis and its estimated prevalence in the United States. Research publications—Association for Research in Nervous and Mental Disease. 1950;28:15–24.

[62] World Health Organization [Internet]. Atlas Multiple Sclerosis resources in the World. 2008. Available from: http://www.who.int/mental_health/neurology/Atlas_MS_WEB.pdf [Accessed: 2016-02-128]

[63] Browne P, Chandraratna D, Angood C, Tremlett H, Baker C, Taylor BV, Thompson AJ. Atlas of Multiple Sclerosis 2013: a growing global problem with widespread inequity. Neurology. 2014;83:1022–1024. DOI: 10.1212/WNL.0000000000000768

[64] Beretich BD and Beretich TM. Explaining multiple sclerosis prevalence by ultraviolet exposure: a geospatial analysis. Multiple Sclerosis. 2009;15:891–898. DOI: 10.1177/1352458509105579

[65] Sundström P and Salzer J. Vitamin D and multiple sclerosis—from epidemiology to prevention. Acta Neurologica Scandinavica. 2015:132:56–61. DOI: 10.1111/ane.12432

[66] Schwarz A, Navid F, Sparwasser T, Clausen BE, Schwarz T. 1,25-dihydroxyvitamin D exerts similar immunosuppressive effects as UVR but is dispensable for local UVR-induced immunosuppression. The Journal of Investigative Dermatology. 2012;132:2762–2769. DOI: 10.1038/jid.2012.238

[67] Breuer J, Schwab N, Schneider-Hohendorf T, Marziniak M, Mohan H, Bhatia U, Gross CC, Clausen BE, Weishaupt C, Luger TA, Meuth SG, Loser K, Wiendl H. Ultraviolet B light attenuates the systemic immune response in central nervous system autoimmunity. Annals of Neurology. 2014;75(5):739–758. DOI: 10.1002/ana.24165

[68] Kampman MT, Wilsgaard T, Mellgren SI. Outdoor activities and diet in childhood and adolescence relate to MS risk above the Arctic Circle. Journal of Neurology. 2007;254:471–477. DOI: 10.1007/s00415-006-0395-5

[69] Munger KL, Zhang SM, O'Reilly E, Hernán MA, Olek MJ, Willett WC, Ascherio A. Vitamin D intake and incidence of multiple sclerosis. Neurology. 2004;62:60–65. DOI: 10.1212/01.WNL.0000101723.79681.38

[70] Cortese M, Riise T, Bjørnevik K, Holmøy T, Kampman MT, Magalhaes S, et al. Timing of use of cod liver oil, a vitamin D source, and multiple sclerosis risk: the EnvIMS study. Multiple Sclerosis Journal. 2015;21:1856–1864. DOI: 10.1177/1352458515578770

[71] Karampoor S, Zahednasab H, Ramagopalan S, Mehrpour M, Safarnejad Tameshkel F, Keyvani H. 25-hydroxyvitamin D levels are associated with multiple sclerosis in Iran: a cross-sectional study. Journal of Neuroimmunology. 2016;290:47–48. DOI: 10.1016/j.jneuroim.2015.11.017

[72] Smolders J, Menheere P, Kessels A. Association of vitamin D metabolite levels with relapse rate and disability in multiple sclerosis. Multiple Sclerosis Journal. 2015;14:1220–1224. DOI: 10.1177/1352458508094399

[73] Muris AH, Rolf L, Broen K, Hupperts R, Damoiseaux J, Smolders J. A low vitamin D status at diagnosis is associated with an early conversion to secondary progressive multiple sclerosis. The Journal of Steroid Biochemistry and Molecular Biology. 2015;pii:S0960-0760:30136-30139. DOI: 10.1016/j.jsbmb.2015.11.009

[74] Simpson S Jr, Taylor B, Blizzard L. Higher 25-hydroxyvitamin D is associated with lower relapse risk in multiple sclerosis. Annals of Neurology. 2010;68:193–203. DOI: 10.1002/ana.22043

[75] Ascherio A, Munger KL, White R, Köchert K, Simon KC, Polman CH, et al. Vitamin D as an early predictor of multiple sclerosis activity and progression. JAMA Neurology. 2014;71:306–314. DOI: 10.1001/jamaneurol.2013.5993

[76] Rotstein DL, Healy BC, Malik MT, Carruthers RL, Musallam AJ, Kivisakk P, et al. Effect of vitamin D on MS activity by disease-modifying therapy class. Neurology: Neuroimmunology & Neuroinflammation. 2015;2:e167. DOI: 10.1212/NXI.0000000000000167

[77] Cree BA. 2014 multiple sclerosis therapeutic update. Neurohospitalist. 2014;4(2):63–65.

[78] Åivo J, Lindsröm BM, Soilu-Hänninen M. A randomised, double-blind, placebo-controlled trial with vitamin D3 in MS: subgroup analysis of patients with baseline disease activity despite interferon treatment. Multiple Sclerosis International. 2012;2012:802796. DOI: 10.1155/2012/802796

[79] Røsjø E, Steffensen LH, Jørgensen L, Lindstrøm JC, Šaltytė Benth J, Michelsen AE, et al. Vitamin D supplementation and systemic inflammation in relapsing-remitting multiple sclerosis. Journal of Neurology. 2015;262:2713–2721. DOI: 10.1007/s00415-015-7902-5

[80] Naghavi Gargari B, Behmanesh M, Shirvani Farsani Z, Pahlevan Kakhki M, Azimi AR. Vitamin D supplementation up-regulates IL-6 and IL-17A gene expression in multiple

sclerosis patients. International Immunopharmacology. 2015;28:414–419. DOI: 10.1016/j.intimp.2015.06.033

[81] Toghianifar N, Ashtari F, Zarkesh-Esfahani SH, Mansourian M. Effect of high dose vitamin D intake on interleukin-17 levels in multiple sclerosis: a randomized, double-blind, placebo-controlled clinical trial. Journal of Neuroimmunology. 2015;285:125–128. DOI: 10.1016/j.jneuroim.2015.05.022

[82] Golan D, Halhal B, Glass-Marmor L, Staun-Ram E, Rozenberg O, Lavi I, et al. Vitamin D supplementation for patients with multiple sclerosis treated with interferon-beta: a randomized controlled trial assessing the effect on flu-like symptoms and immunomodulatory properties. BMC Neurology. 2013;13:60. DOI: 10.1186/1471-2377-13-60

[83] Bushnell SE, Zhao Z, Stebbins CC, Cadavid D, Buko AM, Whalley ET, et al. Serum IL-17F does not predict poor response to IM IFNbeta-1a in relapsing-remitting MS. Neurology. 2012;79:531–537. DOI: 10.1212/WNL.0b013e318259e123

[84] Kallaur AP, Oliveira SR, Colado Simao AN, de Almeida ER D, Kaminami Morimoto H, Lopes J, et al. Cytokine profile in relapsing remitting multiple sclerosis patients and the association between progression and activity of the disease. Molecular Medicine Reports. 2013;7:1010–1020. DOI: 10.3892/mmr.2013.1256

[85] Sotirchos ES, Bhargava P, Eckstein C, Van Haren K, Baynes M, Ntranos A, et al. Safety and immunologic effects of high- vs low-dose cholecalciferol in multiple sclerosis. Neurology. 2016;86:382–390. DOI: 10.1212/WNL.0000000000002316

[86] Ganesh A, Apel S, Metz L, Patten S. The case for vitamin D supplementation in multiple sclerosis. Multiple Sclerosis and Related Disorders. 2013;2:281–306. DOI: 10.1016/j.msard.2012.12.008

[87] Bell DA, Crooke MJ, Hay N, Glendenning P. Prolonged vitamin D intoxication: presentation, pathogenesis and progress. Internal Medicine Journal. 2013;43:1148–1150. DOI: 10.1111/imj.12269

[88] Zittermann A, Prokop S, Gummert JF, Börgermann J. Safety issues of vitamin D supplementation. Anti-Cancer Agents in Medicinal Chemistry. 2013;13:4–10. DOI: 10.2174/1871520611307010004

[89] Wrzosek M, Łukaszkiewicz J, Wrzosek M, Jakubczyk A, Matsumoto H, Piątkiewicz P, et al. Vitamin D and the central nervous system. Pharmacological Reports. 2013;65:271–278.

[90] Brum DG, Comini-Frota ER, Vasconcelos CC, Dias-Tosta E. Supplementation and therapeutic use of vitamin D in patients with multiple sclerosis: consensus of the Scientific Department of Neuroimmunology of the Brazilian Academy of Neurology. Arquivos de Neuro-Psiquiatria. 2014;72:152–156. DOI: 10.1590/0004-282X20130252

[91] Robinson AP, Harp CT, Noronha A, Miller SD. The experimental autoimmune encephalomyelitis (EAE) model of MS: utility for understanding disease pathophysiology

and treatment. Handbook of Clinical Neurology. 2014;122:173–189. DOI: 10.1016/B978-0-444-52001-2.00008-X

[92] Lemire JM, Archer DC. 1,25-dihydroxyvitamin D3 prevents the in vivo induction of murine experimental autoimmune encephalomyelitis. The Journal of Clinical Investigation. 1991;87:1103–1107.

[93] Lemire JM, Archer DC, Reddy GS. 1,25-Dihydroxy-24-OXO-16ene-vitamin D3, a renal metabolite of the vitamin D analog 1,25-dihydroxy-16ene-vitamin D3, exerts immunosuppressive activity equal to its parent without causing hypercalcemia in vivo. Endocrinology. 1994;135:2818–2821.

[94] Mattner F, Smiroldo S, Galbiati F, Muller M, Di Lucia P, Poliani PL, Martino G, Panina-Bordignon P, Adorini L. Inhibition of Th1 development and treatment of chronic-relapsing experimental allergic encephalomyelitis by a non-hypercalcemic analogue of 1,25-dihydroxyvitamin D(3). European Journal of Immunology. 2000;30:498–508.

[95] Nataf S, Garcion E, Darcy F, Chabannes D, Muller JY, Brachet P. 1,25 Dihydroxyvitamin D3 exerts regional effects in the central nervous system during experimental allergic encephalomyelitis. Journal of Neuropathology and Experimental Neurology. 1996;55:904–914.

[96] Meehan TF, DeLuca HF. The vitamin D receptor is necessary for 1alpha,25-dihydroxyvitamin D(3) to suppress experimental autoimmuneencephalomyelitis in mice. Archives of Biochemistry and Biophysics. 2002;408:200–204.

[97] Nashold FE, Miller DJ, Hayes CE. 1,25-dihydroxyvitamin D3 treatment decreases macrophage accumulation in the CNS of mice with experimental autoimmune encephalomyelitis. Journal of Neuroimmunology. 2000;103:171–179.

[98] Pedersen LB, Nashold FE, Spach KM, Hayes CE. 1,25-dihydroxyvitamin D3 reverses experimental autoimmune encephalomyelitis by inhibiting chemokine synthesis and monocyte trafficking. Journal of Neuroscience Research. 2007;85:2480–2490.

[99] Waddell A, Zhao J, Cantorna MT. NKT cells can help mediate the protective effects of 1,25-dihydroxyvitamin D3 in experimental autoimmuneencephalomyelitis in mice. International Immunology. 2015;27:237–244. DOI: 10.1093/intimm/dxu147

[100] Farias AS, Spagnol GS, Bordeaux-Rego P, Oliveira CO, Fontana AG, de Paula RF, Santos MP, Pradella F, Moraes AS, Oliveira EC, Longhini AL, Rezende AC, Vaisberg MW, Santos LM. Vitamin D3 induces IDO+ tolerogenic DCs and enhances Treg, reducing the severity of EAE. CNS Neuroscience & Therapeutics. 2013;19:269–277. DOI: 10.1111/cns.12071

[101] Meehan TF, DeLuca HF. CD8(+) T cells are not necessary for 1 alpha,25-dihydroxyvitamin D(3) to suppress experimental autoimmune encephalomyelitis in mice. Proceedings of the National Academy of Sciences of the United States of America. 2002;99:5557–5560.

[102] Cantorna MT, Woodward WD, Hayes CE, DeLuca HF. 1,25-dihydroxyvitamin D3 is a positive regulator for the two anti-encephalitogenic cytokines TGF-beta 1 and IL-4. Journal of Immunology. 1998;160:5314–5319.

[103] Cantorna MT, Humpal-Winter J, DeLuca HF. In vivo upregulation of interleukin-4 is one mechanism underlying the immunoregulatory effects of 1,25-dihydroxyvitamin D(3). Archives of Biochemistry and Biophysics. 2000;377:135–138.

[104] Spach KM, Nashold FE, Dittel BN, Hayes CE. IL-10 signaling is essential for 1,25-dihydroxyvitamin D3-mediated inhibition of experimental autoimmune encephalomyelitis. Journal of Immunology. 2006;177:6030–6037.

[105] Joshi S, Pantalena LC, Liu XK, Gaffen SL, Liu H, Rohowsky-Kochan C, Ichiyama K, Yoshimura A, Steinman L, Christakos S, Youssef S. 1,25-dihydroxyvitamin D(3) ameliorates Th17 autoimmunity via transcriptional modulation of interleukin-17A. Molecular and Cellular Biology. 2011;31:3653–3669. DOI: 10.1128/MCB.05020-11

[106] Penna G, Roncari A, Amuchastegui S, Daniel KC, Berti E, Colonna M, Adorini L. Expression of the inhibitory receptor ILT3 on dendritic cells is dispensable for induction of CD4+Foxp3+ regulatory T cells by 1,25-dihydroxyvitamin D3. Blood. 2005;106:3490–3497.

[107] McGeachy MJ, Stephens LA, Anderton SM. Natural recovery and protection from autoimmune encephalomyelitis: contribution of CD4+CD25+ regulatory cells within the central nervous system. Journal of Immunology. 2005;175:3025–3032.

[108] Nashold FE, Nelson CD, Brown LM, Hayes CE. One calcitriol dose transiently increases Helios+ FoxP3+ T cells and ameliorates autoimmune demyelinating disease. Journal of Neuroimmunology. 2013;263:64–74. DOI: 10.1016/j.jneuroim.2013.07.016

[109] Spanier JA, Nashold FE, Mayne CG, Nelson CD, Hayes CE. Vitamin D and estrogen synergy in Vdr-expressing CD4(+) T cells is essential to induce Helios(+)FoxP3(+) T cells and prevent autoimmune demyelinating disease. Journal of Neuroimmunology. 2015;286:48–58. DOI: 10.1016/j.jneuroim.2015.06.015

[110] Shirazi HA, Rasouli J, Ciric B, Rostami A, Zhang GX. 1,25-Dihydroxyvitamin D3 enhances neural stem cell proliferation and oligodendrocyte differentiation. Experimental and Molecular Pathology. 2015;98:240–245. DOI: 10.1016/j.yexmp.2015.02.004

[111] Zhen C, Feng X, Li Z, Wang Y, Li B, Li L, Quan M, Wang G, Guo L. Suppression of murine experimental autoimmune encephalomyelitis development by 1,25-dihydroxyvitamin D3 with autophagy modulation. Journal of Neuroimmunology. 2015;280:1–7. DOI: 10.1016/j.jneuroim.2015.01.012

[112] Gold R, Linington C, Lassmann H. Understanding pathogenesis and therapy of multiple sclerosis via animal models: 70 years of merits and culprits in experimental autoimmune encephalomyelitis research. Brain. 2006;129:1953–1971. DOI: http://dx.doi.org/10.1093/brain/awl075

[113] Jiang Z, Li H, Fitzgerald DC, Zhang GX, Rostami A. MOG(35-55) i.v suppresses experimental autoimmune encephalomyelitis partially through modulation of Th17 and JAK/STAT pathways. European Journal of Immunology. 2009;39:789–799. DOI: 10.1002/eji.200838427

[114] Peron JP, Yang K, Chen ML, Brandao WN, Basso AS, Commodaro AG, Weiner HL, Rizzo LV. Oral tolerance reduces Th17 cells as well as the overall inflammation in the central nervous system of EAE mice. Journal of Neuroimmunology. 2010;227:10–17. DOI: 10.1016/j.jneuroim.2010.06.002

[115] Levy Barazany H, Barazany D, Puckett L, Blanga-Kanfi S, Borenstein-Auerbach N, Yang K, Peron JP, Weiner HL, Frenkel D. Brain MRI of nasal MOG therapeutic effect in relapsing-progressive EAE. Experimental Neurology. 2014;255:63–70. DOI: 10.1016/j.expneurol.2014.02.010

[116] Yeste A, Nadeau M, Burns EJ, Weiner HL, Quintana FJ. Nanoparticle-mediated codelivery of myelin antigen and a tolerogenic small molecule suppresses experimental autoimmune encephalomyelitis. Proceedings of the National Academy of Sciences of the United States of America. 2012;109:11270–11275. DOI: 10.1073/pnas.1120611109

[117] Tseveleki V, Tselios T, Kanistras I, Koutsoni O, Karamita M, Vamvakas SS, Apostolopoulos V, Dotsika E, Matsoukas J, Lassmann H, Probert L. Mannan-conjugated myelin peptides prime non-pathogenic Th1 and Th17 cells and ameliorate experimental autoimmune encephalomyelitis. Experimental Neurology. 2015;267:254–267. DOI: 10.1016/j.expneurol.2014.10.019

[118] Fissolo N, Costa C, Nurtdinov RN, Bustamante MF, Llombart V, Mansilla MJ, Espejo C, Montalban X, Comabella M. Treatment with MOG-DNA vaccines induces CD4+CD25+FoxP3+ regulatory T cells and up-regulates genes with neuroprotective functions in experimental autoimmune encephalomyelitis. Journal of Neuroinflammation. 2012;9:139. DOI: 10.1186/1742-2094-9-139

[119] Chiuso-Minicucci F, Ishikawa LL, Mimura LA, Fraga-Silva TF, França TG, Zorzella-Pezavento SF, Marques C, Ikoma MR, Sartori A. Treatment with Vitamin D/MOG Association Suppresses Experimental Autoimmune Encephalomyelitis. PLoS One. 2015;10:e0125836. DOI: 10.1371/journal.pone.0125836

[120] Steinman L. Inverse vaccination, the opposite of Jenner's concept, for therapy of autoimmunity. Journal of Internal Medicine. 2010;267:441–451. DOI: 10.1111/j.1365-2796.2010.02224.x

[121] Mansilla MJ, Sellès-Moreno C, Fàbregas-Puig S, Amoedo J, Navarro-Barriuso J, Teniente-Serra A, Grau-López L, Ramo-Tello C, Martínez-Cáceres EM. Beneficial effect of tolerogenic dendritic cells pulsed with MOG autoantigen in experimental autoimmune encephalomyelitis. CNS Neuroscience & Therapeutics. 2015;21:222–230. DOI: 10.1111/cns.12342

[122] Cappellano G, Woldetsadik AD, Orilieri E, Shivakumar Y, Rizzi M, Carniato F, Gigliotti CL, Boggio E, Clemente N, Comi C, Dianzani C, Boldorini R, Chiocchetti A, Renò F, Dianzani U. Subcutaneous inverse vaccination with PLGA particles loaded with a MOG

peptide and IL-10 decreases the severity of experimental autoimmune encephalomyelitis. Vaccine. 2014;32:5681–5689. DOI: 10.1016/j.vaccine.2014.08.016

[123] Li B, Baylink DJ, Deb C, Zannetti C, Rajaallah F, Xing W, Walter MH, Lau KH, Qin X. 1,25-Dihydroxyvitamin D3 suppresses TLR8 expression and TLR8-mediated inflammatory responses in monocytes in vitro and experimental autoimmune encephalomyelitis in vivo. PLoS One. 2013;8:e58808. DOI: 10.1371/journal.pone.0058808

[124] Grishkan IV, Fairchild AN, Calabresi PA, Gocke AR. 1,25-Dihydroxyvitamin D3 selectively and reversibly impairs T helper-cell CNS localization. Proceedings of the National Academy of Sciences of the United States of America. 2013;110:21101–21106. DOI: 10.1073/pnas.1306072110

[125] Becklund BR, Hansen DW Jr, Deluca HF. Enhancement of 1,25-dihydroxyvitamin D3-mediated suppression of experimental autoimmune encephalomyelitis by calcitonin. Proceedings of the National Academy of Sciences of the United States of America. 2009;106:5276–5281. DOI: 10.1073/pnas.0813312106

[126] van Etten E, Gysemans C, Branisteanu DD, Verstuyf A, Bouillon R, Overbergh L, Mathieu C. Novel insights in the immune function of the vitamin D system: synergism with interferon-beta. The Journal of Steroid Biochemistry and Molecular Biology. 2007;103:546–551. DOI: 10.1016/j.jsbmb.2006.12.094

[127] van Etten E, Branisteanu DD, Overbergh L, Bouillon R, Verstuyf A, Mathieu C. Combination of a 1,25-dihydroxyvitamin D3 analog and a bisphosphonate prevents experimental autoimmune encephalomyelitis and preserves bone. Bone. 2003;32:397–404. DOI: 10.1016/S8756-3282(03)00030-9

[128] Branisteanu DD, Mathieu C, Bouillon R. Synergism between sirolimus and 1,25-dihydroxyvitamin D3 in vitro and in vivo. Journal of Neuroimmunology. 1997;79:138–147. DOI: 10.1016/S0165-5728(97)00116-1

[129] Branisteanu DD, Waer M, Sobis H, Marcelis S, Vandeputte M, Bouillon R. Prevention of murine experimental allergic encephalomyelitis: cooperative effects of cyclosporine and 1 alpha, 25-(OH)2D3. Journal of Neuroimmunology.1995;61:151–160. DOI: 10.1016/0165-5728(95)00076-E

[130] Kang Y, Xu L, Wang B, Chen A, Zheng G. Cutting edge: immunosuppressant as adjuvant for tolerogenic immunization. The Journal of Immunology. 2008; 180: 5172–5176. DOI: 10.4049/jimmunol.180.8.5172

[131] Kang Y, Zhao J, Liu Y, Chen A, Zheng G, Yu Y, Mi J, Zou Q ,Wang B. FK506 as an adjuvant of tolerogenic DNA vaccination for the prevention of experimental autoimmune encephalomyelitis. The Journal of Gene Medicine. 2009;11:1064–1070. DOI: 10.1002/jgm.1387

[132] Mimura LA, Chiuso-Minicucci F, Fraga-Silva TF, Zorzella-Pezavento SF, França TG, Ishikawa LL, Penitenti M, Ikoma MR, Sartori A. Association of myelin peptide with vitamin D prevents autoimmune encephalomyelitis development. Neuroscience. 2016;317:130–140. DOI: 10.1016/j.neuroscience.2015.12.053

9

Sleep Disorders in Multiple Sclerosis

Montserrat González Platas and
María Yaiza Pérez Martin

Abstract

Patients with multiple sclerosis (MS) have multiple causes of poor sleep and potential triggers may relate to MS-related symptoms, co-morbidities and adverse effects from medication. Sleep disorders may occur independently of demographic factors, gender and clinical condition. The real frequency of sleep disturbances in MS and their impact on the patients' quality of life are unknown. The prevalence of sleep problems in the population with MS ranges between 47 and 62% and is more frequent in women, as well as having a higher risk of mortality. High psychological burden has been associated with poor sleep and with increased risk of co-morbid conditions such as heart disease, obesity, dyslipidemia and diabetes, which may have a profound impact on long-term health. The poor sleeping patients with MS were more likely to report fatigue and sleepiness. Insomnia is present in mood disorders, restless leg syndrome (RLS), pain, nocturia and obstructive sleep apnea (OSA), in patients with MS. All the symptoms are intermixed, and it is not possible to discern the precipitating factor or the perpetuating factor. Clinicians should routinely ask about sleep when forming a comprehensive care plan for patients with MS. Sleep specialty referrals should be considered for management of conditions that require polysomnography (PSG) diagnosis.

Keywords: sleep disorders, insomnia, sleepiness, fatigue, respiratory disorders during sleep, cognitive impairment, cognitive behavioral therapy, multiple sclerosis

1. Introduction

Multiple sclerosis (MS) is a chronic autoimmune disease of the central nervous system that is increasingly prevalent in young adults. Patients with MS have multiple causes of poor sleep, and potential triggers may be related to MS-related symptoms, co-morbidities and adverse effects from drug therapy.

Major sleep disorders have been reported to be associated with numerous co-morbid conditions, including heart disease, obesity, stroke and diabetes [1].

The poor sleepers among patients with MS are more likely to report fatigue (one of the most frequent symptoms in MS) and pain (a co-morbid condition to MS-related fatigue but is confounded by depression and medication for treating pain or pain-induced sleep disorder) [1].

All the symptoms are intermixed, and it is not possible to discern the precipitating factor and the perpetuating factor. In this respect, sleepiness and fatigue may converge in some situations [1].

Insomnia is present in mood disorders (depression and anxiety), restless leg syndrome (RLS), pain, nocturia and others [1]. RLS is also an important cause of pain in patients with MS. Sleep disorders may occur independently of demographic factors such as gender and clinical-demographic factors. High psychological burden has been said to be independently associated with poor sleep patients with increased risk of co-morbid conditions such as heart disease, obesity and diabetes, which may have a profound impact on long-term health. The reverse situation is also possible.

The frequency of sleep disturbances in MS and their impact on the patients' quality of life are unknown. The prevalence of sleep problems in the MS population ranges from 47 to 62%, with a higher prevalence in women [2–5]. Sex hormones and genetic mechanisms, psychosocial factors, certain physical factors that disrupt sleep, such as pain or bladder dysfunction may contribute to sleep differences between women and men [5].

Obstructive sleep apnea (OSA), RLS and chronic insomnia in particular are frequent problems in the MS population, and play a key role in the development of debilitating fatigue and other poor functional outcomes in MS. Yet, despite their impact, sleep disorders in MS remain critically under-recognized in most clinical settings. A recommended approach to the fatigued patient with MS is also highlighted [6].

Sleep disorders during the course of MS may be secondary to numerous symptoms arising from the disease itself or can be primary with a common biological link. In either of the two cases, a bidirectional relationship exists between these co-morbid conditions [7].

Sleep disturbances have been associated with increased risk of mortality, cardiac disease, obesity and diabetes [8] and can contribute to the depression, pain and fatigue symptoms that are commonly seen in MS patients, which are often disabling [3, 9].

Sleep disorders are under-recognized in persons with MS. These sleep disorders can contribute significantly to fatigue, other daytime dysfunction and poor quality of life. A systematic, practical approach that takes into account clinical features of MS is recommended to enhance recognition of these conditions and facilitate appropriate treatment. Clinicians caring for patients with MS should routinely screen for sleep disturbances and initiate diagnostic workups, if clinically indicated.

Sleep specialty referrals should be considered for management of conditions that require polysomnography (PSG) diagnosis, for complex patients who present a diagnostic challenge and for patients who do not respond to first-line treatments. Clinicians should also routinely ask about sleep when forming a comprehensive care plan for patients with MS.

2. Effect or influence of multiple sclerosis in sleep disorders

2.1. Insomnia

Sleeplessness or insomnia is an inability to fall asleep or to stay asleep as long as desired. Insomnia is described as a complaint of prolonged sleep-onset latency, disturbance of sleep maintenance or the experience of non-refreshing sleep [10]. Episodic insomnia can usually be traced to an acute psychological stressor or an environmental change. Chronic insomnia may be related to a combination of factors including depression, poor sleep hygiene, learned sleeplessness, sleep-disordered breathing, nocturia, drugs or extrinsic factors such as noise [6, 11].

Patients with MS face a high risk of insomnia of around 40% [6] compared to roughly 10–15% in the general population [12]. Awakening too early in the morning is the most common symptom (58%) [13].

Primary symptoms of MS that can condition the onset of insomnia are neurogenic bladder (nocturia), spasticity, sexual dysfunction, neuropathic pain, paroxysmal phenomena, depression and anxiety [7].

Insomnia affects daytime activities, because of fatigue, mood disturbances (depression and anxiety), attention, concentration and memory impairment [7]. Higher fatigue scores have also been found to correlate with insomnia, especially middle insomnia [13].

2.1.1. Diagnostic approach

Patients with insomnia may complain of difficulty falling asleep, difficulty staying asleep or waking up sooner than desired [10]. There are screening tools to identify such patients.

The Pittsburgh Sleep Quality Index (PSQI) measures seven domains: subjective sleep quality, latency, duration, habitual efficiency, disturbances, use of sleep medication and daytime dysfunction over the last month. Each of these seven domains is self-rated by the individuals. The score of each question is based on a scale from 0 to 3, in which a score of 3 demonstrates the negative extreme on the Likert Scale. A global sum of 5 or greater indicates a poor sleeper (sensitivity of almost 100% for insomnia) [14, 15].

Insomnia Severity Index (ISI): a seven item questionnaire designed to assess the nature, severity, and impact of insomnia in adults. Scores >15 reflect moderate clinical insomnia. It is also a useful tool to monitor the effects of insomnia interventions [6].

Athens Insomnia Scale (AIS): a psychometric instrument designed for quantifying sleep difficulty. It consists of eight items: the first five pertain to sleep induction, awakenings during the night, final awakening, total sleep duration and sleep quality; while the last three refer to well-being, functioning capacity and sleepiness during the day. Either the entire eight-item scale (AIS-8) or the brief five-item version (AIS-5), which contains only the first five items, can be used. The score of each question is based on a scale from 0 to 3, where a score of 3 indicates the negative or normal extreme on the Likert Scale. A cut-off score of ≥6 on the AIS is used to establish the diagnosis of insomnia [16].

2.1.2. *Management*

After detecting insomnia, amelioration of any precipitating causes of insomnia is a cardinal step in its management. Medications or substances that may contribute to insomnia should be reduced or discontinued, if possible, there should be a check on which drugs the patient is taking (medications used to alleviate MS-related symptoms, including over-the-counter medications).

Selective serotonin reuptake inhibitors, while helpful for depressive symptoms, may worsen insomnia.

Stimulants and wake-promoting agents, which are commonly used for fatigue, may interfere with sleep initiation if taken during the late afternoon or early evening hours.

Antihistamines, which are used as sleep aids by up to 25% of patients with MS, have the potential to worsen RLS, and thereby worsen sleep-onset insomnia [6].

Co-morbid symptoms must be identified and treated: neuropathic pain (tricyclic antidepressants and the α-2-δ ligand pregabalin), spasticity (baclofen or tizanidine) and urinary urgency (anticholinergics) [6].

Cognitive behavioral therapy (CBT) is an innovative psychotherapy approach. CBT treatment could reduce anxiety and depression by changing thoughts and beliefs and consequently reduce the symptoms of insomnia [6, 17].

Pharmacological therapies can be considered if more conservative strategies have been exhausted or are not fully effective: benzodiazepines, benzodiazepine agonists, melatonin receptor agonists and orexin receptor antagonists.

2.2. Hypersomnia

Excessive daytime sleepiness (EDS)/excessive daytime drowsiness disrupt daily performance.

Hypersomnia may be due to acute thalamus injuries, mental disorders, especially depressive symptoms, sleep deprivation or as a consequence of received treatments.

2.2.1. *Diagnostic approach*

The Epworth Sleepiness Scale (ESS) is a screening tool that assesses sleepiness and has eight items. ESS values equal to or greater than 10 indicate excessive daytime sleepiness (EDS), and in this case, patients should undergo polygraphy or PSG (screening for sleep apnea) [18].

All fatigued patients should be asked about sleepiness and fill in the Epworth Sleepiness Scale (ESS) as these are not always associated with sleepiness.

Magnetic resonance imaging (MRI) should be performed because of the need to identify structural lesions in the brain.

2.2.2. *Management*

After detecting hypersomnia, the physician should check for any medications involved and withdraw them if possible, treat acute lesions of multiple sclerosis with corticosteroids, indicate adequate sleep hygiene and assess whether specific treatment is needed to improve daily performance.

2.3. Restless leg syndrome

The four main criteria for diagnosis of RLS are: (1) unpleasant sensations in the legs; (2) worsening of the symptoms during rest; (3) relief of the symptoms by movement and (4) exacerbation of the symptoms in the evening or at night [19].

The periodic limb movement disorder (PLMD) includes repetitive periodic shaking episodes lasting between 0.5 and 5 seconds that occur during sleep every 20–40 seconds; mainly in the legs, but sometimes in the arms.

RLS and PLMD are motor disorders of sleep considered separate clinical entities, both conditions have the potential to cause disrupted sleep, share similar pathogenesis and have an increased prevalence among persons with MS. PLMD also frequently occur in the absence of RLS.

Most RLS patients (80–90%) have periodic leg movements PLM during sleep. They can cause arousals or micro-arousals leading to non-refreshing sleep, daytime sleepiness and fatigue. The prevalence of RLS in the general population ranges from 1 to 12% [20]. The prevalence of RLS in MS patients is two to five times higher than in the general population [21–24].

Differentiating RLS from other sensory and motor symptoms of MS can be difficult, as MS patients frequently suffer from spasms, dysesthesia, paraesthesia and spasticity in the legs, which worsen with immobility [25].

Predictive factors for RLS in MS patients include: older age, longer disease duration, progressive primary forms, greater disability as measured by the Expanded Disability Status Scale (EDSS), especially in the pyramidal and sensory subscales and shaking of the legs before onset of sleep [26]. Furthermore, RLS symptoms are more severe when associated with MS than when not associated with MS.

MS patients with RLS have more cervical cord lesions than those patients without RLS. These lesions possibly disrupt the ascending and descending pathways with cerebrospinal disconnection leading to these symptoms [10].

Primary RLS is a genetic form of RLS with autosomal dominant transmission [27]. Four genes have been associated with this syndrome [28] but no crossing over of those involved in MS [10].

Pathogenesis of RLS and PRLS shows dysfunction of downstream dopaminergic pathways, namely diencephalospinal and reticulospinal pathways, that project to the spinal cord. These pathways, *via* dopaminergic transmission, are responsible for the suppression of sensory inputs and motor excitability, and are susceptible to damage from diseases affecting the spinal cord. Impaired iron metabolism is also thought to contribute to the pathogenesis of RLS, as iron is a cofactor for a rate-limiting step in the synthesis of dopamine [6, 10].

Certain medications used in the management of persons with MS, such as antiemetic drugs, antipsychotic dopamine antagonists, antidepressants and antihistamines can also cause or worsen RLS [6, 10].

2.3.1. *Diagnostic approach*

Many descriptors can be used by patients to describe the restless sensation, including creeping, crawling, itching, burning, tightening, tingling or pain.

Symptoms of leg tightness relieved by voluntary movement suggest RLS, whereas involuntary spasms, even if a circadian component is endorsed, suggest spasticity. Rhythmic involuntary movements triggered by stretching or certain leg positions suggest clonus.

The Restless Legs Syndrome Diagnostic Index (RLS-DI) is a 10-item questionnaire. Scores range from −22 (no RLS) to +20 (definite RLS). A score of +11 yields 93.0% sensitivity and 96.1% specificity to accurately diagnose RLS [6].

Diagnosis of PLMD requires overnight PSG to assess for the presence of leg movements [6, 10].

The RLS Rating Scale is a useful tool to track treatment response and is a 10-item self-administered scale. Scores of 11–20 reflect moderate RLS.

2.3.2. *Management*

Iron supplementation should be implemented for a ferritin level of less than 50 ng/ml.

Reduction or discontinuation of medications and substances that can cause or worsen RLS or PLMD (dopamine antagonists, lithium, selective serotonin reuptake inhibitors, serotonin-norepinephrine reuptake inhibitors, antihistamines, tricyclic antidepressants, alcohol, tobacco and caffeine) is recommended.

Dopamine agonists (pramipexole, ropinirole and rotigotine), and the α-2-δ ligand gabapentin and anticonvulsants are first-line treatments.

Benzodiazepines and opioid agents (oxycodone and methadone) are second line treatments.

Treatment for refractory RLS, or augmentation in response to dopaminergic therapy, is also likely to be optimized by sleep specialty care [6].

2.4. Respiratory disorders during sleep

Sleep-disordered breathing is characterized by episodes of nocturnal hypopnea and apnea resulting in a reduction or a cessation of airflow in the upper airway.

Patients with sleep-disordered breathing may complain of "fatigue," decreased concentration, mood changes, erectile dysfunction, nocturia and mood changes, all these complaints are similar to those experienced in MS [29].

2.4.1. *Apnea and hypopnea*

Apneas and hypopneas may be caused by a collapse of the tissues and muscles in the pharynx (obstructive apnea/hypopnea) or a failure in the medullary respiratory signal (central apnea/hypopnea) [10].

Maintenance of upper airway patency during sleep requires an increase in pharyngeal tone that is primarily mediated by efferent motor output from cranial nerves X and XII to the palatal and genioglossus muscles, respectively. This process is largely influenced by afferent sensory input from pressure receptors in the upper airway, peripheral chemoreceptors in the aortic and carotid bodies, and brainstem respiratory generators. Pathophysiological processes that disrupt these tightly regulated brainstem pathways have the potential to impair nocturnal respiration. The medullary reticular formation is responsible for controlling automatic breathing during sleep [10].

Causative factors include obesity, craniofacial abnormalities, enlarged tonsils, congestive heart disease and degenerative central nervous system (CNS) disorders, to name a few [10].

Such apnea and hypopnea episodes may lead to nocturnal hypoxemia, frequent awakenings and daytime somnolence. When the apneas are associated with respiratory effort, the term obstructive apnea is used, and central apnea is used when there is a lack of respiratory effort [10].

Central sleep apnea is diagnosed when more of 50% of the events are central in patients with both central and obstructive apneas.

2.4.2. Obstructive sleep apnea

Obstructive sleep apnea is characterized by repeated episodes of upper airway obstruction and hypoxia during sleep [6].

The incidence of OSA in patients with MS is 2–21% and is one of the most common respiratory disorders [10].

Patients with MS who have a diagnosis of OSA and those at an elevated risk of OSA have increased fatigue and diminished quality life compared with undiagnosed or low-risk patients [6].

Sleepiness is primarily a result of acutely or chronically reduced sleep time, or poor sleep quality. Apnea severity may correlate with impaired cognition in MS [6].

2.4.2.1. Diagnostic approach

Questions must be asked about symptoms of snoring, pauses in breathing witnessed by a bed partner, gasping or choking upon awakening, non-restorative sleep, excessive daytime hypersomnolence or fatigue, cognitive disturbances and nighttime awakenings, any of which may arise in part from underlying OSA [6].

Dysarthria or dysphagia, obesity, increased neck circumference, crowded oropharyngeal inlet, retrognathia, or micrognathia are common physical exam findings [6].

The STOP-Bang questionnaire is a screening tool consisting of eight questions and measures that form the acronym snoring, tired, observed apnea, Blood Pressure-Body Mass Index, age, neck circumference and gender. Scores of 3 or higher indicate an elevated risk of OSA [6].

A full-night PSG is necessary to demonstrate the presence of obstructive respiratory events during sleep to confirm the diagnosis of OSA. These events may be partial (hypopneas) or complete (apneas), but must demonstrate evidence of a reduction in airflow during sleep, despite continued effort to breathe [6].

2.4.2.2. Management

Management strategies for sleep-disordered breathing should take into account the patient's primary apnea subtype, apnea severity, co-morbidities and behaviors, and other MS-specific symptoms or limitations. Guidance by a sleep medicine physician is often helpful [6]. Discontinuation of medication, such as opiates, antispasmodics or CNS depressants medications [6].

Positive airway pressure (PAP) therapy is delivered by a mechanical device and mask to splint the upper airway open during sleep. Supplemental oxygen, bi-level PAP and adaptive servo ventilation are other improvements that these devices have [6].

Oral appliances work by repositioning the mandible in the anterior and inferior position [6]. By improving nocturnal oxygen saturation and sleep quality, PAP therapy effectively reduces fatigue and can be effective in the treatment of depression. This is especially important given the link between fatigue and depression in MS [6, 18].

Disease-modifying therapy use, in particular emerged as a strong predictor of *reduced* apnea severity, raising interesting possibilities about the role of local and/or systemic inflammation in OSA [6].

2.4.3. Central sleep apnea

Central sleep apnea (CSA) is rare, and the prevalence is unclear in the general population. CSA involves repeated complete or partial reduction of airflow, caused by an intermittent lack of respiratory effort by failure in the medullary respiratory signal [10].

While the prevalence of CSA is less than that of OSA, patients with CNS disorders that affect pontine and medullary respiratory generators, including MS, may be at increased risk for this condition as well even nocturnal death (Ondine's curse) [6, 10].

CNS and brain stem-related nocturnal respiratory abnormalities such as central sleep apnea, paroxysmal hyperventilation, hypoventilation, respiratory muscle weakness and respiratory arrest have all been described and should be considered in this patient population in the evaluation of symptoms of daytime somnolence, increased fatigue and non-refreshing sleep [11].

2.4.3.1. Diagnostic approach

In patients with symptoms of daytime somnolence, increased fatigue and non-refreshing sleep, the physician must ask about nocturnal respiratory abnormalities [11] and look for evidence of reduction in airflow in the absence of respiratory effort in an overnight PSG.

In patients with both central and obstructive apneas, central sleep apnea is diagnosed when more than 50% of the events are central. The coexistence of OSA or CSA and MS has been described by several authors [2, 10, 30].

2.4.3.2. Management

In the cases of central sleep apnea not symptomatic or central sleep apnea during sleep-wake transition (20% of central sleep apnea cases resolve spontaneously) observation is recommended.

In other cases, PAP treatment, adaptive servo ventilation, oxygen, added dead space, carbon dioxide inhalation and overdrive atrial pacing are needed.

2.4.4. Nocturnal urinary disorders

Sleep disturbance is associated with outcomes such as increased risk of falls and mortality. Nocturia may both precipitate poor sleep and perpetuate insomnia (awakenings associated with nocturia may themselves be perpetuating factors) [31].

Overactive bladder (OAB) syndrome is a condition that accompanies urgency (a significant factor for sleep disruption), with or without incontinence, frequently with increased daytime frequency and nocturia [32]).

Nocturia is defined by the International Continence Society as the complaint that an individual has to wake at night one or more times to void. It reflects the relationship between the amount of urine produced while asleep, and the storage by the bladder of urine received. Nocturia is a symptom rather than a disease and causative categories have been proposed and is the most common storage symptom in the general population [32].

Nocturia can occur as part of lower urinary tract dysfunction (LUTD), notably in overactive bladder syndrome (OAB). Nocturia can also occur in association with other forms of LUTD, such as bladder outlet obstruction or chronic pelvic pain syndrome [33].

Nocturia is due to nocturnal polyuria, a decreased nocturnal bladder capacity or a mixture of the two. Various duplicating factors for nocturia have been reported, including pathological conditions such as diabetes, LUTD, cardiovascular disease, primary sleep disorders and sleep apnea [32].

Nocturia is a feature of systemic conditions affecting water and salt balance, leading to excessive production of urine at all times (global polyuria) or primarily at night (nocturnal polyuria), so that nocturia can be a systemic symptom such as cardiovascular, endocrine and renal disease can affect water and salt homeostasis, leading to an increased rate of urine production [33].

Nocturia can significantly influence quality of life, efficiency, vigor and awareness of health, primarily due to sleep disruption.

2.4.4.1. Diagnostic approach

Asking how many times the patient wakes up at night because of nocturia, whether urinary urgency exists and the characteristics of urination, quantity of fluid intakes, physical exercise, medication being taken, etc. is also necessary *for the diagnosis of urinary problems.*

The use of specific questionnaires such as the PSQ, ISI and ASI for the diagnosis of insomnia or the ESS for the diurnal hypersomnia helps the physician to approach the functional repercussion of the problem.

The study occasionally needs to be completed with ultrasound studies, urodynamics, MRI and urinary sediment to identify LUTD or OAB problems.

2.4.4.2. Management

Interventions targeting nocturia may potentially improve sleep quality [31].

Hygienic measures such as reduced fluid intake at the end of the evening and frequently going to the bathroom during the day can help. Adequate treatment of co-morbid conditions such as diabetes mellitus, congestive heart failure or sleep apnea requires direct intervention for improvement nocturia.

Anticholinergics, mirabegron, a-blockers, 5-a reductase inhibitors, oral phosphodiester-ase-5 inhibitors, desmopressin, diuretics, sleep-promoting agents and phytotherapy are used to treat urinary problems [33]. Half of MS patients with moderate to severe overactive bladder symptoms are treated with an anticholinergic medication [18].

Antimuscarinic drugs (Solifenacin), the most appropriate treatment for OAB, inhibited bladder stimulation may originate a decrease of drive to the brain stem, improve urination urgency and frequency and effectively reduce involuntary contractions and increase bladder capacity in patients with storage symptoms. The night time dosing of antimuscarinic drugs may improve tolerance compared to daytime dosing [32].

Antidiuretic therapy using clinician-directed dose titration has been reported to be more effective than placebo in terms of reduced nocturnal voiding frequency and duration of undisturbed sleep [33].

Nocturia severity improvement contributes to overall improvements in health-related quality of life [33].

The impact of treatment for nocturia in MS fatigue is unknown [18]. Non-pharmacological therapies such as cognitive behavioral therapy for nocturia (CBT-N) act on the abovementioned perpetuating factors. Sleep restriction entails reducing the excessive time in bed (a common occurrence in insomnia) and thereby improves sleep efficiency.

3. Effect of the quality of sleep in multiple sclerosis

Sleep disturbances have been associated with increased risk of mortality, cardiac disease, obesity and diabetes [8] and can contribute to the depression, pain and fatigue symptoms that are commonly seen in MS patients, which are often disabling [3, 9, 10].

3.1. Fatigue

Fatigue is defined as a subjective lack of physical or mental energy perceived by the patients or their caregivers which interferes with desired activities of daily living and it is the most frequent symptom in MS [18].

Between 80 and 97% [6] of patients report chronic fatigue, and more than 33% of patients rate this symptom as the most disabling [34–36].

Fatigue may occur at any stage of the disease and can even precede MS onset by several years. Fatigue affects the social and professional capabilities of patients, is a major reason for early retirement, reduced employment and is considered to be one of the main causes of impaired quality of life among MS patients, regardless of depression or disability [18].

Fatigue starts early in the morning and increases during the day. The perception of fatigue is exacerbated with environmental temperature and humidity [25], with age, [36] greater EDSS, mental or physical activity, infections and food ingestion [37].

Fatigue also deteriorates cognitive domains, such as information processing, memory and attention, [35] and it has significant socioeconomic consequences, including loss of work hours and in some instances, loss of employment, as well as family relationships and leisure time [36].

Fatigue is a symptom in MS patients and may have multi-factorial causes such as immunologic abnormalities (pro-inflammatory cytokines such as INF-α), endocrine influences (cortisol and dehydroepiandrosterone (DHEA)), axonal loss, altered patterns of cerebral activation, sleep disorders (RLS, chronic insomnia, sleep-disordered breathing and altered sleep microstructure), depression and medications used to treat MS symptoms or immunomodulatory and immunosuppressive treatments [7, 38, 39].

"Primary" fatigue is related to the pathological changes of the disease itself, and results from a spectrum where one pole is the inability to generate the force required to perform the task due to a failure of force production at the muscle level *"peripheral fatigue"*; and the other pole is the inability to sustain the required neural drive to muscle because of supraspinal, spinal and even peripheral nerve contribution *"central fatigue."*

"Central fatigue" can be the result of both cognitive and physical exertion and can reflect either a subjective sensation (fatigue) or an objective change in performance (fatigability) [37]. Dopamine imbalance plays a major role in developing fatigue. Central fatigue is a failure of the non-motor functions of the basal ganglia.

The subjective feeling of fatigue is related to inflammation and increased levels of cytokines such as interleukin-1 (IL-1), IL-6 and TNF-alpha [40].

"Secondary" fatigue attributed to mimicking symptoms, co-morbid sleep, irritable bowel syndrome, migraine, mood disorders, depression and anxiety and medication side effects [36, 37]. Persons with secondary fatigue report greater levels of fatigue than those with isolated primary fatigue [36].

There is a great variability in MS lesions from extensive areas of destruction during MS attacks, healing processes of and neuroplasticity. The clinical manifestations of fatigue do not seem to exclusively depend on the structural damage, but rather on the balance between restorative and inflammatory/degenerative processes and the rupture of the neural network [37].

In this respect, there is evidence that supports these hypotheses, linking fatigue with structural or functional abnormalities (atrophy in the thalamus, corpus callosum, cortical gray matter regions: superior frontal and inferior parietal gyrus, parietal lobe) within various brain networks (the cortico-subcortical circuit as a substrate for MS fatigue and the involvement of a "fronto-striatal network"), greater activation of the premotor area ipsilateral to the movement with functional MRI (fMRI), decreased N-acetylaspartate-creatine ratio (NAA/Cr) as a marker of axonal dysfunction. Resting-state fMRI studies show changes in functional connectivity (FC) of the basal ganglia including reward processing and motivation. In addition to motor functions, the abovementioned aspects are involved in the pathophysiology of fatigue [18].

3.1.1. Diagnostic approach

Patients with MS report being fatigued very often, sometimes it is just the feeling of lack of energy but in others it interferes with their work or their daily life. There are tools that help quantify the degree of fatigue which are described below.

Severity Scale (FSS): is a self-administered questionnaire with nine items (questions) investigating the severity of fatigue in different situations during the previous week. Grading of each item ranges from 1 to 7, where 1 indicates strong disagreement and 7 strong agreement and the final score represents the mean value of the 9 items. A total score of less than 36 suggests that you may not be suffering from fatigue [24].

Modified Fatigue Impact Scale (MFIS): The full-length MFIS consists of 21 items (total score 0–84, 38 as a cutoff to discriminate fatigued from non-fatigued individuals) while the abbreviated version has 5 items (0–20.). The abbreviated version can be used if time is limited but the full-length version has the advantage of generating physical, cognitive and psychosocial functioning subscales. The MFIS is one of the components of the MS quality life inventory [37].

MS patients, regardless of their fatigue level, have a significantly high frequency of RLS, higher Epworth sleepiness scale (ESS) scores, and higher PSQI scores. The time in bed, wake time after sleep onset %, total arousal index, limb movement arousal index and periodic limb movement arousal index are abnormal. The sleep efficiency index and sleep continuity index are lower in fatigued MS patients than non-fatigued MS patients. The PSQI results also suggest more disrupted sleep in fatigued MS patients. For all of the reasons above, quality of sleep studies should be performed with fatigued MS patients.

Once the patient has been identified with fatigue, it is necessary to investigate whether other co-morbidities are present (depression, anxiety, sleep disturbance, diabetes, heart disease, obesity, anemia, thyroid disease and nocturnal urinary disorders), what factors influence perpetuating fatigue and what situations can be modified in their lifestyle [6].

3.1.2. Management

Interventions targeting fatigue may potentially improve sleep quality and quality of life [31].

Pharmacological interventions are also reviewed and if there is evidence that a drug is involved in fatigue, it should be suppressed or the dose decreased [18]. Disease-modifying treatments (DMTs) are generally used to reduce relapses and progression and they occasionally cause an increase in fatigue, and in these circumstances it is important to change the medication for another DMTs [40].

Hygienic measures such as energy conservation programs, specific rehabilitation interventions physical (endurance, resistance, aerobic and combined training), aquatic therapy, cooling therapies, Tai chi, stretching, mindfulness-based interventions, yoga, acupuncture, progressive muscle relaxation and sleep hygiene advice (dependent on the nature of the sleep disorder) are more effective than pharmacological interventions [41].

Adequate treatment of co-morbid conditions such as diabetes mellitus, congestive heart failure, obesity, sleep apnea and other sleep disorders, depression and anxiety with pharmacological, psychological, behavioral and educational interventions is recommended [40, 41]. Pharmacological interventions for fatigue that are effective for reducing fatigue in patients with MS include amantadine, pemoline, prokarin (1 pilot study, side effects not reported), modafinil and pemoline combined with aspirin are efficacious for reducing fatigue in patients with multiple sclerosis. Carnitine has a discreet effectiveness. In general, the risk benefit of the drugs used for fatigue makes their recommendation be evaluated in each patient, highlighting them to the amantadine [37, 41]. Aminopyridines and coenzyme Q10 have an effect on fatigue by improving nerve conduction.

Nowadays, non-invasive brain stimulation (NIBS) techniques are gaining interest in the treatment of MS fatigue [37].

Promotion of health behaviors such as quitting smoking, physical activity (a high level of physical activity was borderline significantly associated with a decrease in co-morbidity) [42] and healthy eating may prevent some co-morbidities which were slow to show improvement in fatigue after the intervention, but they are effective [36].

3.2. Cognition

Cognitive impairment is a frequent feature of MS affecting up to 65% of patients [43] at both the earlier and later stages of the disease [44] and it tends to worsen over time [45].

MS negatively affects several aspects of cognitive functions, including attention, information processing [46], learning and memory, executive function and visuospatial abilities [47], having an important impact on quality of life [48], employment status [49], daily functioning, independence [50] and participation in social activities [51, 52].

Several factors have a negative influence on cognition in MS patients, such as depression [53], fatigue and sleep disturbances. Proper sleep is important for memory consolidation [54], and sleep deprivation has been related to impaired functioning in various cognitive domains [55].

Sleep disturbance causes a decrease in sustained attention [56], interferes with information processing and executive functioning [52]. Sleep disturbed patients reported higher levels of subjective cognitive problems compared to patients with normal sleep [52].

OSA and sleep disturbance are significantly associated with diminished visual memory, verbal memory, executive function (as reflected by response inhibition), attention, processing speed and working memory [52].

Excessive daytime sleepiness can lead to poor attention, poor memory, mood disturbances and increased risk of accidents [29].

In subjects with insomnia, a functional magnetic resonance imaging (fMRI) showed hypoactivation of the medial and inferior prefrontal areas during a cognitive task, in relation to the control subjects, which returned to normal values after treatment. Insomnia or superficial sleep produces less activation of the hippocampus and less connectivity is observed in the thalamus than in the control subjects. Damage to the hippocampus and thalamus (e.g., lesions and atrophy) in MS is associated with worse cognition. In controls, both regions may be related to sleep and cognition [52].

MS patients performed worse on all cognitive tests compared to controls. MS patients had less normalized gray matter (GM) volume, normalized white matter (WM) volume, hippocampal volume and thalamic volume. The hippocampus and thalamus showed increased functional connectivity (FC) in patients compared to controls, but lower FC was observed in patients with sleep disturbances (32%) [52].

3.2.1. Diagnostic approach

Neuropsychological manifestations can even be detected in patients during early stages of the disease. The Brief Repeatable Battery-Neuropsychology (BRB-N) [57] test was developed as a short and sensitive test to identify disturbances of cognitive domains in MS patients. The BRB-N has become the most widely used neuropsychological battery for MS, [58] and it is now being applied in clinical trials to monitor cognitive changes.

Different cognitive impairment criteria have been used: <1.0 SD, <1.5 SD and <2.0 SD in one, two or three subtests of the battery, respectively [59, 60].

3.2.2. Management

Strategies to optimize sleep could improve cognitive function in patients with MS.

In the case of insomnia, relaxation techniques such as autogenic training or progressive muscle relaxation can help the patient fall asleep earlier and have a longer sleep. But they do not improve sleep, so it has no sleep recovery effect. Behavioral therapies can improve sleep, but not prolong it. A combination of relaxation techniques and behavior therapy could be the most appropriate therapy for certain sleep disorders.

The general strategies for insomnia treatment include aspects of sleep hygiene such as extensions of night time in bed and frequent naps during the day. Pharmacological treatment is usually administered with stimulants such as amphetamines, methylphenidates, pemoline and modafinil [61].

As regards sleep hygiene, it is often necessary to make some lifestyle changes such as dinner should not be too late, nor too spicy or copious, maintain a regular sleep schedule, do not spend too much time in bed other than bedtime, do not drink caffeinated beverages such as coffee, black tea or cola, or caffeine medications, 4–6 hours before bedtime, do not smoke before going to bed or during the night, try to get enough rest and darken the bedroom, ventilate the bedroom, the temperature should not exceed 18°, do not do any physically demanding sport immediately before sleep because otherwise it will stimulate too much circulation, do not drink alcohol before going to bed or avoid sleeping too much during the day.

Patients with fatigue should organize daily routine and workloads. The physician also needs to improve the efficiency of information processing and working memory in these patients with fatigue [40].

Anxiety, depression, difficulty in sleeping and fatigue may have an impact on cognitive problems. If a person with MS experiences these symptoms and has problems with memory and cognition, they need to be provided with assessment and treatment (occupational therapist and neuropsychologist).

The concept of mental toughness (MT) has recently been recognized for its psychological importance not just in coping with stress but also for its association with increased physical activity (PA), and for its impact on both stress and objective sleep quality. MT consists of four key factors such as control (of own life and emotions), commitment, challenge and confidence (in own abilities and in other people); thus covering a range of cognitive-emotional processes closely involved in coping with stress, emotions, unexpected events and social setting [62].

3.3. Depression

Patients who suffer from problematic sleep and/or fatigue (with or without anxiety) may be more likely to experience higher depressive symptoms [63].

Depression is a mental illness that causes feelings of sadness and loss of hope, changes in sleeping and eating habits, loss of interest in your usual activities and pains that have no physical explanation.

3.3.1. Diagnostic approach

A trans-diagnostic approach to symptoms may be more effective than targeting each symptom separately, such as depression treatment or pain treatment alone. Trans-diagnostic models explain how multiple co-morbid symptoms or disorders develop rather than create disorder or symptom specific models [63].

3.3.2. Management

A trans-diagnostic treatment is an intervention that targets a range of diagnoses or problems through the use of treatment strategies targeting psychological processes that are common across disorders. It may be useful to consider all five factors such as depression, pain, anxiety, sleep and fatigue in designing a treatment plan. Treatments for the constellation of biopsychosocial concerns affecting many people living with MS.

The beneficial effects on depression of CBT targeting insomnia highlight a need for a comprehensive assessment of multiple concerns such as depression, anxiety, sleep problems or fatigue when treating people with MS who report higher levels of pain [63].

3.4. Trigger for an acute multiple sclerosis exacerbation

The mechanism by which sleep disorders trigger an acute MS relapse might be multi-factorial. Normal sleeping plays an important role in maintaining the normal function of the immune system. Various studies have shown that sleep disorders are associated with elevated serum levels of pro-inflammatory cytokines and markers of oxidative stress [15].

The circadian regulation of cytokine output produces a daily rhythm in the inflammatory profile, with a pro-inflammatory state occurring at night. Disrupted sleep can interfere with this pattern leading to prolonged periods of inflammation throughout the day, thereby exacerbating symptoms. Furthermore, the circadian rhythmicity of key components of the immune system has been shown to be dysregulated in MS patients [64].

The central circadian pacemaker, located in the hypothalamic suprachiasmatic nuclei, is responsible for regulating the timing and expression of various circadian rhythms [65].

Sleep dysfunction and disruption in the circadian system alter the synchrony between these transcriptional and translational feedback loops, resulting in increased cellular permeability, which is thought to be an important underlying mechanism for initiating the inflammatory cascades causing a disease flare. In addition, the presence of pro-inflammatory cytokines has been proven to suppress the activity of circadian genes [65].

Melatonin is produced by the pineal gland that regulates circadian and seasonal rhythms. Secretion of melatonin is suppressed during daylight and enhanced during the night, promotes sleep by reducing sleep latency, decreasing wake time and increasing overall sleep quality [65].

Melatonin promotes anti-inflammatory states: it inhibits nitric oxide production, nuclear factor-κB activation and tumor necrosis factor- α, it reduces COX-2 expression and matrix metalloproteinase activity (modulating apoptosis) [65].

Circadian sleep disorders are common in MS patients and could be linked to a disruption in melatonin production, which is important in sleep-wake cycle regulation. Melatonin helps dampen the overactive immune system and low levels are associated with relapse [64].

According to studies on an animal model, sleep deprivation is associated with an accelerated autoantibody production rate and increases oxidative stress (toxic effect on oligodendrocytes causing oligodendrocyte death and myelin damage). Chronic sleep deprivation breaks down blood-brain barrier (BBB) thereby increasing permeability [15].

Sleep disorders also result in an elevated serum concentration of interleukin-6 (IL-6), which further activates polyclonal B cells and triggers an autoimmune reaction. The serum concentration of IL-6 is significantly associated with the number of relapses in female patients with relapsing-remitting multiple sclerosis (RRMS) [15]. In the study of Sahraian et al. [15], the group in relapse had worse scores of global PSIQI for the previous month than remission group (87.5% were poor quality sleepers). Age, gender, EDSS and disease duration did not associate with sleep quality in either group.

4. Co-morbidity condition

Co-morbidities have been shown to affect MS progression, time to initiation of the disease-modifying therapy (DMT), as well as treatment compliance, which may be related to the increased mortality of these patients as compared to the general population.

Co-morbidities can negatively impact sleep in MS patients, which can, in turn, lead to a worsening of symptoms, especially fatigue and pain.

Patients with sleep disorders are at risk of co-occurrence of other problems like vascular diseases, obesity and diabetes that would threaten the health of patients in the long term [17].

Circadian disruptions occur in shift workers and appear to contribute to hypertension, diabetes, breast cancer, lung cancer and elevated prostate-specific antigen. Shift work entails changes in diet, exercise and tobacco use, which can confound circadian rhythm and sleep disturbance studies [65].

4.1. Narcolepsy

Narcolepsy is classified as a chronic sleep disorder associated with sleep attacks and other features attributed to abnormalities of rapid eye movement sleep, such as hypnagogic/hypnopompic hallucinations, cataplexy, sleep paralysis and disrupted nocturnal sleep. The usual PSG features include a mean sleep latency of less than or equal to 8 minutes and two or more sleep onset rapid eye movement periods [6]. There is a high variability in the prevalence across different geographic areas, which is thought to be related to differences between the populations and current study methods [10].

Narcolepsy is estimated to affect 0.02–0.05% of the general population, the overall prevalence of narcolepsy among persons with MS is unknown [6, 10].

There are two subtypes of primary narcolepsy which are described below.

Narcolepsy type 1(immune-mediated loss of hypocretin-secreting cells in the lateral hypothalamus) [6, 10] is characterized by the presence of cataplexy (a reliable clinical marker for hypocretin deficiency) and hypocretin deficiency in CSF (<110 pg./dl).

Narcolepsy type 2: normal hypocretin levels [6, 10].

The secondary causes of narcolepsy show that MS is the fourth most common cause of narcolepsy after inherited disorders, CNS tumors and brain injury, and it has been found that 12% of the cases of secondary narcolepsy were due to MS [6, 10, 66].

In terms of genetics, 95% of narcoleptic patients and 50–60% of MS patients are positive for DR2 haplotype. The human leukocyte antigen (HLA) DQB1*0602, a known genetic risk factor for narcolepsy, also influences the presence and severity of MS. Therefore, both diseases are closely related to the same genes of the human leukocyte antigen (HLA) system, which is the basis for labeling for most autoimmune diseases. This relationship suggests that similar autoimmune factors may be at work in the development of each disorder and might be partially responsible for symptoms of fatigue and sleepiness [6, 10, 67].

The aforementioned findings merit further attention given the potential impact of sleep disorders on the health and quality of life of MS patients [10].

4.1.1. Diagnostic approach

A diagnosis of narcolepsy requires PSG and CSF hypocretin assays (only performed at a few academic institutions).

Narcolepsy cannot be established in the presence of concomitant OSA, insufficient sleep, shift work or another circadian sleep disorder [10].

In such cases, adequate treatment of concomitant sleep disorders must be confirmed prior to the multiple sleep latency testing.

The usual PSG features include a mean sleep latency of less than or equal to 8 minutes and two or more sleep onset rapid eye movement periods [6].

It is necessary to perform MRI studies to rule out secondary causes of narcolepsy [6].

4.1.2. Management

Patients with suspected narcolepsy are usually referred for diagnosis and management by sleep specialists: wake-promoting agents or stimulants may be used to increase wakefulness and vigilance.

Sodium oxybate (an endogenous metabolite of gamma-aminobutyric acid (GABA) may be used in selected cases.

REM-suppressing antidepressants may be useful for cataplexy and sleep paralysis.

In cases of secondary narcolepsy when new hypothalamic lesions are identified, a trial of high-dose steroids should be considered [6].

4.2. Overweight and obesity

Being overweight is having more body fat than is optimally healthy. The degree to which a person is overweight is generally described by the body mass index (BMI). Overweight is defined as a BMI above or equal to 25 and below 30.

Obesity is defined as a BMI over 30. The prevalence of overweight and obesity in patients with multiple sclerosis ranges from 19 to 55%. These differences are due to the distinct prevalence in the general population, differences in geographic origin, population type (military veterans or hospital users) and/or age group. It is notable that the American population has the highest numbers of obesity. Besides which, it is worth mentioning the different methodology used, including overweight with obesity in some studies [42, 68].

Spanish data (NARCOMS study) have shown that overweight people with MS had lower general and mental health scores compared to those with normal weight and found no differences in other quality of life scales of the SF-36 [69].

Depression levels were higher in the overweight versus normal weight MS Spanish patients. This finding is due to pathophysiological mechanisms common to both depression and obesity, given that chronic low-grade pro-inflammatory states can generate various abnormalities in different neural networks [69].

BMI was significantly related to levels of disability, with obese participants 1.4 times more likely to have moderate/severe disability while controlling for age, gender, time since diagnosis and number of co-morbidities. As the BMI increases, the number of co-morbidities increases with higher odds for disability and prior relapse and lower health-related quality of life [42].

Central obesity, as defined by increased waist circumference, absolute waist circumference >102 cm in men and >88 cm in women or waist-hip ratio (the circumference of the waist divided by that of the hips) of >0.9 for men and >0.85 for women, is often indicative of metabolic syndrome, and is suggested to be a more potent risk factor (cardiovascular disease, Alzheimer's diseases and type 2 diabetes) than body mass index alone.

4.2.1. Diagnostic approach

Weight, height, BMI = weight (kg)/height (m^2), waist circumference and waist-hip ratio.

4.2.2. Management

Patients who are overweight and obese are usually referred for diagnosis and management by a multidisciplinary team such as specialist nutritionist, physiotherapists, surgeons and neuropsychologists.

Gradual weight loss and gentle physical exercise and stretching are recommended. Small meals and small amounts of food, low in animal fats and fresh fruits. Bariatric surgery may be necessary in severe cases of obesity.

Co-morbidities have been shown to be associated with increased hospitalization, rate of progression to disability, decreased quality of life and increased mortality risk which is why they have to be properly treated [42].

Adverse health behavior including being overweight and obese, smoking and sedentary behavior are common in people with MS [42]. These behaviors can be modified and may significantly change the level of health. Health professionals should be focused on achieving these behavioral changes in patients with MS.

5. Influence of the treatment of multiple sclerosis in sleep

The therapeutic approach to multiple sclerosis involves pharmacological, rehabilitative, psychological, lifestyle modifying interventions, etc. These can be used independently or coordinated with each other with a holistic view. This approach involves changes in the structure of sleep, which are not always beneficial.

5.1. Treatment of relapses

Therapeutic options to treat MS relapses include oral glucocorticosteroids [70, 71] or their intravenous administration at a high dose as first line and therapeutic plasma exchange (TPE) and intravenous immunoglobulin (IVIG) as second line treatments in glucocorticosteroids unresponsive patients [72], corticotrophin injection and Acthar [73].

The action mechanisms of glucocorticosteroids in the immune system are pleiotropic, induced apoptosis of peripheral blood leucocytes and down-regulation of T-cell activity delayed for 7–10 days after a 5-day course of administration [72].

TPE is the removal of circulating antibodies, cytokines, immune complexes and complementary factors, all of which are assumed to be involved in immune-mediated neuroinflammation.

IVIG reduces or prevents the activation of inflammatory cells and alters antibody responses.

Optimal treatment of relapses increases the chance of limiting or avoiding residual deficits which have been related to the progression of disability in MS [72].

Sleep disturbance (insomnia) might be one of the side effects of corticosteroid therapy during an acute exacerbation in MS. Benzodiazepines are useful during these periods [74].

5.2. Disease-modifying therapies

Interferons are DMTs that produce major alterations of sleep, mainly by the flulike reaction, fever, headache, alteration of the mood and fatigue. It is imperative to treat these effects to improve the patient's quality of life including finding what time is best to administer the treatment. The monoclonal antibody Natalizumab could reduce fatigue [37].

5.3. Symptomatic treatment

Specific treatment of symptoms of MS manifestations occasionally interferes with sleep quality, leading to insomnia or drowsiness. The treatments the patient is receiving need to be reviewed in the event of any sleep disturbance.

Selective serotonin reuptake inhibitors, while helpful for depressive symptoms, may worsen insomnia. Stimulants and wake-promoting agents, which are commonly used for fatigue, may interfere with sleep initiation if taken during the late afternoon or early evening hours. Antihistamines, which are used as sleep aids by up to 25% of patients with MS, have the potential to worsen RLS, and thereby worsen sleep-onset insomnia.

Patients suffering from fatigue symptoms are often treated with antidepressants due to the strong association between depression and fatigue. Modafinil, amantadine and aminopyridine are known as fatigue treatment options, although the physician must monitor the real effect on sleep and adjust the administration schedules so as not to mask the effect on fatigue.

Medications used to alleviate MS-related symptoms, including over-the-counter medications, also have the potential to interfere with sleep. Given the high frequency use of these medications in this population, the physician should carefully consider screening for these medications and assessing possible effects on sleep.

5.3.1. Management

The first approach includes reviewing the list of drugs being taken by the patient and adjusting doses or suspending them if necessary to avoid interference with other situations of the patient. In this respect, the multidisciplinary approach to the patient is important.

6. Conclusions

Sleep disorders in patients with MS are frequently underdiagnosed. Clinicians caring for patients with MS should routinely screen for sleep disturbances.

All the symptoms are related, many of them share the same pathophysiology where it is not possible to identify the precipitating factor and the perpetuating factor. Sleep disturbances increase the risk of mortality, co-morbidities (cardiac disease, obesity and diabetes) and can contribute to the depression, pain, cognitive impairment and fatigue symptoms which are disabling and worsen the prognosis of multiple sclerosis.

The therapeutic approach to sleep disorders in MS involves pharmacological, rehabilitative, physical, psychological, educational and lifestyle modification interventions. These can be used independently in combination, with combined therapies being more effective.

The list of drugs being taken by the patient should always be reviewed and doses should be adjusted or suspended if necessary to avoid interference with sleeps disorders.

Conflict of interest

Montserrat González Platas and María Yaiza Perez Martín report no conflicts of interest concerning the manuscript.

Author details

Montserrat González Platas* and María Yaiza Pérez Martin

*Address all correspondence to: montserrat.gonzalezplatas@gmail.com

Neurology Service, Hospital Universitario de Canarias, La Laguna, Santa Cruz de Tenerife, Spain

References

[1] Ma S, Rui X, Qi P, Liu G, Yang J. Sleep disorders in patients with multiple sclerosis in China. Sleep Breath. 2017;**21**(1):149-154

[2] Tachibana N, Howard RS, Hirsch NP, Miller DH, Moseley IF, Fish D. Sleep problems in multiple sclerosis. European Neurology. 1994;**34**(6):320-323

[3] Merlino G, Fratticci L, Lenchig C, Valente M, Cargnelutti D, Picello M, et al. Prevalence of "poor sleep" among patients with multiple sclerosis: An independent predictor of mental and physical status. Sleep Medicine. Jan 2009;**10**(1):26-34

[4] Bamer AM, Johnson KL, Amtmann D, Kraft GH. Prevalence of sleep problems in individuals with multiple sclerosis. Multiple Sclerosis (Houndmills, Basingstoke, England: Online). Sep 2008;**14**(8):1127-1130

[5] Vitkova M, Rosenberger J, Gdovinova Z, Szilasiova J, Mikula P, Groothoff JW, et al. Poor sleep quality in patients with multiple sclerosis: Gender differences. Brain and Behavior. Nov 2016;**6**(11):e00553

[6] Braley TJ, Chervin RD. A practical approach to the diagnosis and management of sleep disorders in patients with multiple sclerosis. Therapeutic Advances in Neurological Disorders. Nov 2015;**8**(6):294-310

[7] Caminero A, Bartolomé M. Sleep disturbances in multiple sclerosis. Journal of the Neurological Sciences. Oct 15, 2011;**309**(1):86-91

[8] Kripke DF, Garfinkel L, Wingard DL, Klauber MR, Marler MR. Mortality associated with sleep duration and insomnia. Archives of General Psychiatry. Feb 2002;**59**(2):131-136

[9] Kaynak H, Altintaş A, Kaynak D, Uyanik O, Saip S, Ağaoğlu J, et al. Fatigue and sleep disturbance in multiple sclerosis. European Journal of Neurology. Official Journal of European Federation of Neurological Societies. Dec 2006;**13**(12):1333-1339

[10] González-Platas M, González-Platas J, Bermúdez-Hernández M, Pérez-Martín MY, Croissier-Elías C, Pérez-Lorensu PJ. Low prevalence of sleep disorders in demyelinating disease in a Northern Tenerife population. Journal of Clinical Sleep Medicine: JCSM: Official Publication of the American Academy of Sleep Medicine. Jun 15, 2016;**12**(6): 805-811

[11] Fleming WE, Pollak CP. Sleep disorders in multiple sclerosis. Seminars in Neurology. Mar 2005;**25**(1):64-68

[12] Schutte-Rodin S, Broch L, Buysse D, Dorsey C, Sateia M. Clinical guideline for the evaluation and management of chronic insomnia in adults. Journal of Clinical Sleep Medicine: JCSM: Official Publication of the American Academy of Sleep Medicine. Oct 15, 2008;**4**(5):487-504

[13] Stanton BR, Barnes F, Silber E. Sleep and fatigue in multiple sclerosis. Multiple Sclerosis (Houndmills, Basingstoke, England: Online). Aug 2006;**12**(4):481-486

[14] Veauthier C, Gaede G, Radbruch H, Wernecke K-D, Paul F. Poor sleep in multiple sclerosis correlates with Beck depression inventory values, but not with polysomnographic data. Sleep Disorders. 2016;**2016**:8378423

[15] Sahraian MA, Rezaali S, Hosseiny M, Doosti R, Tajik A, Naser Moghadasi A. Sleep disorder as a triggering factor for relapse in multiple sclerosis. European Neurology. 2017;**77**(5–6):258-261

[16] Soldatos CR, Dikeos DG, Paparrigopoulos TJ. Athens insomnia scale: Validation of an instrument based on ICD-10 criteria. Journal of Psychosomatic Research. Jun 2000;**48**(6): 555-560

[17] Abbasi S, Alimohammadi N, Pahlavanzadeh S. Effectiveness of cognitive behavioral therapy on the quality of sleep in women with multiple sclerosis: A randomized controlled trial study. International Journal of Community Based Nursing and Midwifery. Oct 2016;**4**(4):320-328

[18] Veauthier C, Hasselmann H, Gold SM, Paul F. The berlin treatment algorithm: Recommendations for tailored innovative therapeutic strategies for multiple sclerosis-related fatigue. The EPMA Journal. 2016;**7**:25

[19] Allen RP, Picchietti D, Hening WA, Trenkwalder C, Walters AS, Montplaisi J. Restless legs syndrome: Diagnostic criteria, special considerations, and epidemiology. A report from the restless legs syndrome diagnosis and epidemiology workshop at the National Institutes of Health. Sleep Medicine Mar 2003;**4**(2):101-119.

[20] Ondo WG. Restless legs syndrome. Neurologic Clinics. Aug 2009;**27**(3):779-799, vii

[21] Auger C, Montplaisir J, Duquette P. Increased frequency of restless legs syndrome in a French-Canadian population with multiple sclerosis. Neurology. Nov 22, 2005;**65**(10):1652-1653

[22] Gómez-Choco MJ, Iranzo A, Blanco Y, Graus F, Santamaria J, Saiz A. Prevalence of restless legs syndrome and REM sleep behavior disorder in multiple sclerosis. Multiple Sclerosis (Houndmills, Basingstoke, England: Online). Jul 2007;**13**(6):805-808

[23] Manconi M, Ferini-Strambi L, Filippi M, Bonanni E, Iudice A, Murri L, et al. Multicenter case-control study on restless legs syndrome in multiple sclerosis: The REMS study. Sleep. Jul 1, 2008;**31**(7):944-952

[24] Deriu M, Cossu G, Molari A, Murgia D, Mereu A, Ferrigno P, et al. Restless legs syndrome in multiple sclerosis: A case-control study. Movement Disorders Official Journal of Movement Disorders Society. Apr 15, 2009;**24**(5):697-701

[25] Crayton H, Heyman RA, Rossman HS. A multimodal approach to managing the symptoms of multiple sclerosis. Neurology. Dec 14, 2004;**63**(11 Suppl 5):S12-S18

[26] Manconi M, Rocca MA, Ferini-Strambi L, Tortorella P, Agosta F, Comi G, et al. Restless legs syndrome is a common finding in multiple sclerosis and correlates with cervical cord damage. Multiple Sclerosis (Houndmills, Basingstoke, England: Online). Jan 2008;**14**(1):86-93

[27] Bonati MT, Ferini-Strambi L, Aridon P, Oldani A, Zucconi M, Casari G. Autosomal dominant restless legs syndrome maps on chromosome 14q. Brain. Jan 6, 2003;**126**(6):1485-92

[28] Trenkwalder C, Paulus W. Restless legs syndrome: Pathophysiology, clinical presentation and management. Nature Reviews Neurology. Jun 2010;**6**(6):337-346

[29] Caples SM, Gami AS, Somers VK. Obstructive sleep apnea. Annals of Internal Medicine. Feb 1, 2005;**142**(3):187-197

[30] Ferini-Strambi L, Filippi M, Martinelli V, Oldani A, Rovaris M, Zucconi M, et al. Nocturnal sleep study in multiple sclerosis: Correlations with clinical and brain magnetic resonance imaging findings. Journal of the Neurological Sciences. Sep 1994;**125**(2):194-197

[31] Fung CH, Vaughan CP, Markland AD, Huang AJ, Mitchell MN, Bliwise DL, et al. Nocturia is associated with poor sleep quality among older women in the study of osteoporotic fractures. J Am Geriatr Soc. 2017;**65**(11):2502-2509

[32] Kwon T, Oh TH, Choi S, Cho WY, Min K, Lee JZ, et al. Influence of daytime or nighttime dosing with solifenacin for overactive bladder with nocturia: Impact on nocturia and sleep quality. Journal of Korean Medical Science. Sep 2017;**32**(9):1491-1495

[33] Sakalis VI, Karavitakis M, Bedretdinova D, Bach T, Bosch JLHR, Gacci M, et al. Medical treatment of nocturia in men with lower urinary tract symptoms: Systematic review by the European Association of Urology Guidelines panel for male lower urinary tract symptoms. European Urology. Nov 2017;**72**(5):757-769

[34] Krupp L. Fatigue is intrinsic to multiple sclerosis (MS) and is the most commonly reported symptom of the disease. Multiple Sclerosis (Houndmills, Basingstoke, England: Online). Aug 2006;**12**(4):367-368

[35] Bakshi R. Fatigue associated with multiple sclerosis: Diagnosis, impact and management. Multiple Sclerosis (Houndmills, Basingstoke, England: Online). Jun 2003;**9**(3):219-227

[36] Fiest KM, Fisk JD, Patten SB, Tremlett H, Wolfson C, Warren S, et al. Fatigue and comorbidities in multiple sclerosis. International Journal of MS Care. Apr 2016;**18**(2):96-104

[37] Chalah MA, Riachi N, Ahdab R, Créange A, Lefaucheur J-P, Ayache SS. Fatigue in multiple sclerosis: Neural correlates and the role of non-invasive brain stimulation. Frontiers in Cellular Neuroscience. 2015;**9**:460

[38] Veauthier C. Younger age, female sex, and high number of awakenings and arousals predict fatigue in patients with sleep disorders: A retrospective polysomnographic observational study. Neuropsychiatric Disease and Treatment. 2013;**9**:1483-1494

[39] Pokryszko-Dragan A, Bilińska M, Gruszka E, Biel Ł, Kamińska K, Konieczna K. Sleep disturbances in patients with multiple sclerosis. Neurological Sciences: Official Journal of the Italian Neurological Society and of the Italian Society of Clinical Neurophysiology. Aug 2013;**34**(8):1291-1296

[40] Dettmers C, DeLuca J. Editorial: Fatigue in multiple sclerosis. Frontiers in Neurology. 2015;**6**:266

[41] Miller P, Soundy A. The pharmacological and non-pharmacological interventions for the management of fatigue related multiple sclerosis. Journal of the Neurological Sciences. Oct 15, 2017;**381**:41-54

[42] Marck CH, Neate SL, Taylor KL, Weiland TJ, Jelinek GA. Prevalence of comorbidities, overweight and obesity in an international sample of people with multiple sclerosis and associations with modifiable lifestyle factors. PLoS One. 2016;**11**(2):e0148573

[43] Amato MP, Zipoli V, Portaccio E. Multiple sclerosis-related cognitive changes: a review of cross-sectional and longitudinal studies. Journal of the Neurological Sciences. Jun 15, 2006;**245**(1–2):41-46

[44] Piras MR, Magnano I, Canu EDG, Paulus KS, Satta WM, Soddu A, et al. Longitudinal study of cognitive dysfunction in multiple sclerosis: Neuropsychological, neuroradiological, and neurophysiological findings. Journal of Neurology, Neurosurgery, and Psychiatry. Jul 2003;**74**(7):878-885

[45] Reuter F, Zaaraoui W, Crespy L, Faivre A, Rico A, Malikova I, et al. Cognitive impairment at the onset of multiple sclerosis: Relationship to lesion location. Multiple Sclerosis (Houndmills, Basingstoke, England: Online). Jun 2011;**17**(6):755-758

[46] Beatty WW, Monson N. Problem solving by patients with multiple sclerosis: Comparison of performance on the Wisconsin and California card sorting tests. Journal of the International Neuropsychological Society. Mar 1996;**2**(2):134-140

[47] Calabrese P. Neuropsychology of multiple sclerosis – An overview. Journal of Neurology. Feb 2006;**253**(Suppl 1):I10-I15

[48] Putzki N, Fischer J, Gottwald K, Reifschneider G, Ries S, Siever A, et al. Quality of life in 1000 patients with early relapsing-remitting multiple sclerosis. European Journal of Neurology. Jun 2009;**16**(6):713-720

[49] Schiavolin S, Leonardi M, Giovannetti AM, Antozzi C, Brambilla L, Confalonieri P, et al. Factors related to difficulties with employment in patients with multiple sclerosis: A review of 2002–2011 literature. International Journal of Rehabilitation Research. (Internationale Zeitschrift Fur Rehabilitationsforschung. Revue Internationale De Recherches De Readaptation). Jun 2013;**36** (2):105-111

[50] Engel C, Greim B, Zettl UK. Diagnostics of cognitive dysfunctions in multiple sclerosis. Journal of Neurology. May 2007;**254**(Suppl 2):II30-II34

[51] Rao SM, Leo GJ, Ellington L, Nauertz T, Bernardin L, Unverzagt F. Cognitive dysfunction in multiple sclerosis. II. Impact on employment and social functioning. Neurology. May 1991;**41**(5):692-696

[52] van Geest Q, Westerik B, van der Werf YD, Geurts JJG, Hulst HE. The role of sleep on cognition and functional connectivity in patients with multiple sclerosis. Journal of Neurology Jan 2017;**264**(1):72-80

[53] Arnett PA, Rao SM, Bernardin L, Grafman J, Yetkin FZ, Lobeck L. Relationship between frontal lobe lesions and Wisconsin card sorting test performance in patients with multiple sclerosis. Neurology. Mar 1994;**44**(3 Pt 1):420-425

[54] Walker MP. The role of sleep in cognition and emotion. Annals of the New York Academy of Sciences. Mar 2009;**1156**:168-197

[55] Lo JC, Groeger JA, Santhi N, Arbon EL, Lazar AS, Hasan S, et al. Effects of partial and acute total sleep deprivation on performance across cognitive domains, individuals and circadian phase. PLoS One. 2012;**7**(9):e45987

[56] Lehmann P, Eling P, Kastrup A, Grothues O, Hildebrandt H. Self-reported sleep problems, but not fatigue, lead to decline in sustained attention in MS patients. Multiple Sclerosis (Houndmills, Basingstoke, England: Online). Apr 2013;**19**(4):490-497

[57] Rao SM, Leo GJ, Bernardin L, Unverzagt F. Cognitive dysfunction in multiple sclerosis. I. Frequency, patterns, and prediction. Neurology. May 1991;**41**(5):685-691

[58] Huijbregts SCJ, Kalkers NF, de Sonneville LMJ, de Groot V, Reuling IEW, Polman CH. Differences in cognitive impairment of relapsing remitting, secondary, and primary progressive MS. Neurology. Jul 27, 2004;**63**(2):335-339

[59] Sepulcre J, Vanotti S, Hernández R, Sandoval G, Cáceres F, Garcea O, et al. Cognitive impairment in patients with multiple sclerosis using the brief repeatable battery-neuropsychology test. Multiple Sclerosis (Houndmills, Basingstoke, England: Online). Apr 2006;**12**(2):187-195

[60] Pérez-Martín MY, Eguia-Del Río P, González-Platas M, Jiménez-Sosa A. Cognitive status in patients with multiple sclerosis in Lanzarote. Neuropsychiatric Disease and Treatment. 2016;**12**:1553-1559

[61] Happe S. Excessive daytime sleepiness and sleep disturbances in patients with neurological diseases: Epidemiology and management. Drugs. 2003;**63**(24):2725-2737

[62] Sadeghi Bahmani D, Gerber M, Kalak N, Lemola S, Clough PJ, Calabrese P, et al. Mental toughness, sleep disturbances, and physical activity in patients with multiple sclerosis compared to healthy adolescents and young adults. Neuropsychiatric Disease and Treatment. 2016;**12**:1571-1579

[63] Amtmann D, Askew RL, Kim J, Chung H, Ehde DM, Bombardier CH, et al. Pain affects depression through anxiety, fatigue, and sleep in multiple sclerosis. Rehabilitation Psychology. Feb 2015;**60**(1):81-90

[64] Mills EA, Mirza A, Mao-Draayer Y. Emerging approaches for validating and managing multiple sclerosis relapse. Frontiers in Neurology. 2017;**8**:116

[65] Parekh PJ, Oldfield Iv EC, Challapallisri V, Ware JC, Johnson DA. Sleep disorders and inflammatory disease activity: Chicken or the egg? American Journal of Gastroenterology. Apr 2015;**110**(4):484-488

[66] Nishino S, Kanbayashi T. Symptomatic narcolepsy, cataplexy and hypersomnia, and their implications in the hypothalamic hypocretin/orexin system. Sleep Medicine Reviews. Aug 2005;**9**(4):269-310

[67] Iseki K, Mezaki T, Oka Y, Terada K, Tomimoto H, Miki Y, et al. Hypersomnia in MS. Neurology. Dec 24, 2002;**59**(12):2006-2007

[68] Marrie R, Horwitz R, Cutter G, Tyry T, Campagnolo D, Vollmer T. High frequency of adverse health behaviors in multiple sclerosis. Multiple Sclerosis (Houndmills, Basingstoke, England: Online). Jan 2009;**15**(1):105-113

[69] Cambil-Martín J, Galiano-Castillo N, Muñoz-Hellín E, Díaz-Rodríguez L, Laguarta-Val S, Fernández-de-Las-Peñas C, et al. Influence of body mass index on psychological and functional outcomes in patients with multiple sclerosis: A cross-sectional study. Nutritional Neuroscience 2016;**19**(2):79-85

[70] Grau-López L, Teniente-Serra A, Tintoré M, Rovira A, Ramió-Torrenta L, Brieva L, et al. Similar biological effect of high-dose oral versus intravenous methylprednisolone in multiple sclerosis relapses. Multiple Sclerosis (Houndmills, Basingstoke, England: Online). Apr 2015;**21**(5):646-650

[71] Ramo-Tello C, Grau-López L, Tintoré M, Rovira A, Ramió i Torrenta L, Brieva L, et al. A randomized clinical trial of oral versus intravenous methylprednisolone for relapse of MS. Multiple Sclerosis (Houndmills, Basingstoke, England: Online). May 2014;**20**(6):717-725

[72] Ehler J, Blechinger S, Rommer PS, Koball S, Mitzner S, Hartung H-P, et al. Treatment of the first acute relapse following therapeutic plasma exchange in formerly glucocorticosteroid-unresponsive multiple sclerosis patients-a multicenter study to evaluate glucocorticosteroid responsiveness. Intl J Mol Sci. 2017;**18**(8):1749

[73] Gold LS, Suh K, Schepman PB, Damal K, Hansen RN. Healthcare costs and resource utilization in patients with multiple sclerosis relapses treated with H.P. Acthar Gel®. Advances in Therapy. 2016;**33**:1279-1292

[74] Perrin Ross A, Williamson A, Smrtka J, Flemming Tracy T, Saunders C, Easterling C, et al. Assessing relapse in multiple sclerosis questionnaire: Results of a pilot study. Multiple Sclerosis International. 2013;**2013**:470476

10

HERVs in Multiple Sclerosis: From Insertion to Therapy

Belén de la Hera and Elena Urcelay

Abstract

Genome-wide association studies (GWAS) have not been able to completely elucidate the genetic background of complex diseases. Part of it could lie in repetitive sequences not studied in the GWAS, as those corresponding to Human Endogenous Retroviruses (HERVs). In the present work, we aim to review the potential role of HERVs in the etiology of autoimmune diseases, especially in multiple sclerosis (MS); their potential pathogenic role and their putative consideration as a good target for new treatments. For this purpose, we carried out an in-depth literature review on HERVs, and we integrated our previous findings about HERV-W, HERV-K18, and HERV-Fc1 and MS susceptibility. The study was carried out by a systematic search from electronic databases using the keywords "HERV," "Multiple sclerosis," "HERV-W," "MSRV," "HERV-K," "HERV-Fc1," and "GNbAC1."

Keywords: Multiple sclerosis, HERV, MSRV, GNbAC1

1. Introduction

1.1. HERVs

The endogenous retroviruses (ERVs) could be defined as "genetic parasites" of vertebrates [1], given that their origin is very different from the one displayed by the rest of the genome. Their existence in the genome of mammals is only known since 1970 [2], although, they resulted from ancestral infections by exogenous retroviruses millions of years ago. During an infection, the exogenous retroviruses are able to integrate one copy of their genome (provirus) into the genome of the host. Thus, they can stay permanently associated with the host and be transmitted horizontally by the creation of new virions (the typical spread of an infectious virus). Only when they infect a germ line cell, the integrated DNA can become part of the gene pool and be transmitted in a Mendelian fashion like ERVs [1, 3-5], as shown in Figure 1. Those who are present in the human genome are named human endogenous retroviruses (HERVs).

The endogenization process profoundly impacts on the survival and evolution of the virus and the host. It results from the balance achieved between the immune surveillance and the virus virulence [6]. In this way, the HERVs must surpass the host's antiviral defense mechanisms and infect the germ cells without causing a cytotoxicity that would prevent persistence in the progeny of the host [6]. Furthermore, from this moment on, all host cells are carriers of an integrated provirus [6].

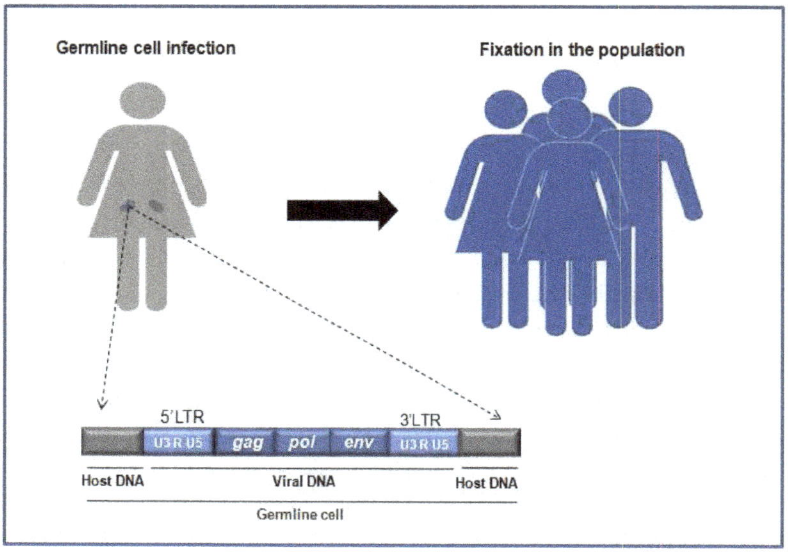

Figure 1. The endogenization process: once the retrovirus infects a germ line cell, vertical transmission in a Mendelian fashion occurs.

The retroviral insertion is aleatory, in the sense that no specific sites for retroviral integration exist in the host genome. Nonetheless, due to the epigenetic chromatin packaging, integrated HERVs elements are more commonly found within the transcriptionally active genome [6]. Currently, HERVs comprise nearly 8% of the human genome [7], distributed in approximately 31 independently acquired multigene families [8]. Even though no standard nomenclature has been defined for HERVs, they have been classified based on their homology with different groups of exogenous retroviruses. They are grouped as class I, class II, or class III retroviruses considering their homology with Gamma and Epsilon retroviruses, Betaretrovirus or Spumavirus, respectively [9, 10]. The family name is usually given by "HERV" followed by a one-letter amino acid code that corresponds to the tRNA specific of the site used to initiate reverse transcription [10]; consequently, the HERV-W family would use a tryptophan.

As mentioned, HERVs have a similar structure to proviruses of infectious retroviruses, with three principal genes, *gag*, *pol*, and *env*, flanked by two long terminal repeats (LTRs) [6]. The *gag* gene codes for the viral assembly proteins, including the nucleocapsid, matrix, and capsid proteins. The *pol* gene codes for the viral replication proteins, yielding the reverse transcriptase, protease, ribonuclease, and integrase proteins. Finally, the *env* gene codes for a viral glycoprotein, with both a surface and a transmembrane subunit. However, important changes are observed in the HERVs expression compared to that of exogenous retroviruses. Most HERVs encode incomplete proteins and accumulate mutations and recombinations. Furthermore, most HERVs with functional LTRs remain in a latent state under homeostatic conditions, owing to the epigenetic silencing of the provirus in heterochromatin [11]. Exceptionally, specific HERVs have been selected during evolution, provided that their biological functions could be beneficial for the host. In these cases, HERVs suffer a "domestication," meaning that a foreign gene can be used for cellular functions of the host [12]. In this group, we find proteins like Syncytin-1 from the HERV-W family, and Syncytin-2 from the HERV-FRD family [13]. These highly fusogenic envelope proteins are necessary to allow the formation of the placental syncytiotrophoblast layer; furthermore, they could be involved in the immune tolerance to the fetus [13].

In addition to these "domestic HERVs," several studies show reactivation of HERVs under pathologic conditions, such as different types of cancer [14-20]; autoimmune diseases including multiple sclerosis (MS) [21-37], rheumatoid arthritis (RA) [38], psoriasis [39], or systemic lupus erythematosus (SLE) [40]; and other diseases like schizophrenia [41, 42]. Nonetheless, we do not know whether their reactivation or increased expression is a causal effect, or conversely, is an underlying consequence of the disease.

1.2. Potential expression mechanisms of HERVs

Many factors can interfere or modulate the expression of HERVs, such as recombination events between two or more replication-defective HERVs [43, 44], infectious agents like Human herpesvirus 6 (HHV6) [34, 45] and Epstein–Barr virus (EBV) [46, 47], several transcription factors [31, 48], and the epigenomic context of the HERVs [6, 49, 50].

- Recombination events

Two or more replication-defective HERVs can restore their own defects through recombination events, resulting in a replication-competent retrovirus [5]. Even though this is an infrequent event, a study in mice points to a significantly increased frequency in specific immune deficiencies [44]. Furthermore, it has been demonstrated that recombination between three HERV-K defective proviruses is possible, leading to an infectious retrovirus [5, 43].

- Infectious agents

A putative explanation about the preferential expression of HERVs found in human brain samples could be the tropism of specific viruses and bacteria to the central nervous system (CNS). Neurotropic agents like herpesvirus [29, 51], Toxoplasma gondii [52], or certain strands of influenza virus [53] are able to cross the hematoencephalic barrier into the CNS. Usually, they are intercepted by cerebral macrophages leading to an abortive infection, but their transient presence in the CNS could activate the HERVs expression as a consequence of their immediate-early (IE) genes expression [4]. The expression of the IE genes of herpes simplex virus type 1 (HSV-1) and its interaction with the transcription factor binding sites situated in the U3 region of the LTR, such as AP-1 [54] and Oct-1 [55], lead to an activation of transcription in HERV-K and HERV-W families.

The herpesviruses are one of the best candidates: they may be neurotropic, remain latent, and can be reactivated. Furthermore, the expression of the Env epitopes in the surface of B cells and monocytes could be a consequence of the interaction between HERVs and herpesviruses [25]. Thus, the herpesviruses could play a dual role in neurodegenerative diseases, acting as pathological entities *per se* and as inducers of HERVs [6].

- Transcription factors

An important component of the antiviral innate immunity is the regulation of the expression and replication of HERVs by different transcription factors [48]. In HERV-W and HERV-K elements, both families previously related to multiple sclerosis (MS), different binding sites for transcription factors such as NF-Kβ [31, 48] are located in their promoter regions and could drive an increased expression of HERVs during inflammation.

- Epigenomic context

The chromatin state as well as the methylation state of GpC islands within the HERV promoter and regulatory regions seem to be crucial factors in the control of HERVs expression [49, 50]. Both play an important role as a part of the defense system against the potential effects of inserted sequences. Previously published studies describe how proviruses and solitary LTRs are densely methylated under physiological conditions, but hypomethylated in placenta [49, 50]. Thus, DNA hypomethylation, as observed in certain types of cancer, could allow reactivation of retroelements. In MS, HERVs have been described as susceptible elements to undergo epigenetic modifications, mainly due to modifications in the methylation state, resulting in activation of their expression and, consequently, inappropriate activation of the immune system.

1.3. Pathogenic mechanisms of HERVs

Even though most inserted copies in the human genome are defective copies, some HERVs could maintain the potential to cause or contribute to disease by different mechanisms [5]. As mentioned, HERVs may alter cellular functions by two ways, either acting as a genetic element or as a viral pathogen [6].

- Gene disruption

HERVs, like transposons, are able to experience transposition, recombination, and integration cycles. Some HERVs families include a high number of copies in the genome. It is believed that these families have been spread around the genome through the reintegration of a provirus. However, each new integration process increases the risk of a harmful insertion. They can disrupt genes present in their integration sites, for example, HERV-K integrations have been identified into tumor suppressor genes like *BRCA2* and into the repair *XRCC1* gene [6, 56].

- Modulation of gene expression

Some HERVs conserve regulatory sequences that can operate as functional promoters, enhancers, or polyadenylation signals, so they could change the expression of adjacent or distal genes [4]. They can also form part of regulatory RNAs: microRNAs (miRNA), small interfering RNAs (siRNA), and long intergenic noncoding RNAs (lincRNAs), contributing to the complex regulatory network of gene expression [5]. Furthermore, HERVs integrated into introns can provide alternative transcription start and termination sites [5].

- Pattern recognition receptors (PRRs)

The HERVs expression products, both nucleic acids and proteins, can modulate immune responses. They have the potential to interact with components involved in the immune innate response and to activate proinflammatory signaling pathways [57, 58]. Therefore, certain HERVs proteins could directly interact with specific toll-like receptors (TLRs), for example with TLR4, resulting in the production of TNFα and proinflammatory cytokines [58-60]. The nucleic acids derived from HERVs may also activate cytosolic PRRs; in this way, both an increased expression of RNA and the presence of cDNA in a nonfamilial compartment like the cytosol could activate PRRs [60]. Nonetheless, the human being has coevolved with endogenous retroelements and this could have shaped the sensibility of DNA sensors of the innate immune system, leading to an increased cDNA detection threshold to avoid an immune response against them. The cDNA levels are restrained by the action of gene products like Trex1 or SAMHD1 [60] and a loss-of-function mutation in these enzymes could result in the cDNA accumulation and the consequent sensors activation. This process would lead to a chronic immune response with release of pathogenic type I IFN and inflammatory mediators, similar to those observed in autoimmune diseases [60].

- Viral proteins: molecular mimicry, superantigen activity, or immunosuppressive proteins

HERVs proteins hold epitopes to B and T cells and molecular mimicry between viral proteins and certain autoantigens may exist, resulting in an autoimmune response. Moreover, some HERVs sequences are able to encode for superantigens. Superantigens combine with MHC class-II molecules to form ligands that stimulate T cells [61], and this may end in an abnormal activation of autoreactive T lymphocytes [62].

Alternatively, evidences exist of the immunosuppressive activity of certain HERVs Env proteins [63, 64]. This activity is reminiscent of their exogenous antecessors, which in this way increased the viability of the virions in the host. This capacity has suffered an adaptation process, and nowadays it might be implicated in the materno-fetal tolerance and could also prevent the immune response to exogen pathogens and tumors [60].

- Retroviral help for B cells

HERVs can also help B cells to quickly produce antibodies directed against pathogenic antigens [65]. The bacterial polysaccharide antigens and the carbohydrates linked to viral glycoproteins have the ability to stimulate B cells in the absence of T-cell help. These antigens are called thymus-independent antigens (TI), and they can be classified into two types: TI-1 or TI-2 antigens. TI-2 antigens cause extensive cross-linking of the BCR, leading to a quick differentiation of B cells into plasma cells. Finally, these plasma cells secrete protective antibodies, IgM and IgG [66]. However, the mechanism by which the TI-2 antigens activate B cells in the marginal zone without the help of T cells still remains poorly understood. It has been recently described that the cross-linking of B cells activates a signaling cascade, including the Bruton Tyrosine Kinase and the nuclear transcription factor NF-Kβ, allowing transcription of endogenous retroviral DNA [66]. The retroviral RNA may activate B cells by two complementary but different pathways: first, it could activate the retinoic-acid-inducible gene 1 receptor (RIG-1), resulting in a mitochondrial antiviral-signaling (MAVS); second, the RNA can be converted into DNA and can activate the cyclic GMP-AMP synthase (cGAS, cGAMP synthase). Finally, both signaling pathways would finish in the antigen-specific B-cell activation [65, 66].

2. HERVs and autoimmune diseases

HERVs represent the immunological limit between the self and the foreign. Their peculiar origin is very different from that of other genome elements, as they can share properties with infectious agents. Indeed, in case they would produce particles, these would not be so different from those originated from exogenous retroviruses. Therefore, they could activate the immune system and would induce autoimmunity [67]. As it has been previously discussed, HERVs have been associated, among other infectious or neurologic diseases, with different autoimmune diseases like MS [21-37], RA [38], psoriasis [39], T1D [68], or SLE [40], as shown in Table 1. Genome-wide association studies (GWAS) showed the existence of a genetic basis shared between different autoimmune diseases, discovering new immunogenic mechanisms implicated, and HERVs could be part of these shared genetic elements.

Class	Family	PBS	Related diseases	Expression mechanisms	Pathogenic mechanisms
I	HERV-W	Trp	MS Schizophrenia HIV Osteoarthitis	Herpesviruses Transcription factors Toxoplasma gondii Influenza A virus	Pro-inflammatory Env protein Superantigen activity OPCs differentiation interference Altered glial function
I	HERV-F	Phe	MS	Demethylating agents	Superantigen activity
I	HERV-H	His	3q13.31 microdeletion syndrome	N/A	Genetic deletion by recombination
I	HERV-E	Glu	SLE	Hypomethylation	Immunosupressor potential of Env
I	HERV-P	Pro	Cancer	Unkown	Unknown
II	HERV-K	Lys	MS ALS HIV	Herpersviruses HTLV-1 Type 1 IFN	Superantigen activity Neoepitopes Genes disruption

Class	Family	PBS	Related diseases	Expression mechanisms	Pathogenic mechanisms
			Schizophrenia T1D RA Juvenil arthitis Cancer	Transcription factors Hypomethylation	

MS, multiple sclerosis; HIV, human immunodeficiency virus; SLE, Systemic lupus erythematosus; ALS, amyotrophic lateral sclerosis; T1D, type 1 diabetes; RA, rheumatoid arthritis, HTLV-1, human T-lymphotropic virus-1; IFN, interferon; Env, envelope; OPCs, olygodendrocyte precursor cells; N/A, not applicable. Based on Douville and Nath, 2014 [6].

Table 1. HERVs families associated with different diseases

3. HERVs and MS

MS is one of the conditions more frequently related with HERVs. It is a chronic progressive disease characterized by neuroinflammation in the CNS accompanied by demyelination, axonal damage, and progressive neurologic dysfunction [69]. It is a complex disease, originated from the interaction of genetic, environmental, and epigenetic factors [70]. Recently, its incidence seems to be increased; at present MS affects 2.3 million people in the world [71]. However, many aspects of its pathogenesis are still poorly understood. GWAS have not completely explained the MS genetic background [72-74], albeit including the ImmunoChip Project [75] a total of 110 single nucleotide polymorphisms (SNPs) have been associated with MS susceptibility. Even considering the strongest risk factor, the HLA-DRB1*15:01 allele, each SNP has a modest effect and all together are able to explain only 20–28% of MS heritability [75]. Part of the missing heritability could reside on HERVs, as repetitive regions were not analyzed in the GWAS. Those repetitive regions were previously considered as "junk DNA" because it was thought that they had little or no physiological role. However, nowadays we know that these sequences could play an important role in the development of autoimmune diseases, including MS.

In 1989, Perron et al. [76] described the presence of extracellular virions associated with reverse transcriptase activity in a culture of leptomeningeal cells (LM7) obtained from the cerebrospinal fluid (CSF) of an MS patient. In the beginning, it was thought that those virions could correspond to the human T-lymphotropic virus (HTLV-1) due to the similarities between the tropical spastic paraparesis (a demyelinating progressive disease) caused by HTLV-1, and MS. However, a new retroviral element called MSRV (Multiple-sclerosis-associated retrovirus) was identified, the founder of the HERV-W family [77]. This multicopy family, consisting of approximately 650 loci around the human genome [35], comprises a total of 311 inserts (more or less complete proviruses or pseudogenes) and 343 additional HERV-W LTRs [78].

Only the *env* gene mapping on chromosome 7, encoding Syncytin, presents a complete open reading frame (ORF) and has been selectively conserved [35]. The MSRV *env* sequence can be differentiated from the one corresponding to Syncytin-1 by a 12-nucleotide insertion in the transmembrane moiety. Both genes are expressed in the brain of MS patients, but the MSRV-type *env* DNA copies were found sixfold more frequently in MS patients than in healthy controls, while comparable copy numbers of Syncytin-1 were observed [79]. Furthermore, Syncytin-1 is originated from the retroviral copy inserted in chromosome 7, and the pathogenic protein MSRV-type Env could be originated from several integrations in the human genome, or it could result from recombination events between insertions in different chromosomes [80, 81]. The genomic origin of HERV-W Env remains unknown although recent works consider the copy mapping to chromosome X one plausible candidate [4, 80, 81]. This copy, located on Xq22.3, would encode for an almost complete MSRV-type protein, truncated on its N-terminal end due to the presence of a stop codon mutation at position 39 [81]. *Ex vivo*, this copy still conserves coding capacity, as it is able to produce a truncated N-terminally Env protein [80]. Furthermore, the reversion of this stop codon would lead to a complete protein with signal peptide, expressed in the cellular surface in the same way that Syncytin [80].

Recently, a genetic screening was performed by specific PCR amplification followed by High Resolution Melting (HRM) analyses of the two MSRV-like env copies which show the ORF with the highest length similarity and homology to Syncytin (1614 bp), inserted in chromosome X (1428 bp) and in chromosome 20 (1419 bp). Both chromosomal origins show similar lengths of their respective ORFs, 10% shorter than the one measured for Syncytin, and could putatively originate functional proteins. The results pointed to the insertion in chromosome X, and not the one in chromosome 20, as an origin of MSRV. One polymorphism identified in chromosome X, rs6622139*T, was associated in women with MS susceptibility and severity [82], and it was also associated with higher MSRV-like *env* levels of expression (Mann–Whitney U test: $p=0.003$), while the two polymorphisms found in chromosome 20 did not show evidence of association [83].

Since it was described, several studies have associated the HERV-W family with MS: the presence of MSRV-type Env protein has been found in demyelinated acute lesions in MS patients [31], as well as an increased number of DNA copies [84] or a higher prevalence of MSRV-type RNA in serum and CSF of MS patients compared with patients suffering from other neurological diseases or healthy controls from all ethnic groups [24, 27, 28, 31, 84-86]. The MSRV presence in serum and CSF is correlated with the clinical progression, severity, and prognosis of MS [28, 46], while the absence of MSRV relates with a more stable course of the disease [28, 36]. The MSRV production is stimulated by cytokines like TNFα, IL6, and IFNγ[87], and current MS therapies like IFN-β and Natalizumab, which are able to reduce MS symptomatology, promote a diminution of MSRV virus load levels in blood [87-89].

HERV-W Env proteins, MSRV-type Env, and Syncytin have proinflammatory and superantigenic properties. They can cause neuroinflammation, neurodegeneration, immune system dysregulation, and endoplasmic reticulum stress [4, 21, 22, 58, 90, 91]. Their pathogenicity has been studied *in vitro* using different types of cell cultures and *in vivo* using a humanized Severe Combined Immunodeficiency Disease (SCID) animal model, showing neurotoxic effects in both settings [22, 92] and a reduced capacity of olygodendrocyte progenitor cells (OPC) differentiation, interfering in the remyelination process [57]. A recent study clarifies the possible pathogenic mechanisms of MSRV. In a human model of BBB, the endothelial cell line

HCMEC/D3, they show that MRSV-type Env interacts with TLR4 and induces a dose-dependent overexpression of ICAM1, as well as an induced IL6 and IL8 production; while the Env protein derived from Syncytin-1 did not show these effects [59]. Furthermore, they also described that the MSRV-type Env presence significantly stimulates the adhesion and migration of activated immune cells through the layer of endothelial cells. These results support the hypothesis that MSRV can be involved in MS pathogenesis, as well as in other chronic inflammatory diseases, at least in the maintenance of the underlying inflammatory condition [59]. Table 2 reflects the possible pathogenic mechanisms described for MSRV.

Cell type	Receptor	Pathogenic mechanisms
T lymphocytes	TCR	Superantigen activity, T lymphocytes proliferation and CK liberation
APC	TLR4	↑ pro-inflammatory CK ↑ costimulatory molecules
HCMEC/D3 endothelial cell line	TLR4	↑ ICAM1 expression IL6, IL8 expression
OPC	TLR4	OPCs differentiation interference (↑ iNOS, oxidative stress)

APC, antigen presenting cell; OPC, olygodendrocyte precursor cell; TCR, T-cell receptor; TLR4, toll-like receptor 4

Table 2. Known pathogenic mechanisms of MSRV

Even though the HERV-W family is one of the HERV families more related to MS, other families like HERV-K18 [37, 93] or HERV-Fc1 [29, 94, 95] have also been associated with MS susceptibility.

HERV-K is a multicopy family including approximately 332 copies dispersed through the human genome. It is the only known retroviral element that codes for all the structural and enzymatic proteins (Gag, Prt, Pol), as well as for the Env protein and for the accessory Rec protein [96]. This family has been related with different autoimmune diseases as MS [37], type-1diabetes (T1D) [68], or juvenile rheumatoid arthritis [38]; and different cancer types [14-17]. One specific member of this family, HERV-K18, has been associated with MS susceptibility and its expression is induced by herpesvirus [97, 98] and by EBV [99-102], both viruses previously proposed as potential environmental factors involved in MS development [45, 51, 97, 103-108]. Three different variants of the HERV-K18 copy mapping to chromosome 1 [37] have been described. They conform haplotypes within the first intron of CD48 that can be defined by two SNPs (18.1 SNP1*A/SNP2*A, 18.2 SNP1*G/SNP2*G, 18.3 SNP1*A/SNP2*G), all of them coding for an Env protein with superantigenic properties. However, only one of these variants (18.3) has been associated with a higher risk to MS [37] and with an overall higher susceptibility to autoimmune diseases, as described by a meta-analysis including a total of 2656 patients and 2016 controls [93].

Considering the HERV-Fc family, a total of 6 HERV-Fc elements and 11 LTRs have been identified across the human genome. Among them, only two elements correspond to a complete HERV-Fc provirus (Fc1env and Fc2master) [109]. Related to MS, it has been observed that the HERV-Fc1 RNA levels were significantly increased in the plasma of patients suffering from active MS, compared to nonactive MS or controls [30]. The HERV-Fc1 is an unusual provirus, because it includes a single copy in the genome, located on Xq21.33. Furthermore, it is a recent acquisition for the genome, only present in humans, chimpanzees, and gorillas [109]. Nexo et al. [94] were the first to describe that rs391745, located in the promoter region of HERV-Fc1, was associated with MS susceptibility in Danish cohorts and, then, a replication study was performed with a Norwegian cohort. The latter study also detailed that the association was only observed in the nonprimary-progressive MS forms [29], results validated in further studies [95]. Regarding the HERV-Fc1 expression mechanisms, it has been observed that the transcriptional expression levels of HERV-Fc1 RNA sequences are negatively correlated with the methylation levels of CpG islands on the 5′ LTR region and, therefore, a higher HERV-Fc1 expression involves DNA demethylation [11, 110].

4. HERVs as future treatment options

An increased expression of HERVs in several autoimmune diseases [21-40, 68] and different types of cancer [14-20], along with the decreased expression levels observed in successfully treated patients with immunomodulatory therapies [88, 89] or chemotherapy [111] point to the potential pathogenic role of HERVs and their putative consideration as a good target for new treatments.

A humanized monoclonal antibody anti-Env-SU MSRV/HERV-W, GNbAC1, has been studied as a putative MS treatment due to its potential neuroprotector effects [112-115]. The results of a phase IIa clinical trial [114] show that the GNbAC1 treatment blocks the transcription of proinflammatory genes mediated by Env, prevents the formation of nitrosantine, and restores OPC differentiation. Furthermore, GNbAC1 has advantages compared to other MS treatments, because the patients retain all their immune capacity. This treatment has also been studied in other diseases like diabetes and schizophrenia.

The proteins encoded by HERV-K *env* have been proposed as therapeutic targets for different types of cancer, due to the fact that a general hypomethylation of HERVs sequences has been observed, as well as an increased expression of Np9 and Rec proteins originating from HERV-K in different cancer cells [116]. Both proteins bind to the PLZF protein, a transcriptional repressor of the C-MYC proto-oncogen. The inflammation and the deregulation of proto-oncogen signaling caused by the HERV-K protein results in a protumorogenic microenvironment, which favors cell proliferation and metastasis [116]. The use of monoclonal antibodies against HERV-K Env protein inhibits tumoral growth and induces apoptosis in breast cancer cells *in vitro* [116]; therefore, it could be considered a good candidate as a therapy used together with other cancer treatments.

In addition to autoimmune diseases and cancer, the human immunodeficiency virus (HIV) has been also related to HERVs, particularly with the HERV-K family, raising the issue of potential beneficial effects of a therapy directed against HERVs in AIDS. Some studies report an increased expression of HERV-K provirus in HIV patients compared to controls [117, 118] and show that the immune responses against HERV-K decrease the HIV-1 viral load. *In vitro*, the use of an antibody directed against the HERV-K transmembrane protein (HML-2), HA-137, was able to eliminate the cells that displayed the antigen in their surface. This was carried out by an antibody-dependent cell-mediated cytotoxicity (ADCC) mechanism by natural killer (NK) cells. It has been described that the HIV-infected cells display this membrane antigen in their surface [119]; therefore, they would be potential targets of the antibody. The possibility of finding a target epitope different from those of the HIV virus could open up opportunities to the development of vaccines against this disease; a field that has been very limited due to the high rate of mutation of the HIV [119].

5. Conclusion

This work aimed to provide a systematic revision of HERVs, with particular emphasis on their potential pathogenic role in MS. Although many aspects of the etiology of this disease remain to be solved, different works support the relevance that HERVs may have in the etiopathogenesis of autoimmune diseases, and specifically in MS. HERVs may contribute to both, disease onset and maintenance, through an exacerbated activation of the immune system. Recently, the results of a phase IIa clinical trial that studies the effectiveness of a human monoclonal antibody (GNbAC1) as a therapeutic target in MS have been published with promising outcome. Thus, evidences support the role of HERVs as potential therapeutic armory in different autoimmune diseases, cancer, and HIV.

Author details

Belén de la Hera and Elena Urcelay*

*Address all correspondence to: elena.urcelay@salud.madrid.org

Instituto de Investigación Sanitaria del Hospital Clínico San Carlos, IdISSC, Madrid, Spain

References

[1] Ribet D, Heidman T. Formation et évolution des rétrovirus endogènes. *Virologie*. 2010;14:141-50. DOI:10.1684/vir.2010.0294.

[2] Coffin JM. Structure, replication, and recombination of retrovirus genomes: some unifying hypotheses. *J Gen Virol.* 1979;42:1-26.

[3] Chuong EB. Retroviruses facilitate the rapid evolution of the mammalian placenta. *Bioessays.* 2013;35:853-61. DOI: 10.1002/bies.201300059.

[4] Perron H, Bernard C, Bertrand JB, Lang AB, Popa I, Sanhadji K, et al. Endogenous retroviral genes, Herpesviruses and gender in Multiple Sclerosis. *J Neurol Sci.* 2009;286:65-72.

[5] Young GR, Stoye JP, Kassiotis G. Are human endogenous retroviruses pathogenic? An approach to testing the hypothesis. *Bioessays.* 2013;35:794-803. DOI: 10.1002/bies.201300049.

[6] Douville RN, Nath A. Human endogenous retroviruses and the nervous system. *Handb Clin Neurol.* 2014;123:465-85. DOI:10.1016/B978-0-444-53488-0.00022-5.

[7] Lander ES, Linton LM, Birren B, Nusbaum C, Zody MC, Baldwin J, et al. Initial sequencing and analysis of the human genome. *Nature.* 2001;409:860-921. DOI: 10.1038/35057062.

[8] Belshaw R, Katzourakis A, Paces J, Burt A, Tristem M. High copy number in human endogenous retrovirus families is associated with copying mechanisms in addition to reinfection. *Mol Biol Evol.* 2005;22:814-7. DOI:10.1093/molbev/msi088.

[9] Voisset C, Weiss RA, Griffiths DJ. Human RNA "rumor" viruses: the search for novel human retroviruses in chronic disease. *Microbiol Mol Biol Rev.* 2008;72:157-96. DOI: 10.1128/MMBR.00033-07.

[10] Gifford R, Tristem M. The evolution, distribution and diversity of endogenous retroviruses. *Virus Genes.* 2003;26:291-315. DOI:10.1023/A:1024455415443.

[11] Laska MJ, Nissen KK, Nexo BA. (Some) cellular mechanisms influencing the transcription of human endogenous retrovirus, HERV-Fc1. *PLoS One.* 2013;8:e53895. DOI: 10.1371/journal.pone.0053895.

[12] Patel MR, Emerman M, Malik HS. Paleovirology - ghosts and gifts of viruses past. *Curr Opin Virol.* 2011;1:304-9. DOI:10.1016/j.coviro.2011.06.007.

[13] Dupressoir A, Heidmann T. [Syncytins – retroviral envelope genes captured for the benefit of placental development]. *Med Sci* (Paris). 2011;27:163-9. DOI:10.1051/medsci/2011272163.

[14] Buscher K, Trefzer U, Hofmann M, Sterry W, Kurth R, Denner J. Expression of human endogenous retrovirus K in melanomas and melanoma cell lines. *Cancer Res.* 2005;65:4172-80. DOI: 10.1158/0008-5472.CAN-04-2983

[15] Herbst H, Kuhler-Obbarius C, Lauke H, Sauter M, Mueller-Lantzsch N, Harms D, et al. Human endogenous retrovirus (HERV)-K transcripts in gonadoblastomas and go-

nadoblastoma-derived germ cell tumours. *Virchows Arch.* 1999;434:11-5. DOI:10.1007/s004280050298

[16] Lower R, Lower J, Frank H, Harzmann R, Kurth R. Human teratocarcinomas cultured in vitro produce unique retrovirus-like viruses. *J Gen Virol.* 1984;65 (Pt 5): 887-98.

[17] Wang-Johanning F, Liu J, Rycaj K, Huang M, Tsai K, Rosen DG, et al. Expression of multiple human endogenous retrovirus surface envelope proteins in ovarian cancer. *Int J Cancer.* 2007;120:81-90. DOI:10.1002/ijc.22256.

[18] Florl AR, Lower R, Schmitz-Drager BJ, Schulz WA. DNA methylation and expression of LINE-1 and HERV-K provirus sequences in urothelial and renal cell carcinomas. *Br J Cancer.* 1999;80:1312-21. DOI: 10.1038/sj.bjc.6690524.

[19] Menendez L, Benigno BB, McDonald JF. L1 and HERV-W retrotransposons are hypomethylated in human ovarian carcinomas. *Mol Cancer.* 2004;3:12. DOI: 10.1186/1476-4598-3-12.

[20] Wentzensen N, Coy JF, Knaebel HP, Linnebacher M, Wilz B, Gebert J, et al. Expression of an endogenous retroviral sequence from the HERV-H group in gastrointestinal cancers. *Int J Cancer.* 2007;121:1417-23. DOI:10.1002/ijc.22826.

[21] Antony JM, Ellestad KK, Hammond R, Imaizumi K, Mallet F, Warren KG, et al. The human endogenous retrovirus envelope glycoprotein, syncytin-1, regulates neuroinflammation and its receptor expression in multiple sclerosis: a role for endoplasmic reticulum chaperones in astrocytes. *J Immunol.* 2007;179:1210-24. DOI: 10.4049/jimmunol.179.2.1210

[22] Antony JM, van Marle G, Opii W, Butterfield DA, Mallet F, Yong VW, et al. Human endogenous retrovirus glycoprotein-mediated induction of redox reactants causes oligodendrocyte death and demyelination. *Nat Neurosci.* 2004;7:1088-95. DOI:10.1038/nn1319.

[23] Antony JM, Zhu Y, Izad M, Warren KG, Vodjgani M, Mallet F, et al. Comparative expression of human endogenous retrovirus-W genes in multiple sclerosis. *AIDS Res Hum Retroviruses.* 2007;23:1251-6. DOI:10.1089/aid.2006.0274..

[24] Arru G, Mameli G, Astone V, Serra C, Huang YM, Link H, et al. Multiple Sclerosis and HERV-W/MSRV: A Multicentric Study. *Int J Biomed Sci.* 2007;3:292-7.

[25] Brudek T, Christensen T, Aagaard L, Petersen T, Hansen HJ, Moller-Larsen A. B cells and monocytes from patients with active multiple sclerosis exhibit increased surface expression of both HERV-H Env and HERV-W Env, accompanied by increased seroreactivity. *Retrovirology.* 2009;6:104. DOI:10.1186/1742-4690-6-104.

[26] Dolei A. MSRV/HERV-W/syncytin and its linkage to multiple sclerosis: the usability and the hazard of a human endogenous retrovirus. *J Neurovirol.* 2005;11:232-5. DOI: 10.1080/13550280590952899.

[27] Dolei A, Perron H. The multiple sclerosis-associated retrovirus and its HERV-W endogenous family: a biological interface between virology, genetics, and immunology in human physiology and disease. *J Neurovirol.* 2009;15:4-13. DOI: 10.1080/13550280802448451.

[28] Dolei A, Serra C, Mameli G, Pugliatti M, Sechi G, Cirotto MC, et al. Multiple sclerosis-associated retrovirus (MSRV) in Sardinian MS patients. *Neurology*. 2002;58:471-3. DOI:10.1212/WNL.58.3.471.

[29] Hansen B, Oturai AB, Harbo HF, Celius EG, Nissen KK, Laska MJ, et al. Genetic association of multiple sclerosis with the marker rs391745 near the endogenous retroviral locus HERV-Fc1: analysis of disease subtypes. *PLoS One*. 2011;6:e26438. DOI:10.1371/journal.pone.0026438.

[30] Laska MJ, Brudek T, Nissen KK, Christensen T, Moller-Larsen A, Petersen T, et al. Expression of HERV-Fc1, a human endogenous retrovirus, is increased in patients with active multiple sclerosis. *J Virol*. 2012;86:3713-22. DOI:10.1128/JVI.06723-11.

[31] Mameli G, Astone V, Arru G, Marconi S, Lovato L, Serra C, et al. Brains and peripheral blood mononuclear cells of multiple sclerosis (MS) patients hyperexpress MS-associated retrovirus/HERV-W endogenous retrovirus, but not Human herpesvirus 6. *J Gen Virol*. 2007;88:264-74. DOI: 10.1099/vir.0.81890-0

[32] Mameli G, Astone V, Khalili K, Serra C, Sawaya BE, Dolei A. Regulation of the syncytin-1 promoter in human astrocytes by multiple sclerosis-related cytokines. *Virology*. 2007;362:120-30. DOI:10.1016/j.virol.2006.12.019.

[33] Rolland A, Jouvin-Marche E, Saresella M, Ferrante P, Cavaretta R, Creange A, et al. Correlation between disease severity and in vitro cytokine production mediated by MSRV (multiple sclerosis associated retroviral element) envelope protein in patients with multiple sclerosis. *J Neuroimmunol*. 2005;160:195-203. DOI:10.1016/j.jneuroim.2004.10.019.

[34] Ruprecht K, Obojes K, Wengel V, Gronen F, Kim KS, Perron H, et al. Regulation of human endogenous retrovirus W protein expression by herpes simplex virus type 1: implications for multiple sclerosis. *J Neurovirol*. 2006;12:65-71. DOI: 10.1080/13550280600614973.

[35] Schmitt K, Richter C, Backes C, Meese E, Ruprecht K, Mayer J. Comprehensive analysis of human endogenous retrovirus group HERV-W locus transcription in multiple sclerosis brain lesions by high-throughput amplicon sequencing. *J Virol*. 2013;87:13837-52. DOI:10.1128/JVI.02388-13..

[36] Sotgiu S, Arru G, Mameli G, Serra C, Pugliatti M, Rosati G, et al. Multiple sclerosis-associated retrovirus in early multiple sclerosis: a six-year follow-up of a Sardinian cohort. *Mult Scler*. 2006;12:698-703. DOI:10.1177/1352458506070773

[37] Tai AK, O'Reilly EJ, Alroy KA, Simon KC, Munger KL, Huber BT, et al. Human endogenous retrovirus-K18 Env as a risk factor in multiple sclerosis. *Mult Scler.* 2008;14:1175-80. DOI:10.1177/1352458508094641.

[38] Sicat J, Sutkowski N, Huber BT. Expression of human endogenous retrovirus HERV-K18 superantigen is elevated in juvenile rheumatoid arthritis. *J Rheumatol.* 2005;32:1821-31.

[39] Moles JP, Tesniere A, Guilhou JJ. A new endogenous retroviral sequence is expressed in skin of patients with psoriasis. *Br J Dermatol.* 2005;153:83-9. DOI:10.1111/j.1365-2133.2005.06555.x.

[40] Wu Z, Mei X, Zhao D, Sun Y, Song J, Pan W, et al. DNA methylation modulates HERV-E expression in CD4+ T cells from systemic lupus erythematosus patients. *J Dermatol Sci.* 2015;77:110-6. DOI:10.1016/j.jdermsci.2014.12.004.

[41] Perron H, Mekaoui L, Bernard C, Veas F, Stefas I, Leboyer M. Endogenous retrovirus type W GAG and envelope protein antigenemia in serum of schizophrenic patients. *Biol Psychiatry.* 2008;64:1019-23. DOI:10.1016/j.biopsych.2008.06.028.

[42] Yao Y, Schroder J, Nellaker C, Bottmer C, Bachmann S, Yolken RH, et al. Elevated levels of human endogenous retrovirus-W transcripts in blood cells from patients with first episode schizophrenia. *Genes Brain Behav.* 2008;7:103-12. DOI:10.1111/j.1601-183X.2007.00334.x.

[43] Lee YN, Bieniasz PD. Reconstitution of an infectious human endogenous retrovirus. *PLoS Pathog.* 2007;3:e10. DOI: 10.1371/journal.ppat.0030010.

[44] Young GR, Eksmond U, Salcedo R, Alexopoulou L, Stoye JP, Kassiotis G. Resurrection of endogenous retroviruses in antibody-deficient mice. *Nature.* 2012;491:774-8. DOI:10.1038/nature11599.

[45] Alvarez-Lafuente R, Garcia-Montojo M, De Las Heras V, Dominguez-Mozo MI, Bartolome M, Benito-Martin MS, et al. Herpesviruses and human endogenous retroviral sequences in the cerebrospinal fluid of multiple sclerosis patients. *Mult Scler.* 2008;14:595-601. DOI:10.1177/1352458507086425.

[46] Mameli G, Madeddu G, Mei A, Uleri E, Poddighe L, Delogu LG, et al. Activation of MSRV-type endogenous retroviruses during infectious mononucleosis and Epstein-Barr virus latency: the missing link with multiple sclerosis? *PLoS One.* 2013;8:e78474. DOI: 10.1371/journal.pone.0078474..

[47] Mameli G, Poddighe L, Mei A, Uleri E, Sotgiu S, Serra C, et al. Expression and activation by Epstein Barr virus of human endogenous retroviruses-W in blood cells and astrocytes: inference for multiple sclerosis. *PLoS One.* 2012;7:e44991. DOI:10.1371/journal.pone.0044991.

[48] Manghera M, Douville RN. Endogenous retrovirus-K promoter: a landing strip for inflammatory transcription factors? *Retrovirology*. 2013;10:16. DOI: 10.1186/1742-4690-10-16.

[49] Matouskova M, Blazkova J, Pajer P, Pavlicek A, Hejnar J. CpG methylation suppresses transcriptional activity of human syncytin-1 in non-placental tissues. *Exp Cell Res*. 2006;312:1011-20. DOI:10.1016/j.yexcr.2005.12.010.

[50] Reiss D, Zhang Y, Mager DL. Widely variable endogenous retroviral methylation levels in human placenta. *Nucleic Acids Res*. 2007;35:4743-54. DOI: 10.1093/nar/gkm455.

[51] Hawkes CH, Giovannoni G, Keir G, Cunnington M, Thompson EJ. Seroprevalence of herpes simplex virus type 2 in multiple sclerosis. *Acta Neurol Scand*. 2006;114:363-7. DOI:10.1111/j.1600-0404.2006.00677.x.

[52] Frank O, Jones-Brando L, Leib-Mosch C, Yolken R, Seifarth W. Altered transcriptional activity of human endogenous retroviruses in neuroepithelial cells after infection with Toxoplasma gondii. *J Infect Dis*. 2006;194:1447-9. DOI:10.1086/508496.

[53] Li F, Nellaker C, Sabunciyan S, Yolken RH, Jones-Brando L, Johansson AS, et al. Transcriptional derepression of the ERVWE1 locus following influenza A virus infection. *J Virol*. 2014;88:4328-37. DOI:10.1128/JVI.03628-13..

[54] Kwun HJ, Han HJ, Lee WJ, Kim HS, Jang KL. Transactivation of the human endogenous retrovirus K long terminal repeat by herpes simplex virus type 1 immediate early protein 0. *Virus Res*. 2002;86:93-100.

[55] Lee WJ, Kwun HJ, Kim HS, Jang KL. Activation of the human endogenous retrovirus W long terminal repeat by herpes simplex virus type 1 immediate early protein 1. *Mol Cells*. 2003;15:75-80.

[56] Misra A, Chosdol K, Sarkar C, Mahapatra AK, Sinha S. Alteration of a sequence with homology to human endogenous retrovirus (HERV-K) in primary human glioma: implications for viral repeat mediated rearrangement. *Mutat Res*. 2001;484:53-9. DOI: 10.1016/S0027-5107(01)00240-8.

[57] Kremer D, Schichel T, Forster M, Tzekova N, Bernard C, van der Valk P, et al. Human endogenous retrovirus type W envelope protein inhibits oligodendroglial precursor cell differentiation. *Ann Neurol*. 2013;74:721-32. DOI: 10.1002/ana.23970..

[58] Rolland A, Jouvin-Marche E, Viret C, Faure M, Perron H, Marche PN. The envelope protein of a human endogenous retrovirus-W family activates innate immunity through CD14/TLR4 and promotes Th1-like responses. *J Immunol*. 2006;176:7636-44. DOI: 10.4049/jimmunol.176.12.7636

[59] Duperray A, Barbe D, Raguenez G, Weksler BB, Romero IA, Couraud PO, et al. Inflammatory response of endothelial cells to a human endogenous retrovirus associat-

ed with multiple sclerosis is mediated by TLR4. *Int Immunol*. 2015;27. DOI:10.1093/intimm/dxv025.

[60] Hurst T, Magiorkinis G. Activation of the innate immune response by endogenous retroviruses. *J Gen Virol*. 2014. DOI:10.1099/jgv.0.000017.

[61] Herman A, Kappler JW, Marrack P, Pullen AM. Superantigens: mechanism of T-cell stimulation and role in immune responses. *Annu Rev Immunol*. 1991;9:745-72. DOI: 10.1146/annurev.iy.09.040191.003525.

[62] Zhang J, Vandevyver C, Stinissen P, Mertens N, van den Berg-Loonen E, Raus J. Activation and clonal expansion of human myelin basic protein-reactive T cells by bacterial superantigens. *J Autoimmun*. 1995;8:615-32. DOI:10.1016/0896-8411(95)90012-8.

[63] Mangeney M, Renard M, Schlecht-Louf G, Bouallaga I, Heidmann O, Letzelter C, et al. Placental syncytins: Genetic disjunction between the fusogenic and immunosuppressive activity of retroviral envelope proteins. *Proc Natl Acad Sci U S A*. 2007;104:20534-9. DOI:10.1073/pnas.0707873105.

[64] Morozov VA, Dao Thi VL, Denner J. The transmembrane protein of the human endogenous retrovirus--K (HERV-K) modulates cytokine release and gene expression. *PLoS One*. 2013;8:e70399. DOI:10.1371/journal.pone.0070399.

[65] Grasset EK, Cerutti A. Immunology. Retroviral help for B cells. *Science*. 2014;346:1454-5. DOI:10.1371/journal.pone.0070399.

[66] Zeng M, Hu Z, Shi X, Li X, Zhan X, Li XD, et al. MAVS, cGAS, and endogenous retroviruses in T-independent B cell responses. *Science*. 2013;346:1486-92. DOI: 10.1126/science.346.6216.1486.

[67] Nexo BA, Villesen P, Nissen KK, Lindegaard HM, Rossing P, Petersen T, et al. Are human endogenous retroviruses triggers of autoimmune diseases? Unveiling associations of three diseases and viral loci. *Immunol Res*. 2015. DOI:10.1007/s12026-015-8671-z.

[68] Marguerat S, Wang WY, Todd JA, Conrad B. Association of human endogenous retrovirus K-18 polymorphisms with type 1 diabetes. *Diabetes*. 2004;53:852-4. DOI: 10.2337/diabetes.53.3.852

[69] Noseworthy JH, Lucchinetti C, Rodriguez M, Weinshenker BG. Multiple sclerosis. *N Engl J Med*. 2000;343:938-52.

[70] Oksenberg JR, Baranzini SE. Multiple sclerosis genetics--is the glass half full, or half empty? *Nat Rev Neurol*. 2010;6:429-37. DOI:10.1038/nrneurol.2010.91.

[71] Browne P, Chandraratna D, Angood C, Tremlett H, Baker C, Taylor BV, et al. Atlas of Multiple Sclerosis 2013: A growing global problem with widespread inequity. *Neurology*. 2013;83:1022-4. DOI:10.1212/WNL.0000000000000768.

[72] IMSGC, Hafler DA, Compston A, Sawcer S, Lander ES, Daly MJ, et al. Risk alleles for multiple sclerosis identified by a genomewide study. *N Engl J Med.* 2007;357:851-62.

[73] IMSGC, Sawcer S, Hellenthal G, Pirinen M, Spencer CC, Patsopoulos NA, et al. Genetic risk and a primary role for cell-mediated immune mechanisms in multiple sclerosis. *Nature.* 2011;476:214-9. DOI:10.1038/nature10251.

[74] Gourraud PA, Harbo HF, Hauser SL, Baranzini SE. The genetics of multiple sclerosis: an up-to-date review. *Immunol Rev.* 2012;248:87-103. DOI: 10.1111/j.1600-065X.2012.01134.x.

[75] IMSGC, Beecham AH, Patsopoulos NA, Xifara DK, Davis MF, Kemppinen A, et al. Analysis of immune-related loci identifies 48 new susceptibility variants for multiple sclerosis. *Nat Genet.* 2013;45:1353-60. DOI:10.1038/ng.2770..

[76] Perron H, Geny C, Laurent A, Mouriquand C, Pellat J, Perret J, et al. Leptomeningeal cell line from multiple sclerosis with reverse transcriptase activity and viral particles. *Res Virol.* 1989;140:551-61.

[77] Perron H, Garson JA, Bedin F, Beseme F, Paranhos-Baccala G, Komurian-Pradel F, et al. Molecular identification of a novel retrovirus repeatedly isolated from patients with multiple sclerosis. The Collaborative Research Group on Multiple Sclerosis. *Proc Natl Acad Sci U S A.* 1997;94:7583-8.

[78] Pavlicek A, Paces J, Elleder D, Hejnar J. Processed pseudogenes of human endogenous retroviruses generated by LINEs: their integration, stability, and distribution. *Genome Res.* 2002;12:391-9. DOI:10.1101/gr.216902

[79] Mameli G, Poddighe L, Astone V, Delogu G, Arru G, Sotgiu S, et al. Novel reliable real-time PCR for differential detection of MSRVenv and syncytin-1 in RNA and DNA from patients with multiple sclerosis. *J Virol Methods.* 2009;161:98-106. DOI: 10.1016/j.jviromet.2009.05.024..

[80] Roebke C, Wahl S, Laufer G, Stadelmann C, Sauter M, Mueller-Lantzsch N, et al. An N-terminally truncated envelope protein encoded by a human endogenous retrovirus W locus on chromosome Xq22.3. *Retrovirology.* 2010;7:69. DOI: 10.1186/1742-4690-7-69.

[81] Laufer G, Mayer J, Mueller BF, Mueller-Lantzsch N, Ruprecht K. Analysis of transcribed human endogenous retrovirus W env loci clarifies the origin of multiple sclerosis-associated retrovirus env sequences. *Retrovirology.* 2009;6:37. DOI: 10.1186/1742-4690-6-37.

[82] Garcia-Montojo M, de la Hera B, Varade J, de la Encarnacion A, Camacho I, Dominguez-Mozo M, et al. HERV-W polymorphism in chromosome X is associated with multiple sclerosis risk and with differential expression of MSRV. *Retrovirology.* 2014;11:2.

[83] Varadé J, García-Montojo M, de la Hera B, Camacho I, García-Martíneza MA, Arroyo R, et al. Multiple sclerosis retrovirus-like envelope gene: Role of the chromosome 20 insertion. *BBA Clin*. 2015;3:162-7. DOI:10.1016/j.bbacli.2015.02.002.

[84] Garcia-Montojo M, Dominguez-Mozo M, Arias-Leal A, Garcia-Martinez A, De las Heras V, Casanova I, et al. The DNA copy number of human endogenous retrovirus-W (MSRV-type) is increased in multiple sclerosis patients and is influenced by gender and disease severity. *PLoS One*. 2013;8:e53623. DOI:10.1371/journal.pone.0053623.

[85] Garson JA, Tuke PW, Giraud P, Paranhos-Baccala G, Perron H. Detection of virion-associated MSRV-RNA in serum of patients with multiple sclerosis. *Lancet*. 1998;351:33. DOI:10.1016/S0140-6736(98)24001-3.

[86] Perron H, Germi R, Bernard C, Garcia-Montojo M, Deluen C, Farinelli L, et al. Human endogenous retrovirus type W envelope expression in blood and brain cells provides new insights into multiple sclerosis disease. *Mult Scler*. 2012;18:1721-36. DOI: 10.1177/1352458512441381..

[87] Serra C, Mameli G, Arru G, Sotgiu S, Rosati G, Dolei A. In vitro modulation of the multiple sclerosis (MS)-associated retrovirus by cytokines: implications for MS pathogenesis. *J Neurovirol*. 2003;9:637-43. DOI:10.1080/13550280390246462.

[88] Mameli G, Serra C, Astone V, Castellazzi M, Poddighe L, Fainardi E, et al. Inhibition of multiple-sclerosis-associated retrovirus as biomarker of interferon therapy. *J Neurovirol*. 2008;14:73-7. DOI:10.1080/13550280701801107.

[89] Arru G, Leoni S, Pugliatti M, Mei A, Serra C, Delogu LG, et al. Natalizumab inhibits the expression of human endogenous retroviruses of the W family in multiple sclerosis patients: a longitudinal cohort study. *Mult Scler*. 2014;20:174-82. DOI: 10.1177/1352458513494957.

[90] Antony JM, Deslauriers AM, Bhat RK, Ellestad KK, Power C. Human endogenous retroviruses and multiple sclerosis: innocent bystanders or disease determinants? *Biochim Biophys Acta*. 2011;1812:162-76. DOI: 10.1016/j.bbadis.2010.07.016..

[91] Perron H, Jouvin-Marche E, Michel M, Ounanian-Paraz A, Camelo S, Dumon A, et al. Multiple sclerosis retrovirus particles and recombinant envelope trigger an abnormal immune response in vitro, by inducing polyclonal Vbeta16 T-lymphocyte activation. *Virology*. 2001;287:321-32. DOI:10.1006/viro.2001.1045.

[92] Firouzi R, Rolland A, Michel M, Jouvin-Marche E, Hauw JJ, Malcus-Vocanson C, et al. Multiple sclerosis-associated retrovirus particles cause T lymphocyte-dependent death with brain hemorrhage in humanized SCID mice model. *J Neurovirol*. 2003;9:79-93. DOI:10.1080/13550280390173328.

[93] de la Hera B, Varade J, Garcia-Montojo M, Lamas JR, de la Encarnacion A, Arroyo R, et al. Role of the human endogenous retrovirus HERV-K18 in autoimmune disease

susceptibility: study in the Spanish population and meta-analysis. *PLoS One*. 2013;8:e62090. DOI:10.1371/journal.pone.0062090..

[94] Nexo BA, Christensen T, Frederiksen J, Moller-Larsen A, Oturai AB, Villesen P, et al. The etiology of multiple sclerosis: genetic evidence for the involvement of the human endogenous retrovirus HERV-Fc1. *PLoS One*. 2011;6:e16652. DOI: 10.1371/journal.pone.0016652.

[95] de la Hera B, Varade J, Garcia-Montojo M, Alcina A, Fedetz M, Alloza I, et al. Human endogenous retrovirus HERV-Fc1 association with multiple sclerosis susceptibility: a meta-analysis. *PLoS One*. 2014;9:e90182. DOI:10.1371/journal.pone.0090182.

[96] Kraus B, Fischer K, Sliva K, Schnierle BS. Vaccination directed against the human endogenous retrovirus-K (HERV-K) gag protein slows HERV-K gag expressing cell growth in a murine model system. *Virol J*. 2014;11:58. DOI:10.1186/1743-422X-11-58.

[97] Turcanova VL, Bundgaard B, Hollsberg P. Human herpesvirus-6B induces expression of the human endogenous retrovirus K18-encoded superantigen. *J Clin Virol*. 2009;46:15-9. DOI:10.1016/j.jcv.2009.05.015.

[98] Tai AK, Luka J, Ablashi D, Huber BT. HHV-6A infection induces expression of HERV-K18-encoded superantigen. *J Clin Virol*. 2009;46:47-8. DOI:10.1016/j.jcv.2009.05.019.

[99] Hsiao FC, Lin M, Tai A, Chen G, Huber BT. Cutting edge: Epstein-Barr virus transactivates the HERV-K18 superantigen by docking to the human complement receptor 2 (CD21) on primary B cells. *J Immunol*. 2006;177:2056-60. DOI: 10.4049/ jimmunol.177.4.2056

[100] Sutkowski N, Conrad B, Thorley-Lawson DA, Huber BT. Epstein-Barr virus transactivates the human endogenous retrovirus HERV-K18 that encodes a superantigen. *Immunity*. 2001;15:579-89. DOI:10.1016/S1074-7613(01)00210-2.

[101] Hsiao FC, Tai AK, Deglon A, Sutkowski N, Longnecker R, Huber BT. EBV LMP-2A employs a novel mechanism to transactivate the HERV-K18 superantigen through its ITAM. *Virology*. 2009;385:261-6. DOI:10.1016/j.virol.2008.11.025.

[102] Sutkowski N, Chen G, Calderon G, Huber BT. Epstein-Barr virus latent membrane protein LMP-2A is sufficient for transactivation of the human endogenous retrovirus HERV-K18 superantigen. *J Virol*. 2004;78:7852-60. DOI:10.1128/JVI.78.14.7852-7860.2004

[103] Buljevac D, van Doornum GJ, Flach HZ, Groen J, Osterhaus AD, Hop W, et al. Epstein-Barr virus and disease activity in multiple sclerosis. *J Neurol Neurosurg Psychiatry*. 2005;76:1377-81. DOI:10.1136/jnnp.2004.048504

[104] Christensen T. The role of EBV in MS pathogenesis. *Int MS J*. 2006;13:52-7.

[105] Nielsen TR, Pedersen M, Rostgaard K, Frisch M, Hjalgrim H. Correlations between Epstein-Barr virus antibody levels and risk factors for multiple sclerosis in healthy individuals. *Mult Scler*. 2007;13:420-3. DOI:10.1177/1352458506071470

[106] DeLorenze GN, Munger KL, Lennette ET, Orentreich N, Vogelman JH, Ascherio A. Epstein-Barr virus and multiple sclerosis: evidence of association from a prospective study with long-term follow-up. *Arch Neurol*. 2006;63:839-44. DOI:10.1001/archneur.63.6.noc50328.

[107] Hollsberg P, Kusk M, Bech E, Hansen HJ, Jakobsen J, Haahr S. Presence of Epstein-Barr virus and human herpesvirus 6B DNA in multiple sclerosis patients: associations with disease activity. *Acta Neurol Scand*. 2005;112:395-402. DOI:10.1111/j.1600-0404.2005.00516.x.

[108] Martinez A, Alvarez-Lafuente R, Mas A, Bartolome M, Garcia-Montojo M, de Las Heras V, et al. Environment-gene interaction in multiple sclerosis: human herpesvirus 6 and MHC2TA. *Hum Immunol*. 2007;68:685-9. DOI:10.1016/j.humimm.2007.05.005.

[109] Benit L, Calteau A, Heidmann T. Characterization of the low-copy HERV-Fc family: evidence for recent integrations in primates of elements with coding envelope genes. *Virology*. 2003;312:159-68. DOI:10.1016/S0042-6822(03)00163-6.

[110] Strissel PL, Ruebner M, Thiel F, Wachter D, Ekici AB, Wolf F, et al. Reactivation of codogenic endogenous retroviral (ERV) envelope genes in human endometrial carcinoma and prestages: Emergence of new molecular targets. *Oncotarget*. 2012;3:1204-19.

[111] Rhyu DW, Kang YJ, Ock MS, Eo JW, Choi YH, Kim WJ, et al. Expression of human endogenous retrovirus env genes in the blood of breast cancer patients. *Int J Mol Sci*. 2014;15:9173-83. DOI: 10.3390/ijms15069173.

[112] Kremer D, Forster M, Schichel T, Gottle P, Hartung HP, Perron H, et al. The neutralizing antibody GNbAC1 abrogates HERV-W envelope protein-mediated oligodendroglial maturation blockade. *Mult Scler*. 2014;21:1200-3. DOI: 10.1177/1352458514560926.

[113] Curtin F, Perron H, Kromminga A, Porchet H, Lang AB. Preclinical and early clinical development of GNbAC1, a humanized IgG4 monoclonal antibody targeting endogenous retroviral MSRV-Env protein. *MAbs*. 2015;7:265-75. DOI: 10.4161/19420862.2014.985021.

[114] Derfuss T, Curtin F, Guebelin C, Bridel C, Rasenack M, Matthey A, et al. A phase IIa randomised clinical study of GNbAC1, a humanised monoclonal antibody against the envelope protein of multiple sclerosis-associated endogenous retrovirus in multiple sclerosis patients. *Mult Scler*. 2014;21:885-93. DOI: 10.1177/1352458514554052.

[115] Curtin F, Lang AB, Perron H, Laumonier M, Vidal V, Porchet HC, et al. GNbAC1, a humanized monoclonal antibody against the envelope protein of multiple sclerosis-

associated endogenous retrovirus: a first-in-humans randomized clinical study. *Clin Ther*. 2012;34:2268-78. DOI:10.1016/j.clinthera.2012.11.006.

[116] Downey RF, Sullivan FJ, Wang-Johanning F, Ambs S, Giles FJ, Glynn SA. Human endogenous retrovirus K and cancer: Innocent bystander or tumorigenic accomplice? *Int J Cancer*. 2014;137:1249-57. DOI: 10.1002/ijc.29003.

[117] van der Kuyl AC. HIV infection and HERV expression: a review. *Retrovirology*. 2012;9:6. DOI:10.1186/1742-4690-9-6.

[118] Bhardwaj N, Maldarelli F, Mellors J, Coffin JM. HIV-1 infection leads to increased transcription of human endogenous retrovirus HERV-K (HML-2) proviruses in vivo but not to increased virion production. *J Virol*. 2014;88:11108-20. DOI:10.1128/JVI.01623-14.

[119] Michaud HA, SenGupta D, de Mulder M, Deeks SG, Martin JN, Kobie JJ, et al. Cutting edge: An antibody recognizing ancestral endogenous virus glycoproteins mediates antibody-dependent cellular cytotoxicity on HIV-1-infected cells. *J Immunol*. 2014;193:1544-8. DOI:10.4049/jimmunol.1302108.

11

HLA Allele Frequencies in Pediatric and Adolescent Multiple Sclerosis Patients

Maria Anagnostouli and Maria Gontika

Abstract

Early-onset (pediatric and adolescent) multiple sclerosis (MS) is a chronic autoimmune and neurodegenerative disorder of the central nervous system, which accounts for 3–5% of all MS cases. The major histocompatibility complex (MHC) with its polymorphisms has been the genetic locus with the most robust association with adult MS, since its first discovery in the 1970s. Nowadays, human leukocyte antigen (HLA) typing studies and genome-wide association studies (GWAS) have tried to provide insight into the genetics of early-onset MS and their role in disease diagnosis, prognosis, and therapeutic decision-making. Fundamental genetic similarities have emerged, supporting the assumption that MS shares similar genetic variants and biological processes in all age groups. In this chapter, we considered it useful to collect all the available data concerning the HLA distribution in early-onset MS, given the absence of a review paper with such an approach. We additionally aimed toward the summarization of the association of the HLA frequencies in early-onset MS and the main acquired demyelinating disorders that are considered in differential diagnosis of early-onset MS, like ADEM, NMO/NMOSD, and anti-MOG encephalopathy, for further understanding and current or future research in this promising field.

Keywords: multiple sclerosis, pediatric, early onset, human leukocyte antigens, immunogenetics, therapy, precision medicine

1. Introduction

Early-onset (pediatric and adolescent) multiple sclerosis (MS), which accounts approximately for 3–5% of all MS cases worldwide, has recently aroused the interest of the scientific community regarding its underlying pathogenetic mechanisms, both autoimmune demyelination and neurodegeneration of the central nervous system (CNS) [1–3]. Additionally, in this specific age, other acquired demyelinating diseases are in the MS differential diagnosis of everyday practice, like ADEM, anti-MOG encephalopathy, and optic neuritis [4]. Recently, anti-NMO, anti-MOG, and other autoantibodies have been established as strong biomarkers of the previously referred newly emerged clinical entities or a key element of classical demyelinating diseases, like MS, especially of early onset [5, 6].

Nevertheless, for four decades now, the HLA alleles have been globally recognized as the core genetic (risk or protective) component in adult MS. Since the early 1970s, the major histocompatibility complex (MHC) with its polymorphisms on chromosome 6p21.3 [7, 8] has been the genetic locus with the most robust association with MS. In specific, DRB1*1501 (split of DR2), along with DRB1*0301 and DRB1*1301, has been found to confer risk for MS, while HLA-A*0201 protection against MS [9]. Genome-wide association studies (GWAS) regarding early-onset MS are still ongoing, in contrast with large-scale cohorts of adult-onset MS patients. However, single nucleotide polymorphisms (SNPs) of more modest effect have been detected that influence the risk of both adult- and early-onset MS, equalizing the genetic burden of these age groups [10–12]. The HLA alleles that have been studied in early-onset MS concern mainly the class II DRB1* and DQB1* loci, although DPB1* alleles confer susceptibility in adult-onset MS as well [13]. Thus, HLA immunogenetics in early-onset MS apart from the lower number of worldwide studies needs an extension to the whole HLA class I and class II systems, given the increased role that was in MS risk and MS association with vitamin D, body mass index (BMI), hormones, estrogen receptor, gender, EDSS score, disease course, MRI findings, cognitive status, and most importantly neutralizing antibody formation and response to treatment [8, 14–18].

In this chapter, we present the available data concerning the HLA distribution in early-onset MS, in parallel with the other acquired demyelinating diseases, given the increased knowledge that has recently emerged in this promising field. We also aimed to include all this useful data in a workable table.

2. HLA allele distribution in early-onset MS worldwide

Regarding HLA alleles, DRB1*15 association with early-onset MS has been noted by a series of studies [12, 19–22]. In 2000, a study of 286 Norwegians MS patients demonstrated that the HLA-DR2, DQ6 haplotype is negatively correlated with age at diagnosis [23]. Since then, many studies came to show that DRB1*15-positive patients have a significantly earlier age at onset than DRB1*15-negative patients [18, 24–30]. Maslova et al. replicated this testimony in a pure pediatric Russian population in 2000 [31]. An Australian study of 978 patients in 2010 went further to prove that carrying DRBI*15 significantly decreases the age of MS onset by 3.2 years in homozygotes and 1.3 years in heterozygotes [32].

On the other hand, a series of studies pleads against these remarks and claims no correlation of DRB1*15 status and age of disease onset [33–39]. In a Korean population, close linkage of DRB3*02, DRB1*13, and DQB1*03 was also associated with the risk of childhood MS, while DRB1*1501 was not as high as in Western children [40].

	MS	NMO	ADEM
HLA alleles	HLA-DRB1*1501 (Caucasian)	HLA-DRB1*03 (adult Caucasian)	HLA-DRB1*01 and HLA-DRB1*017 (Russian)
	HLA-DRB1*0401 (Caucasian)	HLA-DRB1*0501 (adult Japanese)	HLA-DRB1*1501 and HLA-DRB5*0101 (Korean)
	HLA-DRB3*02, HLA-DRB1*13, and HLA-DQB1*03 (Korean)		HLA-DQB1*0602, HLA-DRB1*1501, and HLA-DRB1*1503 (Brazil)
			HLA-DRB1*16 and HLA-DQB1*05 (Caucasian adult)

MS, multiple sclerosis; ADEM, acute disseminated encephalomyelitis; NMO, neuromyelitis optica.

Table 1. Summary of the available data regarding the HLA allele distribution in early-onset multiple sclerosis, ADEM, and NMO [12, 18–41, 46–49].

A remarkable DRB1-genotyping study in Australia in 2010 declared the first results indicative of the significance of the epistatic interactions at the HLA-DRB1 locus. Carriage of the DRB1*1501 risk allele alone was not significantly associated with age at disease onset, while the DRB1*0401 allele was associated with a reduced age at onset when combined with DRB1*1501 [41].

Regarding Greece, Anagnostouli et al. in 2003 noticed for the first time the higher frequency of DRB1*1501 in MS patients [42]. In 2011, Kouri et al. [43] observed no significant correlations among DRB1*1501, DQB1*0602, and DQA1*0102 alleles with age at onset, an observation repeated by Anagnostouli et al. in 2014 [20]. Anagnostouli et al. attributed this discrepancy either to a possible parent of origin effect, relying on Ramagopalan et al.' observation that only maternally transmitted DRB1*15 promotes a lower age of MS [44], or to fluctuations of vitamin D levels among different populations [45]. New findings in this former are the putative predisposing role of DRB1*03 allele and the protective role of the DRB1*16 allele for early-onset MS [20].

While the role of HLA alleles in early-onset MS has been well studied, this is not the case in other young-onset acquired demyelinating diseases, especially acute disseminated encephalomyelitis (ADEM) and neuromyelitis optica (NMO), its main differential diagnoses. In **Table 1**, we summarize the available data regarding the HLA allele distribution in early-onset MS, ADEM, and NMO, and despite the obvious lack of information, the primary results demonstrate clear genetic diversity [12, 18–41, 46–49].

3. Conclusions

The well-established HLA-DRB1*15:01 allele associated with adult-onset MS appears to confer increased susceptibility to early-onset MS too, supporting a fundamental similarity in genetic contribution to MS risk, regardless of age at onset. Regarding whether HLA-DRB1*1501 by itself lowers the age at onset of MS, the results are conflicting and possibly related to both genetic and environmental epistatic mechanisms and in particular those through HLA-DRB1*04. Moreover,

HLA-DRB1*04 also appears to bind with high affinity to myelin oligodendrocyte glycoprotein (MOG) epitopes, whose role in early-onset demyelinating disorders has been widely studied, in both familial MS patients and asymptomatic relatives, indicating that the humoral immune reactivity against MOG is partially under control of certain HLA class II alleles [50–54]. This observation could guide therapy, as HLA-DRB1∗0401 allele is associated with greater risk of developing neutralizing antibodies against interferon beta (IFN-β) in adult studies, resulting in poorer therapeutic outcome [55]. Finally, the putative relation of DRB1*03 allele with early-onset MS is also interesting, as this allele has been associated not only with a presumed better MS prognosis but also with NMO [46], a mainly humoral immunological entity.

Accumulating data highlights the role of HLA-genotype and especially HLA-DRB1*1501 in regulating the immune response to a range of environmental factors, modulating the risk of MS appearance. Research has mainly focused on viral infections, especially EBV [56–58], CMV, and HSV-1 [58]. In specific, Epstein–Barr nuclear antigen-1 seropositivity has been associated with an increased risk of MS, while a remote infection with CMV with a lower risk. A strong interaction has been found between HSV-1 status and HLA-DRB1 in predicting MS, as HSV-1 has been associated with an increased risk of MS only in DRB1*15 carriers. Moreover, obesity and higher body mass index (BMI) during adolescence, rather than childhood, seem to be critical in determining MS risk [59], while tobacco smoke exposure and HLA-DRB1*15 interact to increase risk for MS in children diagnosed with monophasic acquired demyelinating syndromes [60]. Finally, as research regarding the role of gut bacteria in the development of central nervous demyelinating disorders robustly expands, possible protective correlations of specific bacteria through interplay with specific HLA alleles emerge in animal models of MS, expanding our knowledge regarding disease pathogenesis [61, 62]. Larger studies in early-onset MS populations are required in order to clarify these possible correlations which may also expand to other HLA alleles, proving the interplay among cellular activity, humoral activity, and environment in MS and their possible impact in therapeutics.

In conclusion, HLA alleles emerge as a primary biomarker in both early- and adult-onset MS, regarding genetic risk, outcome, and differential diagnosis. We strongly believe that larger HLA-genotyping studies regarding early-onset demyelinating disorders are needed, in different ethnic groups, in order to clarify, replicate, and expand the already limited existing results. We also believe that these future studies will aim toward personalized therapeutics and generally precision medicine in early-onset MS patients.

Author details

Maria Anagnostouli[1,2]* and Maria Gontika[1]

*Address all correspondence to: managnost@med.uoa.gr

1 Immunogenetics Laboratory, 1st Dep. of Neurology, Medical School, National and Kapodistrian University of Athens, Athens, Greece

2 Demyelinating Diseases Clinic, 1st Dep. of Neurology, Medical School, National and Kapodistrian University of Athens, Athens, Greece

References

[1] Renoux C, Vukusic S, Confavreux C. The natural history of multiple sclerosis with childhood onset. Clinical Neurology and Neurosurgery. 2008;**110**(9):897-904

[2] Venkateswaran S, Banwell B. Pediatric multiple sclerosis. The Neurologist. 2010;**16**(2): 92-105

[3] Ferreira ML, Machado MI, Dantas MJ, Moreira AJ, Souza AM. Pediatric multiple sclerosis: Analysis of clinical and epidemiological aspects according to National MS Society consensus 2007. Arquivos de Neuro-Psiquiatria. 2008;**66**(3B):665-670

[4] Hintzen RQ, Dale RC, Neuteboom RF, et al. Pediatric acquired CNS demyelinating syndromes: Features associated with multiple sclerosis. Neurology. 2016;**87**(9 Suppl 2): S67-S73

[5] Chitnis T, Ness J, Krupp L, et al. Clinical features of neuromyelitis optica in children: US network of pediatric MS centers report. Neurology. 2016;**86**(3):245-252

[6] Hennes EM, Baumann M, Lechner C, et al. MOG Spectrum disorders and role of MOG-antibodies in clinical practice. Neuropediatrics. 2018;**49**(1):3-11

[7] Ramagopalan SV, Dyment DA, Ebers GC. Genetic epidemiology: The use of old and new tools for multiple sclerosis. Trends in Neurosciences. 2008;**31**:645-652

[8] Katsavos S, Anagnostouli M. Biomarkers in multiple sclerosis: An up-to-date overview. Multiple Sclerosis International. 2013;**2013**:340508

[9] International Multiple Sclerosis Genetics Consortium; Welcome Trust Case Control Consortium 2, Sawcer S, Hellenthal G, Pirinen M, Spencer CC, et al. Genetic risk and a primary role for cell-mediated immune mechanisms in multiple sclerosis. Nature. 2011;**476**:214-219

[10] Disanto G, Ramagopalan SV. Similar genetics of adult and pediatric MS: Age is just a number. Neurology. 2013;**81**(23):1974-1975

[11] Graves JS, Barcellos LF, Simpson S, et al. The multiple sclerosis risk allele within the AHI1 gene is associated with relapses in children and adults. Multiple Sclerosis Related Disorders. 2018;**19**:161-165

[12] Gianfrancesco MA, Stridh P, Shao X, et al. Genetic risk factors for pediatric-onset multiple sclerosis. Multiple Sclerosis. 2017;**1**:1352458517733551

[13] Patsopoulos NA, Barcellos LF, Hintzen RQ, et al. Fine-mapping the genetic association of the major histocompatibility complex in multiple sclerosis: HLA and non-HLA effects. PLoS Genetics. 2013;**9**(11):e1003926

[14] Sintzel MB, Rametta M, Reder AT, et al. Vitamin D and multiple sclerosis: A comprehensive review. Neurology and Therapy. 2018;**7**(1):59-85

[15] Hedström AK, Lima Bomfim I, Barcellos L, et al. Interaction between adolescent obesity and HLA risk genes in the etiology of multiple sclerosis. Neurology. 2014;**82**(10):865-872

[16] Kikuchi S, Fukazawa T, Niino M, et al. Estrogen receptor gene polymorphism and multiple sclerosis in Japanese patients: Interaction with HLA-DRB1*1501 and disease modulation. Journal of Neuroimmunology. 2002;**128**(1-2):77-81

[17] Katsavos S, Artemiadis A, Davaki P, et al. Familial multiple sclerosis in Greece: Distinct clinical and imaging characteristics in comparison with the sporadic disease. Clinical Neurology and Neurosurgery. 2018;**173**:144-149

[18] Okuda DT, Srinivasan R, Oksenberg JR, et al. Genotype-phenotype correlations in multiple sclerosis: HLA genes influence disease severity inferred by 1HMR spectroscopy and MRI measures. Brain. 2009;**132**(Pt 1):250-259

[19] Stamatelos P, Anagnostouli M. HLA-genotype in multiple sclerosis: The role in disease onset, clinical course, cognitive status and response to treatment: A clear step towards personalized therapeutics. Immunogenetics Open Access. 2017;**2**:116. (review in press)

[20] Anagnostouli M, Manouseli A, Artemiadis A, et al. HLA-DRB1* allele frequencies in pediatric, adolescent and adult-onset multiple sclerosis patients, in a Hellenic sample. Evidence for new and established associations. Multiple Sclerosis Journal. 2014;**1**:1

[21] Banwell B, Bar-Or A, Arnold DL, et al. Clinical, environmental, and genetic determinants of multiple sclerosis in children with acute demyelination: A prospective national cohort study. Lancet Neurology. 2011;**10**(5):436-445

[22] Disanto G, Magalhaes S, Handel AE, et al. HLA-DRB1 confers increased risk of pediatric-onset MS in children with acquired demyelination. Neurology. 2011;**76**(9):781-786

[23] Celius EG, Harbo HF, Egeland T, et al. Sex and age at diagnosis are correlated with the HLA-DR2, DQ6 haplotype in multiple sclerosis. Journal of the Neurological Sciences. 2000;**178**(2):132-135

[24] Masterman T, Ligers A, Olsson T, et al. HLA-DR15 is associated with lower age at onset in multiple sclerosis. Annals of Neurology. 2000;**48**(2):211-219

[25] Hensiek AE, Sawcer SJ, Feakes R, et al. HLA-DR 15 is associated with female sex and younger age at diagnosis in multiple sclerosis. Journal of Neurology, Neurosurgery, and Psychiatry. 2002;**72**(2):184-187

[26] Weatherby SJ, Thomson W, Pepper L, et al. HLA-DRB1 and disease outcome in multiple sclerosis. Journal of Neurology. 2001;**248**(4):304-310

[27] Smestad C, Brynedal B, Jonasdottir G, et al. The impact of HLA-A and -DRB1 on age at onset, disease course and severity in Scandinavian multiple sclerosis patients. European Journal of Neurology. 2007;**14**(8):835-840

[28] Imrell K, Greiner E, Hillert J, Masterman T. HLA-DRB115 and cerebrospinal-fluid-specific oligoclonal immunoglobulin G bands lower age at attainment of important disease milestones in multiple sclerosis. Journal of Neuroimmunology. 2009;**210**(1-2):128-130

[29] Balnyte R, Rastenyte D, Vaitkus A, et al. The importance of HLA DRB1 gene allele to clinical features and disability in patients with multiple sclerosis in Lithuania. BMC Neurology. 2013;**13**:77

[30] Al-Shammri S, Nelson RF, Al-Muzairi I, Akanji AO. HLA determinants of susceptibility to multiple sclerosis in an Arabian gulf population. Multiple Sclerosis. 2004;**10**(4):381-386

[31] Maslova OI, Bykova OV, Guseva MR, et al. Multiple sclerosis with early onset: Pathogenesis, clinical characteristics, possibilities in the treatment of its pathogenesis. Zhurnal Nevrologii i Psikhiatrii Imeni S.S. Korsakova. 2002;(Suppl):46-51

[32] Van der Walt A, Stankovich J, Bahlo M, et al. Heterogeneity at the HLA-DRB1 allelic variation locus does not influence multiple sclerosis disease severity, brain atrophy or cognition. Multiple Sclerosis. 2011;**17**(3):344-352

[33] Villoslada P, Barcellos LF, Rio J, et al. The HLA locus and multiple sclerosis in Spain. Role in disease susceptibility, clinical course and response to interferon beta. Journal of Neuroimmunology. 2002;**130**(1-2):194-201

[34] Barcellos LF, Sawcer S, Ramsay PP, et al. Heterogeneity at the HLA-DRB1 locus and risk for multiple sclerosis. Human Molecular Genetics. 2006;**15**(18):2813-2824

[35] Barcellos LF, Oksenberg JR, Begovich AB, et al. HLA-DR2 dose effect on susceptibility to multiple sclerosis and influence on disease course. American Journal of Human Genetics. 2003;**72**(3):710-716

[36] Silva AM, Pereira C, Bettencourt A, et al. The role of HLA-DRB1 alleles on susceptibility and outcome of a Portuguese multiple sclerosis population. Journal of the Neurological Sciences. 2007;**258**(1-2):69-74

[37] Ouadghiri S, El Alaoui Toussi K, Brick C, et al. Genetic factors and multiple sclerosis in the Moroccan population: A role for HLA class II. Pathologie Biologie. 2013;**61**(6):259-263

[38] Ballerini C, Guerini FR, Rombolà G, et al. HLA-multiple sclerosis association in continental Italy and correlation with disease prevalence in Europe. Journal of Neuroimmunology. 2004;**150**(1-2):178-185

[39] Boiko AN, Gusev EI, Sudomoina MA, et al. Association and linkage of juvenile MS with HLA-DR2(15) in Russians. Neurology. 2002;**58**(4):658-660

[40] Oh HH, Kwon SH, Kim CW, et al. Molecular analysis of HLA class II-associated susceptibility to neuroinflammatory diseases in Korean children. Journal of Korean Medical Science. 2004;**19**:426-430

[41] Wu JS, Qiu W, Castley A, et al. Modifying effects of HLA-DRB1 allele interactions on age at onset of multiple sclerosis in Western Australia. Multiple Sclerosis. 2010;**16**(1):15-20

[42] Bozikas VP, Anagnostouli MC, Petrikis P, et al. Familial bipolar disorder and multiple sclerosis: A three-generation HLA family study. Progress in Neuro-Psychopharmacology & Biological Psychiatry. 2003;**27**(5):835-839

[43] Kouri I, Papakonstantinou S, Bempes V, et al. HLA associations with multiple sclerosis in Greece. Journal of the Neurological Sciences. 2011;**308**(1-2):28-31

[44] Ramagopalan SV, Byrnes JK, Dyment DA, et al. Parent-of-origin of HLA-DRB1*1501 and age of onset of multiple sclerosis. Journal of Human Genetics. 2009;**54**(9):547-549

[45] Ramagopalan SV, Maugeri NJ, Handunnetthi L, et al. Expression of the multiple sclerosis-associated MHC class II allele HLA-DRB1*1501 is regulated by vitamin D. PLoS Genetics. 2009;**5**:e1000369

[46] Gontika M, Anagnostouli M. Human leukocyte antigens immunogenetics of neuromyelitis optica or Devic's disease and the impact on the immunopathogenesis, diagnosis and treatment: A critical review. Neuroimmunology and Neuroinflammation. 2014;**1**:44-50

[47] Imbesi D, Calabrò RS, Gervasi G, et al. Does HLA class II haplotype play a role in adult acute disseminated encephalomyelitis? Preliminary findings from a southern Italy hospital-based study. Archives Italiennes de Biologie. 2012;**150**(1):1-4

[48] Alves-Leon SV, Veluttini-Pimentel ML, Gouveia ME, et al. Acute disseminated encephalomyelitis: Clinical features, HLA DRB1*1501, HLA DRB1*1503, HLA DQA1*0102, HLA DQB1*0602, and HLA DPA1*0301 allelic association study. Arquivos de Neuro-Psiquiatria. 2009;**67**(3A):643-651

[49] Idrissova ZR, Boldyreva MN, Dekonenko EP, et al. Acute disseminated encephalomyelitis in children: Clinical features and HLA-DR linkage. European Journal of Neurology. 2003;**10**(5):537-546

[50] Forsthuber TG, Shive CL, Wienhold W, et al. T cell epitopes of human myelin oligodendrocyte glycoprotein identified in HLA-DR4 (DRB1*0401) transgenic mice are encephalitogenic and are presented by human B cells. Journal of Immunology. 2001;**167**(12):7119-7125

[51] Klehmet J, Shive C, Guardia-Wolff R, et al. T cell epitope spreading to myelin oligodendrocyte glycoprotein in HLA-DR4 transgenic mice during experimental autoimmune encephalomyelitis. Clinical Immunology. 2004;**111**(1):53-60

[52] Khare M, Rodriguez M, David CS. HLA class II transgenic mice authenticate restriction of myelin oligodendrocyte glycoprotein-specific immune response implicated in multiple sclerosis pathogenesis. International Immunology. 2003;**15**(4):535-546

[53] Raddassi K, Kent SC, Yang J, et al. Increased frequencies of myelin oligodendrocyte glycoprotein/MHC class II-binding CD4 cells in patients with multiple sclerosis. Journal of Immunology. 2011;**187**(2):1039-1046

[54] Lutterotti A, Reindl M, Gassner C, et al. Antibody response to myelin oligodendrocyte glycoprotein and myelin basic protein depend on familial background and are partially associated with human leukocyte antigen alleles in multiplex families and sporadic multiple sclerosis. Journal of Neuroimmunology. 2002;**131**(1-2):201-207

[55] Buck D, Cepok S, Hoffmann S, et al. Influence of the HLADRB1 genotype on antibody development to interferon beta in multiple sclerosis. Archives of Neurology. 2011;**68**(4):480-487

[56] Waubant E, Mowry EM, Krupp L, et al. Antibody response to common viruses and human leukocyte antigen-DRB1 in pediatric multiple sclerosis. Multiple Sclerosis. 2013;**19**(7):891-895

[57] Morandi E, Jagessar SA, 't Hart BA, Gran B. EBV infection empowers human B cells for autoimmunity: Role of autophagy and relevance to multiple sclerosis. Journal of Immunology. 2017;**199**(2):435-448

[58] Waubant E, Mowry EM, Krupp L, et al. Common viruses associated with lower pediatric multiple sclerosis risk. Neurology. 2011;**76**(23):1989-1995

[59] Hedström AK, Olsson T, Alfredsson L. Body mass index during adolescence, rather than childhood, is critical in determining MS risk. Multiple Sclerosis. 2016;**22**(7):878-883

[60] Lavery AM, Collins BN, Waldman AT, et al. The contribution of secondhand tobacco smoke exposure to pediatric multiple sclerosis risk. Multiple Sclerosis. 2018;**1**:1352458518757089

[61] Mangalam A, Shahi SK, Luckey D, et al. Human gut-derived commensal bacteria suppress CNS inflammatory and demyelinating disease. Cell Reports. 2017;**20**(6):1269-1277

[62] Lerner A, Matthias T. Rheumatoid arthritis-celiac disease relationship: Joints get that gut feeling. Autoimmunity Reviews. 2015;**14**(11):1038-1047

Permissions

All chapters in this book were first published by InTech Open; hereby published with permission under the Creative Commons Attribution License or equivalent. Every chapter published in this book has been scrutinized by our experts. Their significance has been extensively debated. The topics covered herein carry significant findings which will fuel the growth of the discipline. They may even be implemented as practical applications or may be referred to as a beginning point for another development.

The contributors of this book come from diverse backgrounds, making this book a truly international effort. This book will bring forth new frontiers with its revolutionizing research information and detailed analysis of the nascent developments around the world.

We would like to thank all the contributing authors for lending their expertise to make the book truly unique. They have played a crucial role in the development of this book. Without their invaluable contributions this book wouldn't have been possible. They have made vital efforts to compile up to date information on the varied aspects of this subject to make this book a valuable addition to the collection of many professionals and students.

This book was conceptualized with the vision of imparting up-to-date information and advanced data in this field. To ensure the same, a matchless editorial board was set up. Every individual on the board went through rigorous rounds of assessment to prove their worth. After which they invested a large part of their time researching and compiling the most relevant data for our readers.

The editorial board has been involved in producing this book since its inception. They have spent rigorous hours researching and exploring the diverse topics which have resulted in the successful publishing of this book. They have passed on their knowledge of decades through this book. To expedite this challenging task, the publisher supported the team at every step. A small team of assistant editors was also appointed to further simplify the editing procedure and attain best results for the readers.

Apart from the editorial board, the designing team has also invested a significant amount of their time in understanding the subject and creating the most relevant covers. They scrutinized every image to scout for the most suitable representation of the subject and create an appropriate cover for the book.

The publishing team has been an ardent support to the editorial, designing and production team. Their endless efforts to recruit the best for this project, has resulted in the accomplishment of this book. They are a veteran in the field of academics and their pool of knowledge is as vast as their experience in printing. Their expertise and guidance has proved useful at every step. Their uncompromising quality standards have made this book an exceptional effort. Their encouragement from time to time has been an inspiration for everyone.

The publisher and the editorial board hope that this book will prove to be a valuable piece of knowledge for researchers, students, practitioners and scholars across the globe.

List of Contributors

Juan Espinosa-Parrilla, Marco Pugliese, Nicole Mahy and Manuel J Rodríguez
Department of Biomedical Sciences, Institute of Neuroscience, IDIBAPS, University of Barcelona and Center for Biomedical Research Network in Neurodegenerative Diseases (CIBERNED), Barcelona, Spain

Daisuke Kamimura, Yasunobu Arima, Andrea Stofkova, Naoki Nishikawa, Kotaro Higuchi, Takuto Ohki and Masaaki Murakami
Molecular Neuroimmunology, Graduate School of Medicine, Institute for Genetic Medicine, Hokkaido University, Sapporo, Hokkaido, Japan

Valentina Ignatova
National Heart Hospital-MHAT, Clinic of neurology, Sofia, Bulgaria

Lyudmila Todorova
Institute of Biophysics and Biomedical Engineering, Bulgarian Academy of Sciences, Sofia, Bulgaria

Jivko Surchev
Medical University of Sofia, Department of Neurosurgery, St Ivan Rilski University Hospital, Clinic of Neurosurgery, Sofia, Bulgaria

Ozgul Ekmekci
Ege University, Faculty of Medicine, Department of Neurology, Izmir, Turkey

Daniel Čierny
Department of Clinical Biochemistry, Jessenius Faculty of Medicine and University Hospital Martin, Comenius University in Bratislava, Martin, Slovak Republic

Denisa Zimová
Department of Neurology, 3rd Medical Faculty, Charles University, University Hospital FNKV, Prague, Czech Republic

Jozef Michalik, Ema Kantorová and Egon Kurča
Department of Neurology, Jessenius Faculty of Medicine and University Hospital Martin, Comenius University in Bratislava, Martin, Slovak Republic

Ján Lehotský
Department of Medical Biochemistry and BioMed, Jessenius Faculty of Medicine in Martin, Comenius University in Bratislava, Martin, Slovak Republic

Alena Javůrková
Department of Clinical Psychology, University Hospital FNKV, Prague, Czech Republic
Department of Nursing, 2nd Medical Faculty, Charles University, University Hospital Motol, Prague, Czech Republic

Katarína Tomašovičová
Department of Psychology, Faculty of Arts, Charles University, Prague, Czech Republic

Jaroslava Raudenská
Department of Nursing, 2nd Medical Faculty, Charles University, University Hospital Motol, Prague, Czech Republic
Department of Clinical Psychology, University Hospital Motol, Prague, Czech Republic

Genaro G. Ortiz, Erandis D. Torres–Sánchez, Tanya E. Sorto–Gómez, Erika D. González–Renovato and Angelica L. Sánchez–López
Laboratory of Mitochondria–Oxidative Stress and Pathology, Neurosciences Division, Occidental Biomedical Research Center, The Mexican Social Security Institute, Guadalajara, Jalisco, México

Fermín P. Pacheco–Moisés and Margarita Cid–Hernández
Department of Chemistry, Centre of Exact Sciences and Engineering, University of Guadalajara, Guadalajara, Jalisco, México

Mario Mireles–Ramírez, Alfredo León–Gil and Héctor González–Usigli
Department of Neurology, Sub-specialty Medical Unit, National Occidental Medical Center, The Mexican Social Security Institute, Guadalajara, Jalisco, México

Luis J. Flores–Alvarado
Department of Biochemistry, Health Sciences Center, University of Guadalajara, Guadalajara, Jalisco, México

Irma E. Velázquez–Brizuela
Health Sciences Center, University of Guadalajara, Guadalajara, Jalisco, México

Sofia F.G. Zorzella–Pezavento, Larissa L.W. Ishikawa, Thais F.C. Fraga–Silva, Luiza A.N. Mimura and Alexandrina Sartori
Department of Microbiology and Immunology, Institute of Biosciences of Botucatu, Sao Paulo State University (UNESP), Botucatu, São Paulo, Brazil

Montserrat González Platas and María Yaiza Pérez Martin
Neurology Service, Hospital Universitario de Canarias, La Laguna, Santa Cruz de Tenerife, Spain

Belén de la Hera and Elena Urcelay
Instituto de Investigación Sanitaria del Hospital Clínico San Carlos, IdISSC, Madrid, Spain

Maria Gontika
Immunogenetics Laboratory, 1st Dep. of Neurology, Medical School, National and Kapodistrian University of Athens, Athens, Greece

Maria Anagnostouli
Immunogenetics Laboratory, 1st Dep. of Neurology, Medical School, National and Kapodistrian University of Athens, Athens, Greece
Demyelinating Diseases Clinic, 1st Dep. of Neurology, Medical School, National and Kapodistrian University of Athens, Athens, Greece

Index